# Hegde's
# PocketG
# Assessm
# Speech-Language
# Pathology

Third Edition

# Hegde's PocketGuide to Assessment in Speech-Language Pathology

## Third Edition

M. N. Hegde, Ph.D.
Department of Communicative Sciences and Disorders
California State University–Fresno

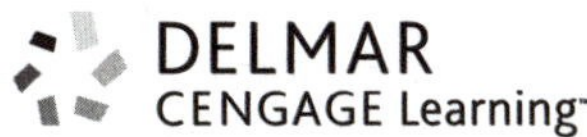


Australia • Brazil • Japan • Korea • Mexico • Singapore Spain • United Kingdom • United States

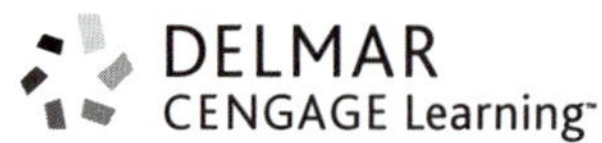

**Hegde's PocketGuide to Assessment in Speech-Language Pathology, Third Edition**
**M. N. Hegde**

Vice President, Health Care Business Unit: William Brottmiller

Director of Learning Solutions: Matthew Kane

Senior Acquisitions Editor: Sherry Dickinson

Senior Product Manager: Juliet Steiner

Editorial Assistant: Angela Doolin

Marketing Director: Jennifer McAvey

Marketing Manager: Chris Manion

Marketing Coordinator: Vanessa Carlson

Production Director: Carolyn Miller

Content Project Manager: Stacey Lamodi

Art Director: Jack Pendlet



For product information and technology assistance, contact us at **Cengage Learning Customer & Sales Support, 1-800-354-9706**

For permission to use material from this text or product, submit all requests online at **www.cengage.com/permissions** Further permissions questions can be emailed to **permissionrequest@cengage.com**

Library of Congress Control Number: 2007012907

ISBN-13: 978-1-4180-1495-7

ISBN-10: 1-4180-1495-8

**Delmar**
Executive Woods
5 Maxwell Drive
Clifton Park, NY 12065
USA

Cengage Learning is a leading provider of customized learning solutions with office locations around the globe, including Singapore, the United Kingdom, Australia, Mexico, Brazil, and Japan. Locate your local office at **www.cengage.com/global**

Cengage Learning products are represented in Canada by Nelson Education, Ltd.

To learn more about Delmar, visit **www.cengage.com/delmar**

Purchase any of our products at your local bookstore or at our preferred online store **www.ichapters.com**



Printed in the United States of America
5 6 7 8 9 16 15 14 13 12

# Major Entries

# About the Author

M. N. (Giri) Hegde, Ph.D., is Professor of Communication Sciences and Disorders at California State University–Fresno. He holds a Master's degree in experimental psychology from the University of Mysore, India; a post-Master's diploma in Medical (Clinical) Psychology from Bangalore University, India; and a doctoral degree in Speech-Language Pathology from Southern Illinois University at Carbondale, Illinois.

Dr. Hegde is a specialist in fluency disorders, language disorders, research methods, and treatment procedures in communicative disorders. He has published many research articles on language and fluency disorders. He has made numerous presentations to national and international audiences on both basic and applied topics in communicative disorders and experimental and applied behavior analysis. With his deep, as well as wide scholarship, Dr. Hegde has authored several highly regarded and widely used scientific and professional books, including: *Treatment Procedures in Communicative Disorders, Clinical Research in Communicative Disorders, Introduction to Communicative Disorders, A Coursebook on Aphasia and Other Neurogenic Language Disorders, Language Disorders in Children: An Evidence-Based Approach to Assessment and Treatment* (with Christine Maul), *Clinical Methods and Practicum in Speech-Language Pathology* (with Deborah Davis), *Treatment Protocols for Stuttering,* the two-volume *Treatment Protocols for Language Disorders in Children, A Coursebook on Scientific and Professional Writing in Speech-Language Pathology, An Advanced Review of Speech-Language Pathology* (with Celeste Roseberry-McKibbin), and *Assessment and Treatment of Articulation and Phonological Disorders in Children* (with Adriana Peña-Brooks). He also has served on the editorial boards of several scientific and professional journals and continues to serve as an editorial consultant to the *American Journal of Speech-Language Pathology* and the *Journal of Fluency Disorders.*

Dr. Hegde is the recipient of various honors, including: the Outstanding Professor Award from California State University–Fresno; CSU–Fresno Provost's Recognition for Outstanding Scholarship and Publication; Distinguished Alumnus Award from the Southern Illinois University Department of Communication Sciences and Disorders; and Outstanding Professional Achievement Award from District 5 of California Speech-Language-Hearing Association. Dr. Hegde is a Fellow of the American Speech-Language-Hearing Association.

# Preface

The third edition of this PocketGuide to assessment procedures in speech-language pathology has been updated and expanded to offer even more detailed and comprehensive coverage of assessment procedures than did the second edition. New entries in this edition include alternative assessment approaches, childhood apraxia of speech, literacy and literacy skills, psychiatric disorders associated with communication disorders, and several newer forms of dementia, including frontotemporal dementia and vascular dementia. Assessment information on cluttering, neurogenic stuttering, and stuttering of early childhood onset has been streamlined and updated under the main entry, Fluency Disorders. Many other entries have been expanded. In most cases, additional and the most current references have been added for clinicians to easily retrieve information from other sources. The companion volume, *Hegde's PocketGuide to Treatment in Speech-Language Pathology* (3rd ed.), has been simultaneously revised to update and expand treatment information.

The publication of the third edition of the two existing PocketGuides has been marked by the simultaneous publication of a new *Hegde's PocketGuide to Communication Disorders*. Because of the ever-expanding knowledge base in communication disorders, it was necessary to create this new PocketGuide that describes research and clinical information on the disorders themselves. The new book includes expanded descriptions of epidemiological and ethnocultural factors, neurophysiological pathology when relevant, associated behavioral disorders, symptomatology of disorders, and theories of major communication disorders—some of which were only briefly sketched in the earlier assessment PocketGuide. The third guide also makes it possible to expand information on assessment procedures and include information on disorders that were excluded in the previous edition because of space limitations.

This third edition of the PocketGuide to assessment procedures is designed for clinical practitioners and students in communicative disorders. The PocketGuide combines the most desirable features of a specialized dictionary of terms, clinical resource book, and textbooks on assessment. It is meant to be a quick reference book like a dictionary because the entries are alphabetized, but it offers more than a dictionary because it specifies assessment procedures in a "do this" format. The PocketGuide is like a resource book in that it concentrates on practical procedures to be used in diagnosing disorders, but it offers more than a resource book by clearly specifying the steps involved in assessing clients with communicative disorders. The PocketGuide is like standard textbooks that describe assessment procedures, but it organizes the information in a manner conducive to more ready use and easier access.

## How the PocketGuide is Organized

All main entries for assessment of communication disorders are printed in bold and green color. Each cross-referenced entry is underlined. Each main disorder of communication is entered in its alphabetical order. Subcategories or types of a given disorder are described under the main entry (e.g., Broca's Aphasia under Aphasia, Ataxic Dysarthria under Dysarthria, or Neurogenic Stuttering under Fluency Disorders).

To avoid repetition under each main entry, common assessment techniques (e.g., case history, interview, hearing screening, orofacial examination) are described as one main entry (Common/Standard Assessment Procedures). However, certain aspects of these common/standard procedures that are unique to a given disorder are described under the main entry for that disorder.

## How to Use This PocketGuide

The guide may be used very much like a dictionary. There are two basic ways in which a clinician can find information of interest. First, a clinician who wants to read about assessment of a particular disorder will find it by its main alphabetical entry. The table of contents quickly directs the clinician to the major entries in the book; most of these are names of various disorders. Under each main entry, the clinician may be referred to certain concepts, assessment techniques, or assessment tools that are cross-referenced. All cross-referenced entries are underlined. Thus, throughout the guide, an underlined term means that the reader can find more about it in its own main alphabetical entry.

Second, the clinician also may look up certain assessment methods by name. Two such entries, Speech and Language Sample and Standard/Common Assessment Procedures, have been noted. Other such entries that are not disorders but assessment targets, concepts, or techniques include Augmentative and Alternative Communication (AAC), Phonological Processes, Grammatical Morphemes of Language, Computerized Axial Tomography, Maximum Phonation Duration, and so forth.

## A Caveat

Serious attempts have been made to include most assessment techniques described in the literature. However, the author is aware that not all techniques have been included. The author did not set for himself the impossible goal of including all assessment techniques. The practical goal was to describe assessment techniques that are most commonly used in the context of frequently encountered disorders.

# Acknowledgments

I would like to thank several anonymous reviewers of the earlier editions of this book. Their thoughtful and detailed comments have been invaluable in making revisions for this third edition. I would also like to thank Francine Pomaville, my colleague and friend at California State University–Fresno, who reviewed and offered excellent suggestions to revise the section on laryngectomy. Finally, I am thankful to Juliet Steiner, Senior Product Manager at Delmar, Cengage Learning, for her excellent, friendly, and sustained support to complete the revision.

# A

**Abductor Spasms.** To assess this type of voice disorder of neurological origin (laryngeal dystonia) or a voice disorder with no demonstrated neurophysiological impairment (see Spasmodic Dysphonia), consider the following special features of assessment:

- Take a careful case history to document reported phonation breaks in social conversation
- Measure the frequency of sudden, intermittent, and fleeting cessation of voice during conversational speech
- Note that the problem may be absent for days, so if not observed during an initial session, repeat the clinical observation and measurement; ask the client to submit a taped sample of voice taken on a day he or she experiences it the most
- Note the presence of excessive effort in voice production, because this is a hyperfunctional voice disorder (the reason why some clinicians classify it as spasmodic dysphonia)
- Note whether the client coughs, tries to clear the throat, or requests a drink of water to restore voice that is temporarily lost; such efforts to restore voice are a sign of abductor spasms
- Observe any signs of vocal fatigue, which is a part of the problem
- Rule out vocal nodules because they, too, can cause intermittent phonation breaks due to reduced subglottal air pressure
- See the companion volumes: *Hegde's PocketGuide to Communication Disorders, Hegde's PocketGuide to Treatment in Speech-Language Pathology (3rd ed.),* and the cited source

Boone, D. R., McFarlane, S. C., & Von Berg, S. L. (2005). *The voice and voice therapy* (7th ed.). Boston, MA: Allyn and Bacon.

**Adaptation Effect.** An aspect of stuttering assessment, adaptation effect is a measure of stuttering under repeated oral reading of a brief printed passage; there is a typical decrease in the frequency of Stuttering from the first through the fifth reading; may be a part of the assessment of stuttering because of its diagnostic significance; to assess adaptation:

- Ask the client who stutters to read aloud a printed passage (e.g., *My Grandfather* or the *Rainbow*) up to five times
- Count both the number and the loci of dysfluencies on each oral reading and calculate the percent dysfluency rate
- Note the loci (specific words or locations between words) on which dysfluencies occurred
- Note the specific words and sounds on which dysfluencies were more consistent (dysfluencies on the same loci on three or more readings) and those on which dysfluencies occurred only during the first three readings
- Words or sounds on which dysfluencies occurred more consistently across the five readings suggest more severe stutterings than those that adapted (disappeared) on the third and subsequent readings; more severe stutterings, so identified, may persist longer in treatment and probably need special attention during treatment
- Adaptation effect is more typically found in stuttering of early onset and it may be absent or less remarkable in case of neurogenic stuttering

**Agnosia.** Assessment of agnosia, which is a difficulty in recognizing the meaning of various sensory stimuli in the absence of sensory deficits, is part of a comprehensive evaluation of clients with central nervous system dysfunction; includes many varieties that need to be assessed:

*Auditory Agnosia*

- Have the client's peripheral hearing tested; the hearing should be within the normal limits
- Check awareness of auditory stimuli, including speech; the client should be aware of sound
- Check visual recognition of objects; there should be no problem
- Ask the client to match objects or animal pictures with the sounds they make; the performance is expected to be poor

*Auditory Verbal Agnosia (Pure Word Deafness)*

- Check whether the client can hear spoken words; the client should hear them and be aware of them
- Ask the client to point to objects or pictures you name; expect errors
- Check comprehension of words during conversation by asking questions; expect many wrong responses
- Ask the client to recognize printed or written words; there should be no problem
- Ask the client to recognize nonverbal sounds; expect no problems
- Check spontaneous speech, reading, and writing; expect no significant problems

*Tactile Agnosia*

- Ask client to touch and name objects when blindfolded; expect difficulty in correct tactile recognition of objects
- Remove the blindfold and ask the client to name the objects; expect improved performance
- Present the characteristic sounds associated with the objects; expect improved performance

*Prosopagnosia*

- Present pictures of family members and ask the client to name them; expect errors
- Ask the client to name individuals within the room while they remain silent; expect mistakes or no responses
- Ask the client to recognize when the individuals say something; expect mostly correct recognition
- Verify right hemisphere damage through medical records, including neurological and neuroimaging examination results

*Visual Agnosia*

- Present objects or pictures visually and ask the client to name them; expect a high error rate
- Ask the client to touch and feel objects and then name each; expect much improved performance
- Present sounds associated with the objects and ask the client to name them; expect improvement performance

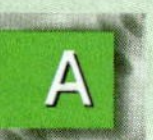



- Verify bilateral occipital lesions, posterior parietal lobe lesions, or other visual cortex-related damage through medical records
- See the companion volumes: *Hegde's PocketGuide to Communication Disorders* and *Hegde's PocketGuide to Treatment in Speech-Language Pathology* (3rd ed.)

**Agrammatism.** Assessment of agrammatism, which is deficient grammar, characterized by telegraphic speech is important in clients with Aphasia and dementia; short phrases, limited sentence structures and varieties, found especially in clients with nonfluent aphasias, are described as *agrammatic speech*; to assess:

- Record a conversational speech sample and have the client describe pictures and pictured story scenes
- Analyze missing grammatical morphemes, typical phrase or sentence lengths, and the number of different sentence types used
- Administer selected standardized tests described under Aphasia
- See Aphasia for more detailed assessment information

**Agraphia.** Assessment of writing problems in clients with neurological impairments or diseases is essential to develop a comprehensive treatment program; agraphia is a general term to describe writing problems that are due to recent cerebral pathology; to be distinguished from writing problems children may exhibit because of poor instruction or learning disabilities; includes a few varieties; to assess them:

- Assess associated disorders, including Aphasia, Cerebral Palsy, Dementia, and other neurological disorders that may be present
- Verify left, right, or bilateral hemispheric lesions though medical records, neurological examinations, and results of radiographic or scanning procedures
- Apraxic Agraphia: To assess these writing problems associated with apraxia:
  - Obtain samples of spontaneous writing, copying, and dictation; analyze for errors in letter formation, spelling errors, repletion of words and phrases, and such other writing problems—all diagnostic of apraxia
  - Check whether the writing includes only capital letters, a positive sign of apraxic agraphia
- Motor Agraphia: To assess writing problems due to impaired neuromotor control:
  - Obtain spontaneous, dictated, and copied writing samples
  - Look for writing extremely small letters (micrographia) or letters that get progressively smaller
  - Look for extreme difficulty writing or disorganized writing due to tremors, tics, chorea, and dystonia
  - Observe obvious neuromuscular problems in the hand and verify them in medical records
- Pure Agraphia: To assess writing problems with no other language dysfunctions:
  - Obtain spontaneous, dictated, and copied writing samples
  - Look for extreme difficulty writing anything at all
  - Check whether copying or automatic writing is nearly normal but spontaneous writing is full of errors—both are diagnostic features

  - Check medical records for evidence of lesions in the premotor cortex and superior parietal lobe
- Generally, relate morphologic and syntactic errors and neologistic writing to predominantly left hemisphere lesions; compare writing problems with expressive language problems for similarities (except for clients with pure agraphia)
- Generally, relate such spatial writing errors as failure to give margins, erratic spacing between words and sentences, and left neglect to right hemisphere lesions
- See the companion volumes: *Hegde's PocketGuide to Communication Disorders* and *Hegde's PocketGuide to Treatment in Speech-Language Pathology* (3rd ed.)

**AIDS Dementia Complex.** Assessment of progressive physical and intellectual deterioration associated with Acquired Immune Deficiency Syndrome (AIDS) is essential to distinguish it from other forms of dementia; AIDS dementia complex resembles subcortical dementia in the beginning and cortical dementia in the advanced stages. See Dementia. Also, see the companion volume: *Hegde's PocketGuide to Communication Disorders*, for etiological factors and symptomatology of AIDS dementia complex.

### *Assessment Objectives/General Guidelines*

- To assess language, cognitive skills, memory, and emotional reactions (e.g., apathy or depression)
- To diagnose dementia associated with AIDS
- To develop a plan for communication treatment or rehabilitation
- To make periodic assessment to evaluate changes in the symptom complex

### *Case History/Interview Focus*

- See **Case History** and **Interview** under Standard/Common Assessment Procedures
- Concentrate on history of AIDS and general symptoms that support its diagnosis
- Examine medical evidence that supports the diagnosis of AIDS
- Get information on the client's health and various diseases clients with AIDS are vulnerable to
- Get information that helps establish the premorbid skills, intellectual levels, hobbies, and general behavior patterns
- Pay special attention to changes in skills, behavior, and intellectual level that the family members may have noticed

### *Ethnocultural Considerations*

- See Ethnocultural Considerations in Assessment
- Assess the family's resources and needed support system because the treatment and rehabilitation of AIDS and dementia associated with it are expensive and drawn out
- Seek such additional services as counseling and medical management if warranted
- Counsel the family and work closely with the caregivers

## AIDS Dementia Complex

### Assessment

- Take note of the neurological symptoms associated with AIDS dementia (e.g., gait disturbances, tremors, seizures, and facial nerve paralysis)
- Use procedures described under Dementia and Alzheimer's Disease to assess:
  - State of awareness, which may range from fully aware to mostly sleeping; use the *Mini-Mental State Examination*
  - Mood and affect, which may vary from apathy to clinical depression
  - Speech and language skills: assess both production and comprehension through a conversational speech sample and general picture description;
  - Cognition, memory, and related intellectual skills; use client-specific procedures to assess these and general behavioral deterioration; note that in the final stages, the client may be mute
- Be aware that in some clients, dementia may be the only presenting symptom of undiagnosed AIDS

### Standardized Tests

- Administer one or more tests that sample communication deficits in clients with dementia, including the *Arizona Battery of Communication Disorders of Dementia;* consider administering selected tests of aphasia, especially the *Western Aphasia Battery* and *Communication Abilities in Daily Living* that have been used with clients with dementia
- Administer one or more of the several tests of dementia, including the *Blessed Dementia Rating Scale,* the *Clinical Dementia Rating,* the *Global Deterioration Scale,* or the *Dementia Deficits Scale;* see Dementia for additional tests

### Related/Medical Assessment Data

- Medical diagnosis of HIV infection and AIDS is essential to diagnose AIDS dementia complex
- Neurological evidence of encephalopathy is supportive

### Standard/Common Assessment Procedures

- Complete the Standard/Common Assessment Procedures

### Diagnostic Criteria

- A combination of symptoms of Dementia, medical and laboratory evidence of AIDS infection and encephalopathy, and supportive evidence from assessment of communication, cognition, and behavioral deterioration is essential to diagnose this type of dementia

### Differential Diagnosis

- Relatively early onset of cognitive and behavioral decline (as early as late 20s; unlike dementia associated with degenerative neurological diseases) along with evidence of HIV infection, AIDS, and encephalopathy helps distinguish it from other forms of dementia
- Prominent neurological symptoms associated with AIDS-induced encephalopathy, along with the presence of opportunistic infectious diseases help distinguish it from various forms of aphasia; mutism in the final stages also may be of some significance

### *Prognosis*

- Guarded; although medical treatment of AIDS has improved significantly, encephalopathy and Dementia, once begun, will be irreversible

### *Recommendations*

- Treatment for the client in the early stages of dementia; clinical management of the behavioral and cognitive problems is the main goal
- Working with the family in all stages, and especially in the final stages, is the most critical clinical management concern
- See the two companion volumes: *Hegde's PocketGuide to Communication Disorders* and *Hegde's PocketGuide to Treatment in Speech-Language Pathology* (3rd ed.), and the cited sources

Clark, C. M., & Trojanowski, J. Q. (2000). *Neurodegenerative dementias.* New York: McGraw-Hill.

Larsen, C. (1998). *HIV and communication disorders.* Clifton Park, NY: Thomson Delmar Learning.

**Alexia.** Assessment of reading problems due to recent brain injury or disease is a part of a comprehensive evaluation of adults who have aphasia, dementia, and other neurological disorders; to be distinguished from dyslexia, which is commonly diagnosed in children with learning disabilities but with no obvious neurological impairments; includes *Alexia With Agraphia; Alexia Without Agraphia; Deep Dyslexia*, and *Frontal Dyslexia*; for additional assessment procedures, see Aphasia. See the companion volume: *Hegde's PocketGuide to Communication Disorders* for etiological factors and symptomatology.

***Alexia With Agraphia.*** Coexistence of reading and writing problems often found in clients with aphasia; also called parietal-temporal alexia; see Agraphia for associated writing problems; due to lesions in the dominant parietal and temporal lobes.

#### Assessment

- Review the client's history to establish a recent episode of strokes, tumors, and trauma including gunshot wounds
- Examine the client's medical records to document lesions in the angular gyrus and the dominant parietal and temporal lobes and for diagnosis of Wernicke's aphasia or Broca's aphasia (see Aphasia: Specific Types)
- Tape-record the client's oral language sample; analyze the oral language problems as you would with clients with Aphasia
- Tape-record one or more oral reading samples; select reading materials that are appropriate for the individual's education, interest, and ethnocultural background
- Obtain the client's spontaneous, dictated, and copied writing samples; also, the client's premorbid writing samples
- Administer such tests of reading skills as the *Reading Comprehension Battery for Aphasia* or the *Gates-MacGinitie Reading Tests;* see Aphasia for additional tests
- Administer selected aphasia tests that include writing subtests (e.g., *Communication Abilities of Daily Living*); some of these also include reading subtests

- Analyze the reading and writing difficulties in light of the oral language problems
- Note that the reading comprehension deficits will be prominent in clients with Wernicke's aphasia and oral reading difficulties will be prominent in clients with Broca's aphasia
- Compare the reading and writing problems of the same client; generally, reading and writing problems will be similar
- Compare the client's premorbid writing skills with those of the current skills; analyze the kinds of errors that are not shared by the two samples to assess deterioration due to recent cerebral pathology

#### Differential Diagnosis

- Rule out visual problems and left visual neglect, because alexia with agraphia is not due to such problems
- Rule out reading and writing problems due to poor premorbid literacy skills or persistent childhood dyslexia, because these are not the same as adult alexia with agraphia
- Rule out peripheral motor problems (such as paralyzed preferred hand or weakness in the hand) that may make it difficult to write
- Distinguish reading comprehension problems from motor speech difficulties in expressing what may have been comprehended well
- Rule out attention deficits and fatigue as the potential variables related to reading and writing skills; such variables are not a strong basis to diagnose alexia with agraphia in clients with brain injury or pathology
- Do not diagnose alexia in children whose reading difficulties are a part of their learning disorders; most children with reading problems are diagnosed with dyslexia; there usually is no evidence of recent brain injury in most children with dyslexia; if there is such evidence, it may be alexia

*Alexia Without Agraphia.* Assessment of reading difficulties with relatively intact writing skills is necessary in some clients with neuropathologies; such reading problems are commonly associated with Aphasia and, more specifically, a disassociation between the occipital association cortex and the dominant angular gyrus.

#### Assessment

- Assess reading skills more extensively than the writing skills; generally, use the procedures described for alexia with agraphia; writing subtests included in tests of aphasia are sufficient to rule out writing problems in clients thought to have alexia without agraphia; a brief premorbid writing sample will help rule out current writing problems
- Compare the reading and writing skills with oral language problems; compare premorbid writing skills with the current skills
- Assess color naming, because it is a diagnostically significant impairment associated with alexia without agraphia, although it may not be found in all clients
- Assess visual field deficits to diagnose right or left hemianopia; present visual stimuli (small objects) in the right and left visual field and have the client recognize them

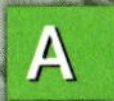



### Differential Diagnosis

- Distinguish pure alexia from alexia with agraphia; document writing skills comparable to those at the premorbid levels in clients with pure alexia to make this differential diagnosis; see also Agraphia
- Distinguish alexia without agraphia from frontal alexia by documenting symptoms of Broca's aphasia associated with the latter
- Distinguish pure alexia from deep dyslexia by documenting semantic errors in oral reading associated with the latter; see *Deep Dyslexia* in this section
- Document visual field deficits and color naming problems (if present)

***Deep Dyslexia.*** Assessment of a variety of reading disorders in which the client makes semantic reading errors is a part of evaluating clients with aphasia; called as such because the meaning of the misread words are related to the error types (e.g., the client may read the printed word *close* as *shut*).

### Assessment

- Select reading material that is appropriate to the individual's education, interest, ethnocultural background, and gauged premorbid reading skill level
- Tape record one or more samples of the client's oral reading
- Analyze the types of errors; the client may exhibit general semantic errors (e.g., reading *pen* as *pencil*), derivational errors (e.g., misreading the printed word *wise* as *wisdom*), deletion of grammatical suffixes (e.g., misreading the printed word *hardest* as *hard* or *walking* as *walk*), and so forth

### Differential Diagnosis

- Diagnose deep dyslexia on the basis of the highest number of errors on grammatical function words, followed by adjectives, verbs, and abstract nouns; and the lowest number of errors on concrete nouns
- Distinguish aphasia without deep dyslexia by documenting an absence of semantic errors in the former and their predominance in the latter
- Distinguish deep dyslexia from frontal alexia by documenting the association of Broca's aphasia with the latter

***Frontal Alexia.*** These types of reading disorders that are associated with frontal lobe pathology may be necessary, especially in clients with Broca's aphasia, although not all clients with this type of aphasia have frontal alexia; also called the third alexia or anterior alexia.

### Assessment

- Select reading material that is appropriate to the individual's education, interest, ethnocultural background, and gauged premorbid reading skill level
- Tape record one or more samples of the client's oral reading
- Analyze the types of errors (e.g., omission of grammatical morphemes, refusal to read, greater difficulty with abstract words)

### Differential Diagnosis

- Document not only reading problems, but reluctance to read or complete avoidance of reading, a differential diagnostic feature of frontal alexia

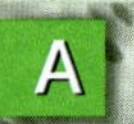



- Document the absence of letter-by-letter reading, another diagnostic feature of the disorder
- Distinguish frontal alexia from deep dyslexia by documenting semantic errors in the latter
- Distinguish frontal alexia from alexia with agraphia by a lack of significant writing problems in the former
- See the two companion volumes: *Hegde's PocketGuide to Communication Disorders* and *Hegde's PocketGuide to Treatment in Speech-Language Pathology* (3rd ed.)

**Alternating Motion Rates (AMRs).** Assessment of AMRs, also known as diadochokinetic rates, is one of the standard assessment procedures in speech-language pathology; both are a measure of the speed and regularity with which repetitive movements of the articulatory structures are made; help assess the functional and structural integrity of the lips, jaw, and tongue; of special diagnostic value in assessing motor speech disorders; in assessment, usually followed by Sequential Motion Rates (SMRs), which require rapid movement from one articulatory posture to another by having the client produce different syllables as rapidly and as steadily as possible; see also Diadochokinetic Rates and Standard/Common Assessment Procedures.

### *Assessment*

- Ask the client to take a deep breath and say "**pʌh-pʌh-pʌh-pʌh**" for as long and as steadily as possible
- Model the response for 2 to 3 seconds
- Ask the client to "stop" when a 3- to 5-second sample has been recorded
- Ask the client to take a deep breath and say "**tʌh-tʌh-tʌh-tʌh**" for as long and as steadily as possible; model if necessary; record a 3- to 5-second sample
- Ask the client to take a deep breath and say "**kʌh-kʌh-kʌh-kʌh**" for as long and as steadily as possible; model if necessary; record a 3- to 5-second sample
- Move on to measure the SMRs by asking the client to say "**pʌh-tʌh-kʌh-pʌh-tʌh-kʌh-pʌh-tʌh-kʌh-pʌh-tʌh-kʌh**" for as long and as steadily as possible; reinstruct or model if necessary; record the sample
- Observe the range of motion of the jaw and lips
- Observe the rhythmicity of the jaw and lip movements

### *Analysis*

- Analyze the response rates in relation to normative data
- The normative data for AMRs (**pʌh**, **tʌh**, or **kʌh**):
  - Range from 5 to 7 repetitions per second in normally speaking adults
  - Range from about 4 repetitions to 6 repetitions in normally speaking children
  - Show a slower rate in children under 9 (generally 4 or more repetitions), compared to those above 9 (generally fewer than 4 repetitions)
- The normative data for SMRs (**pʌh-tʌh-kʌh**):
  - Range from 3.6 to 7.5 repetitions per second in normally speaking adults
  - Range from 1 to 2.5 repetitions per second in normally speaking children

- Inadequate AMRs and SMRs may be due to inadequate breath support for speech; phonatory abnormalities also may be suggested
- Slowness or accelerated speech may suggest neuromotor problems of the kind seen in clients with Dysarthria
- Arrhythmic and irregular movements of the jaw and lips also suggest neuromotor problems that are associated with Dysarthria
- The range of motion is significantly reduced in clients with certain types of Dysarthria
- Although the significance of AMRs and SMRs in the assessment of clients with neuromotor control problems is evident, their significance in assessing clients with no such problems is not clear

Fletcher, S. G. (1972). Time-by-count measurement of diadachokinetic syllable rate. *Journal of Speech and Hearing Disorders, 15*, 763–770.

Kent, R. D., Kent, J. F., & Rosenbek, J. C. (1987). Maximum performance rates of speech production. *Journal of Speech and Hearing Disorders, 52*, 367–371.

**Alternative (Nonbiased) Assessment Approaches.** To assess communication disorders without making reference to norms derived from standardized tests, consider one of several alternative nonbiased approaches; note that the traditional assessment approach is heavily dependent on norm-referenced standardized tests; limitations of standardized tests, which include their inappropriateness to assess many minority and ethnoculturally different clients, has prompted the development of alternative assessment approaches; thoughtfully designed alternative approaches may be appropriate for all children, including children from the mainstream society because they avoid many other limitations of standardized tests; consider one or more of the following alternative approaches:

***Authentic Assessment.*** An alternative to assessment based on standardized tests and norm-referencing in diagnosing communication disorders; more appropriate in assessing clients of varied ethnocultural background because it avoids tests that are not standardized on specific minority groups; requires the use of meaningful and worthwhile tasks during assessment to make connection between assessment activities and real-world affairs; more often used in education than in speech-language pathology, although its use in the latter is appropriate and has been advocated; consider the following in conducting an authentic assessment of communication disorders:

- Construct assessment items derived from the child's academic curricula (e.g., select words, phrases, syntactic structures, and so forth from the child's grade books) instead of using standardized test items
- Derive assessment items from the child's home environment (e.g., child's storybooks may provide plenty of assessment materials to test narrative skills, reading comprehension, writing skills)
- Select assessment items that are useful and functional (e.g., assess a child's language skills as the child holds a conversation with a peer and his or her teacher, instead of administering a standardized test); assess abstract reasoning skills from the child's textbooks; assess literacy skills that are also the teacher's targets in classroom instruction

- Observe the child as he or she interacts in naturalistic settings (e.g., a brief observation of the child on the playground, in the school cafeteria)
- Seek information on the child's communication patterns from adults who are familiar with the child (e.g., parents and teachers may provide information that cannot be obtained from standardized tests)
- Analyze the results of authentic assessment in terms of criterion-based standards or minimum competency core concepts, not age-based norms; in consultation with teachers and parents, set the skill levels the child should attain
- Recommend treatment to have the child meet the selected skill levels

Schraeder, T., Quinn, M., Stockman, I. & Miller, J. (1999). Authentic assessment as an approach to preschool speech-language screening. *American Journal of Speech-Language Pathology, 8,* 195–200.

***Client-Specific Assessment Procedures.*** Assessment tools or procedures that a clinician specifically designs for a given client; needed when standard, standardized, or readily available procedures are judged not appropriate or found to be ineffective with a given client; both individual uniqueness and diverse ethnocultural background may necessitate such procedures; consider the following in designing client-specific procedures:

- See Ethnocultural Considerations in Assessment
- Use the case history information to understand the cultural background, bilingual/multilingual status, education, occupation, and general level of sophistication of the client and family
- Make initial judgments about potential assessment tools, standardized tests, and the need for client-specific procedures based on the case history information
- During the interview, ask questions about the client's interests, hobbies, social activities, and literacy; in the case of children, ask questions about favorite toys, books, and activities
- To design client-specific procedures, select target behaviors or skills to be assessed in the specific child or adult client
  - Specific grammatical morphemes produced in words, phrases, or sentences (e.g., the regular and irregular plural morphemes, past tense inflections, the verbal auxiliary and the copula, the present progressive *ing*)
  - Specific syntactic structures (e.g., active declarative sentences, questions, requests, complex sentences)
  - Narrative skills (telling a story or retelling a story the clinician narrates)
  - Frequency of dysfluencies of stuttering in conversational exchanges
  - Conversational repair strategies during a conversational episode involving the clinician (e.g., request for clarification, response to request for clarification)
  - General conversational skills (e.g., topic initiation, turn taking, topic maintenance)
  - Specific speech sound productions (e.g., fricatives, affricates, blends of specific types)

  - Breakdown in speech production with increasingly complex phonetic sequences (bisyllabic to multisyllabic words, or words involving common to uncommon phoneme sequences)
  - Naming skills (naming selected objects, photographs of family members, or line drawings to evoke the names within such categories as *animals* or *vegetables*)
  - Writing skills (writing to dictation, spontaneous writing, copying a printed paragraph, copying geometric shapes)
  - Reading skills (reading printed passages)
- Prepare the stimulus materials, taking the information gathered about the client into consideration
  - Write words, phrases, or sentences that help assess the various targets
  - Take into consideration the client's interests, hobbies, literacy levels, cultural background, and linguistic variation
  - Select gestures or signs that will be useful in evaluating the target behaviors or skills; select gestures that are ethnoculturally appropriate and familiar to the client
  - Select assessment stimulus items that are used in the home, familiar in the culture, accepted by the client or the family; avoid using stimuli that are irrelevant to the client's cultural and linguistic background
  - Whenever practical, select the stimulus items from everyday sources, familiar magazines, and colorful pictures
  - Select stimuli from the client's home environment; request the family members to bring the child's favorite books, a few favorite toys; request the spouse of the client to bring photographs of family members; request the client to bring his or her own favorite storybooks
  - Gradually create your own collection of stimuli by cutting out colorful pictures from magazines; include three-dimensional, naturalistic pictures; select toys and objects; before their administration, assess their familiarity and appropriateness to the client
  - Design multiple stimulus items or exemplars for each target (e.g., four items that evoke the same sound in the same position, five phrases in which the plural /s/ is produced)
  - Freely substitute stimuli that are found to be inappropriate for the client
- During the assessment, make each task specific to the client
  - Have the client name his or her own family member's pictures or items in his or her own room as shown in a photograph
  - Let the client narrate a personal experience
  - Tell a story to the client that is selected from the client's own storybook or a story that is specific to the client's culture
  - Introduce conversational topics that are client-specific or let the client suggest topics for conversation
  - Have the client write a paragraph about his or her personal experience; dictate a paragraph from the client's books unless the objective is to assess writing skills when the material is unfamiliar to the client
  - Have the client read a passage from his or her own book; have the client read unfamiliar books if that suits the assessment purpose

- Include additional exemplars of target behavior to be assessed if time permits to counteract inadequate sampling of target behaviors inherent to standardized tests
- Note that the flexibility involved in client-specific procedures is typically absent in the use of standardized tests (e.g., you cannot expand exemplars or substitute stimulus items)
- Analyze and interpret the results of client-specific assessment procedures the way you would the outcome of Criterion-Referenced Testing; do not evaluate the results in relation to standardized test norms; consider the results as informative of the client's current skill level
- Make judgments whether the present skill level is adequate to meet the oral, gestural, or written communication needs of the client; if not, recommend treatment

Hegde, M. N. (1998). *Treatment procedures in communicative disorders* (3rd ed.). Austin, TX: Pro-Ed.

***Criterion-Referenced Assessment.*** An alternative form of assessment in which the results are not compared against norms derived from the performance of a representative sample; an approach that is useful in avoiding the pitfalls of standardized tests; appropriate in assessing all kinds of skills in all clients, but especially useful in assessing children and adults from ethnoculturally diverse backgrounds for whom the standardized tests may be unsuitable; to perform criterion-reference assessment:

- Select target behaviors to be assessed in view of the child's communication needs and academic and social demands made on the child; in essence, assess functional communication skills regardless of age-based norms
- Set performance standards the child is expected to meet; for instance, reading and writing at a certain level; mastery of certain language structures at 80% accuracy; mastery of speech sounds at 90% accuracy; narrative skills or other conversational skills at 80% accuracy, and so forth
- Prepare stimulus materials that are effective, specific to the client, appropriate from the standpoint of the child's ethnocultural background; select materials from the child's academic curricula and from the child's natural environment; see Client-Specific Assessment Procedures for additional details; prepare an adequate number of stimulus items for each target skill (e.g., 10 opportunities to produce a grammatical morpheme or a sound in the initial position of words versus one or two opportunities typically afforded on standardized tests)
- Administer the selected stimulus materials, modify the stimuli as you see fit, and repeat and modify the instructions to effectively evoke responses (strategies that would not be appropriate in standardized test-based assessment)
- Analyze and summarize the results in terms of the skills that are present, mastered, not yet mastered, absent, and so forth; state the quantitative level at which the skills are produced (e.g., the child produced the regular plural morpheme at 75% accuracy) without evaluating the results in terms of standardized test norms; compare the different skills and their level of

production within the child, versus comparing a child's performance with the performance of other children

- Recommend treatment based on the desired skill levels that fall below the performance criterion
- Use criterion-referenced assessment to periodically evaluate a clients' progress under treatment.

McCauley, R. J. (1996). Familiar strangers: Criterion-referenced measures in communication disorders. *Language, Speech, and Hearing Services in Schools, 27,* 122–131.

***Dynamic Assessment.*** An alternative assessment procedure that may be more appropriate for all children, and especially to children of ethnoculturally diverse backgrounds, than the traditional standardized test-based assessment; the basic approach is to find out whether the child can learn the skills he or she lacks during assessment, versus during treatment offered only after an assessment is completed; to perform this kind of assessment that is relatively bias-free:

- Structure the dynamic assessment session to teach the skills the child lacks; it is not essential to teach all the skills to the full extent, but to informally experiment with a few to see whether the child can learn what he or she lacks; in essence, this approach is similar to stimulability testing, but is done more intensively
- While testing a skill, give feedback on the child's performance to see whether such feedback (reinforcement) would improve performance; tell the child why a response was correct and why another was incorrect; note that such a practice would invalidate the results of a standardized test
- Ask the child why he or she thinks a response was correct or incorrect to promote better self-evaluation of responses given during assessment
- Even if you use standardized tests, modify the test items or instructions; select a stimulus picture that is different from what is given in the manual but more suitable to the child's ethnocultural background; repeat instructions or modify the words; but when you do this, do not interpret the results in terms of the test norms
- Use the test-teach-retest format; informally teach the deficient skills by prompts, reinforcement, and corrective feedback to assess learnability; but do not conclude that a child who had difficulty learning the skills has a poor prognosis for mastering them in more systematic and extended treatment sessions—a potential weakness of the approach

Gutierrez-Clellen, V. F., & Pena, E. (2001). Dynamic assessment of diverse children: A tutorial. *Language, Speech, and Hearing Services in Schools, 32*, 212–224.

Lidz, C. S., & Pena, E. D. (1996). Dynamic assessment: The model, its relevance, as a nonbiased approach, and its application to Latino American preschool children. *Language, Speech, and Hearing Services in Schools*, *27*, 367–372.

Ukrainetz, T. A., Harpell, S., Walsh, C., & Coyle, C. (2000). A preliminary investigation of dynamic assessment with Native American Kindergartners. *Language, Speech, and Hearing Services in Schools, 31*, 142–154.

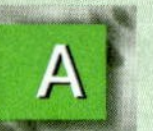



*Portfolio Assessment.* An assessment approach that offers an alternative to a standardized test-based assessment of a child's skills, including speech and language skills; it is especially relevant to make a comprehensive assessment of all related skills in the context of academic demands placed on the child and the performance standards the child needs to meet; standardized test results may be a part of the portfolio developed for a child, although they will be only one of several pieces of assessment data that help make clinical and academic decisions; in making a portfolio assessment:

- Consider the assessment of a child a continuous process in which data are gathered as they become available and placed in the portfolio; in this sense, an assessment database is constantly expanded; such a portfolio provides a good historical perspective on the student's problems and progress
- Obtain multiple measures that are valid, reliable, and nondiscriminatory; with such measures, construct a portfolio for the student, which is a collection of a student's multiple work samples
- Note that a portfolio is developed as a team effort and will contain information from different professionals, including the child's teacher, special education teacher, educational psychologist, and other specialists
- As a speech-language pathologist, contribute portfolio items that are relevant to the child's communication strengths and needs, assessment results, treatment plans, progress in treatment, results of parent participation in treatment, home assessment or treatment activities, and so forth
- Include a specific statement about the child's problem, typically written by the team serving the student
- Participate in the team discussion that will determine the items to be added to the portfolio; generally, different specialists will include items relevant to their work with the child; as a speech-language pathologist, you may include the following:
    - Case history and referral forms; reasons for referral, a problem statement, and main concerns the specialists and family members have about the child's performance
    - Language sample, preferably transcribed; a brief report that describes how the child interacts with the teacher and peers will be especially useful because it reflects naturalistic communication; a home sample, if practical, will be relevant as well
    - Narrative samples, recorded verbatim; how the child narrates his or her experiences or tells or retells stories will be useful in relating more advanced language skills to demanding academic tasks
    - Conversational skills, summaries of weaknesses; a description of such skills as topic initiation, topic maintenance, and turn taking will be useful items in the portfolio
    - Clinician's observational reports; periodically completed reports on the clinician's observation of the child's communication patterns, treatment progress as seen in naturalist contexts (e.g., increased fluency while talking to the teacher, improved turn taking while taking part in a class discussion) will help evaluate the child's changing (improving) skills

- Various kinds of work samples; child's writing samples, drawings, paintings, and other artwork samples, math work samples, and other kinds of work a student does in the classroom may be a part of the portfolio; in such cases, write your comments on relevant pieces of work (e.g., writing samples) to point out errors, improvement over time, need for additional intervention strategies, and so forth
- Interview data; interview teachers about the child's speech and language skills and specific disorders (e.g., stuttering or a voice problem) and place a brief summary of the interview in the portfolio; also place similar summaries of the interview with the parents and the student himself or herself
- Standard test results; if standardized test administration is required in the particular school setting, place the results and summaries of the administered speech and language tests in the child's portfolio
- Periodically summarize and evaluate the content of the portfolio, because a mere collection of items will be of no help to the child; make clinical decisions based on periodic reviews and consultations with other team members; recommend changes in intervention strategies as the child's skills and the demands made on the child change over time

Kratcoski, A. M. (1998). Guidelines for using portfolios in assessment and evaluation. *Language, Speech, and Hearing Services in Schools, 29*, 3–10.

**Alzheimer's Disease (AD).** Assessment of this degenerative neurological disorder that terminates in a severe form of dementia requires a sampling of a client's varied cognitive, behavioral, and neurological symptoms that get progressively worse; see the sources cited at the end of this main entry and the companion volume, *Hegde's PocketGuide to Communication Disorders,* for etiological factors and symptomatology; see also Dementia.

### *Assessment Objectives/General Guidelines*

- To document communication deficits including memory problems
- To substantiate a diagnosis of dementia with an assessment of communication problems
- To help plan a communication intervention program and a family support program
- To coordinate the assessment results with those of other members of the professional team working with the client and family members

### *Case History/Interview Focus*

- See **Case History** and **Interview** under Standard/Common Assessment Procedures
- Review the results of medical examinations and special laboratory tests including the results of brain scanning procedures
- In interviewing the family, consider using the Alzheimer Dementia Risk Questionnaire by J. C. Breitner and M. Folstein, which facilitates a systematic gathering of information from the family members
- Concentrate on changes in cognition, general behavior, and communication skills; consider using the Alzheimer Dementia Risk Questionnaire during case history taking and interview

- Concentrate also on how the family members view the client's problems, onset of symptoms, and progression
- Obtain information on the family's living conditions, coping strategies, financial and personal resources needed to manage the client on a long-term basis, and the family members' ability to care for the client at home and the support systems they may need
- Pay special attention to information that helps gauge the client's premorbid intellectual level and general behavioral patterns; for instance, education, occupation, hobbies, reading and writing skills, special talents, typical behaviors and routines, and so forth; such information will help evaluate potential changes in behavior and cognition
- Get information that may suggest previous strokes, infections (especially AIDS), alcoholism, vitamin deficiencies, neurological symptoms (e.g., tics, tremor, rigidity), psychiatric problems (e.g., history of schizophrenia, paranoia, depression)
- Concentrate on changes in behaviors, skills, and especially memory because they are the early signs of dementia

## Ethnocultural Considerations

- During the interview of the family, pay special attention to the cultural and family views of this lifelong disability; assess whether the family members distinguish intellectual limitations associated with the normal aging process from limitations that may be signs of dementia
- Assess access to health care and support systems the family has (or does not have) because these may be particularly problematic and complicate rehabilitation efforts with certain ethnic minority groups
- Assess the degree to which the family members may need counseling about health care and other resources and client management strategies at home
- See also Ethnocultural Considerations in Assessment

## Assessment

### General Considerations and Global Assessment Concerns

- The various intellectual, communicative, and general behavioral symptoms may be subtle or mild in the beginning stages of the disease; distinguishing them from changes associated with normal aging will be a main objective of the assessment
- The number and severity of symptoms increase gradually and intensify in the later stages
- Assessment requires more careful analysis of communication skills in the beginning stages; symptoms of advanced stage dementia are quite obvious
- Communication assessment cannot be done in a vacuum; the clinician will have to consider all aspects of the client, including the client's intellectual, behavioral, psychiatric, neurological, and general health status
- Family members or other caregivers play an important role in providing information on subtle or gross behavioral changes that is valuable in making a diagnosis (e.g., inappropriate social behavior, forgetting to pay the bills, disorientation and confusion, depression, or avoidance of actions previously well performed)

- While assessing communication disorders, the clinician should observe other behavioral symptoms of dementia; the clinician may take note of neglected self-care, irritability or hostility, frustration with assessment tasks presented, confusion and disorientation, hyperactivity, ritualistic handling of objects, and so forth
- The clinician should take note of the neurological symptoms associated with Alzheimer's disease (e.g., gait disturbances, rigidity and spasticity, ideational and ideomotor apraxia, seizures, incontinence)
- The clinician should assess the state of awareness, which may range from fully aware to mostly sleeping; use the Mini-Mental State Examination; further testing and assessment may depend on the results of the awareness evaluation
- The clinician also should assess visuospatial problems unless other professionals have done it; for instance, the clinician should have the client copy three-dimensional drawings, construct block designs, or lace one's own shoes
- The clinician may also assess such other difficulties as problems in calculations and mathematical skills (acalculia) and Agnosia of various sorts

### Assess Speech

- Record a Speech and Language Sample (see Standard/Common Assessment Procedures) to analyze articulation or phonological disorders
- Be aware that no significant errors of articulation are noted in the early or middle stages of the disease
- Errors of sound production may be noted in the late stages, but no sound combinations that are alien to the language of the client
- Analyze speech production to diagnose a possible Hypokinetic Dysarthria (see under Dysarthria: Specific Types) and Apraxia of Speech

### Assess Language

- Record the client's description of pictures that depict a story sequence; analyze the client's description to assess memory for words, temporal sequences, logical connections, causes and effects, production of grammatical morphemes and sentence types, and topic maintenance
- Use the recorded speech and language sample to analyze language problems including the length of utterances, production of grammatical morphemes, and sentence types
- Assess language comprehension in conversational speech; take note of the number of utterances the client correctly and incorrectly comprehends
- Assess sentence comprehension by orally presenting a series of simple and progressively more complex sentences; use the *Auditory Comprehension Test for Sentences or* the *Revised Token Test* (see Aphasia)
- Assess such Pragmatic Language Skills as turn taking, topic initiation, topic maintenance, eye contact, and conversational repair during conversation; assess narrative skills by telling brief stories and having the client retell it; ask the client to narrate an experience; judge whether the client is inattentive during conversation, makes irrelevant and inappropriate comments, or offers offensive jokes

- Assess comprehension of word meaning; present a series of client-specific words and ask the client to define or give meanings for; also, use the *Peabody Picture Vocabulary Test (PPVT)*
- Assess confrontation naming by presenting a series of common objects or pictures and asking the client to name them; use the *Boston Naming Test* (see Aphasia)
- Assess short-term and long-term memory; ask client-specific questions about the recent and remote events in his or her life; in addition, administer a memory test (e.g., the *Wechsler Memory Scale—Revised,* or the *Memory Assessment Scale*)
- Administer standardized tests of aphasia such as the *Boston Diagnostic Aphasia Examination* (BDAE), the *Porch Index of Communicative Ability*, and the *Western Aphasia Battery* for an overall analysis of language problems associated with cerebral pathology (see Aphasia)
- Note that in the final stages, the client may be mute

### Assess Fluency

- Analyze the conversational speech sample to count all the Dysfluencies; count the number of words spoken to calculate the percent dysfluency rates (divide the number of dysfluencies by the number of words spoken and multiply it by 100)
- Assess word fluency by asking the client to say as many words as possible that begin with a certain letter, or belong to a certain category (e.g., animals, food items, furniture); use the Word Fluency Measure

### Assess Voice

- Make a routine analysis of voice quality, pitch, and intensity; make clinical judgments based on the interview
- Take note of any voice disorders, although no specific kinds of voice disorders are characteristic of Alzheimer's dementia

## *Standardized Tests*

- Administer one or more of the following tests for dementia; the tests allow for an assessment of various aspects of cognition, behavior, communication, and deterioration in measured skills

| Test | Purpose |
|---|---|
| *Activities of Daily Living Questionnaire (ADLQ)* (M. Johnson & associates) | To assess the daily living skills with the help of a knowledgeable informant |
| *Alzheimer Disease Assessment Scale (ADAS)* (Rosen, Mohs, & Davis) | To assess cognitive and noncognitive behaviors and their deterioration; widely used in medial settings |
| *Arizona Battery for Communication Disorders of Dementia* (K. A. Bayles & C. Tomoeda) | To assess dementia through 14 subtests and screen it with 4 subtests |
| *Benton Revised Visual Retention Test* (A. L. Benton) | To assess visual memory with figural recall |

*(continues)*

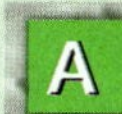



(continued)

| Test | Purpose |
|---|---|
| *The Blessed Dementia Scale* (G. Blessed & associates) | A scale to rate changes in performance in everyday activities and habits |
| *Brief Cognitive Rating Scale* (B. Reisberg) | To assess cognitive decline due to any reason |
| *Clinical Dementia Rating Scale* (C. P. Hughes & associates) | To rate dementia on a 5-point rating scale; does not assess communication skills |
| *Dementia Deficits Scale (DDS)* (A. Snow & associates) | To assess self-awareness deficits that may lead to dangerous behaviors |
| *Discourse Abilities Profile* (B. Terrel & D. Ripich) | To assess various forms of discourse during conversation with the client and conversation between the client, family members, and caregivers |
| *Global Deterioration Scale* (B. Reisberg & associates) | To rate dementia on a 7-point rating scale |
| *Memory Assessment Scales* (J. M. Williams) | To assess memory skills in greater detail than possible with dementia scales |
| *Mini-Mental State Examination* (M. F. Folstein, S. E. Folstein, & P. R. McHugh) | To assess the mental status with 11 items |
| *The Progressive Deterioration Scale (PDS)* (R. Dejong & associates) | To assess deterioration over time in daily living skills |
| *Wechsler Adult Intelligence Scale—III (WAIS—III)* (D. Wechsler) | To assess general intellectual level and intellectual deterioration |
| *Wechsler Memory Scale—Revised* (E. W. Russell) | To assess various memory functions in greater detail than possible with dementia scales |

- Several tests require the participation of family members or caregivers who are familiar with the client and can give reliable information; to evaluate the reliability, validity, and ethnocultural appropriateness of tests to be administered, consult the test manual thoroughly

## Related/Medical Assessment Data

- Integrate available medical, neurological, psychological, behavioral, and diagnostic medical laboratory findings with the results of communication assessment
- Integrate medical and communication assessment results with information obtained from case history, observation of clients, and information gathered from caretakers and family members

## Standard/Common Assessment Procedures

- Complete the Standard/Common Assessment Procedures

## Alzheimer's Disease (AD)

### *Diagnostic Criteria/Guidelines*

- A gradual onset of a progressive and generalized memory and intellectual deterioration is a necessary condition to diagnose AD; significant behavioral changes distinguish dementia of the Alzheimer's type from aphasia
- In the absence of direct pathological evidence, diagnosis is made by exclusion (ruling out dementia due to other causes)
- Agrammatism is not characteristic of the early stage; speech and language are generally better preserved in the early stages; in contrast, language is impaired in the early stage of aphasia

### *Differential Diagnosis*

- Note that the diagnosis of AD is finally established only through an autopsy to document its neuropathology
- Exclude dementia due to such other factors as:
  - Cerebrovascular diseases by ruling out repeated strokes; typical aphasia that results from strokes is not associated with intellectual and behavioral deterioration
  - Parkinson's disease, by its characteristic movement disorders and associated hypokinetic dysarthria, which is more common than in Alzheimer's disease
  - Huntington's disease, by its characteristic chorea and other neurological (movement) disorders and associated hyperkinetic dysarthria
  - Hypothyroidism, by ruling out endocrine disorders in the client
  - Vitamin $B_{12}$ deficiency by ruling out such deficiencies through laboratory tests
  - HIV infection by ruling out laboratory evidence of infection and other symptoms associated with AIDS dementia complex
  - Substance abuse, by ruling out a history of abuse and clinical findings
- Do *not* diagnose AD if:
  - The symptoms are exclusively associated with delirium
  - The cognitive deterioration may be explained on the basis of such other psychiatric disorders as schizophrenia
- Distinguish AD from aphasia
  - AD is likely to be confused with Wernicke's aphasia, anomic aphasia, and transcortical sensory aphasia because of relative fluency in all of them, but not with Broca's aphasia because of nonfluent, agrammatic speech of the latter; (see Aphasia: Specific Types)
  - The greater the severity of dementia of the Alzheimer type, the more it contrasts with aphasia

| Dementia of the Alzheimer's Type | Aphasia |
|---|---|
| Slow onset | Sudden onset |
| Bilateral brain damage | Damage in the left hemisphere |
| Diffuse brain damage | Focal brain lesions; however, some may have more diffuse damage |

*(continues)*

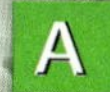




*(continued)*

| Dementia of the Alzheimer's Type | Aphasia (continued) |
|---|---|
| May be moody, withdrawn, agitated | Mood is usually appropriate, though depressed or frustrated at times |
| Impaired cognition, but relatively better preserved language; however, some clients may show greater impairment in language than in cognition | Impaired language, but relatively intact cognition; however, some cognitive impairment may be present in some clients |
| Memory is impaired to various degrees, often severely | Memory typically is intact |
| Often irrelevant, socially inappropriate, and disorganized | Behavior generally is relevant, socially appropriate, and organized |
| Progression of deterioration from semantic to syntactic to phonologic performance | Semantic, syntactic, and phonologic performance simultaneously impaired |
| Fluent until dementia becomes worse | Fluent or nonfluent |
| Relatively poor performance on spatial and verbal recognition tasks | Relatively better performance on spatial and verbal recognition tasks |
| Relatively poor story retelling skills | Relatively better story retelling skills |
| Relatively poor description of common objects | Relatively better description of common objects |
| Relatively poor silent reading comprehension | Relatively better silent reading comprehension |
| Relatively poor pantomimic expression | Relatively better pantomimic expression |
| Relatively poor drawing skills | Relatively better drawing skills |

- Distinguish subtypes of AD
  - AD with early onset (65 years or under)
  - AD with late onset (after age 65 years)
  - AD with Down syndrome (see Syndromes Associated With Communicative Disorders)
  - AD with aphasia
  - AD with such other diseases as Parkinson's Disease
  - Uncomplicated AD (with no associated clinical conditions)

### *Prognosis*

- Poor because dementia is irreversible and there is no effective medical treatment

### *Recommendations*

- Family counseling
- Behavioral management of client's symptoms in the earlier stages
- Family counseling and client management strategies during the latter stages
- See the two companion volumes: *Hegde's PocketGuide to Communication Disorders* and *Hegde's PocketGuide to Treatment in Speech-Language Pathology* (3rd ed.)

American Psychiatric Association (1994). *Diagnostic and statistical manual of mental disorders* (4th ed.). Washington, DC: Author.

Brookshire, R. H. (2003). *An introduction to neurogenic communication disorders* (6th ed.). St. Louis, MO: Mosby Year Book.

Clark, C. M., & Trojanowski, J. Q. (2001). *Neurodegenerative dementias.* New York: McGraw-Hill.

Cummings, J. L., & Benson, D. F. (1983). *Dementia: A clinical approach.* Boston, MA: Butterworth.

Jacques, A., Jackson, G. A. (2000). *Understanding dementia* (3rd ed.). New York: Churchill-Livingstone.

Hegde, M. N. (2006). *A coursebook on aphasia and other neurogenic language disorders* (3rd ed.). Clifton Park, NY: Thomson Delmar Learning.

Weiner, M. F. (1996). *The dementias: Diagnosis, management, and research* (2nd ed.). Washington, DC: American Psychiatric Association.

**Alzheimer Dementia Risk Questionnaire.** A guide to conducting family interviews and obtaining a comprehensive case history; helps obtain information on the client's family, education, work, onset and course of dementia, and communication.

Breitner, J. C., & Folstein, M. (1984). A prevalent disorder with specific clinical features. *Psychological Medicine, 14*, 63–80.

**Anarthria.** Assessment of speechlessness or mutism in clients with severe forms of Dysarthria requires a differential diagnosis of Mutism due to other reasons (e.g., mutism as a psychiatric disorder or mutism due to severe apraxia); to assess anarthria:

- Assess Dysarthria, as it is the main symptom of clients who have severe forms of motor speech disorders; spastic and hypokinetic dysarthria are the most likely types associated with anarthria
- Take note of any residual verbal or nonverbal communication skills because mutism is rarely complete
- Document a history of multiple strokes which may combine with other neurological diseases (e.g., amyotrophic lateral sclerosis and multiple sclerosis)
- Establish severe neuromotor impairments that prevent or seriously impair speech production

**Anomia.** Assessment of naming difficulties is essential to diagnose Aphasia; also important in assessing clients with Dementia, Right Hemisphere Syndrome, and Traumatic Brain Injury; it is the main symptom of anomic aphasia; the client may communicate a word he or she cannot say by gestures, descriptions, circumlocution, and writing; it is not a simple absence of naming; the naming difficulty manifests in various ways as the client who is typically aware of the problem tries to overcome the problem with different strategies; therefore, anomia needs different assessment strategies; see Aphasia. To assess naming difficulties:

- The basic method of assessing anomia is to show a picture or object and ask the client "What is this?" A response to this type of question is called *confrontation naming.*

- Assess reaction time when you ask the client to name a stimulus because slow response is an indication of naming difficulty; the client may eventually name it correctly
- Ask the client to name (verbally list) as many animals, flowers, fruits, vegetables, or pieces of furniture as possible; difficulty in generating a list of category names is evidence of category-specific anomia; some may have more difficulty with certain categories than others; therefore, it is essential to test multiple categories
- During conversation, note the frequency of circumlocution, word substitutions (generally nonspecific words for specific words), and sound substitutions within words; these strategies suggest *paraphasic anomia*
- During conversation, note the frequency of errors that persist; the client may give a wrong name for an object, realize the error, and in an effort to correct it, repeat the error several times
- During conversation, observe the frequency with which the client corrects himself or herself; such self-correction attempts may be fully or only partially successful
- Ask the client to define the meaning of words he or she has difficulty with; difficulty defining or recognizing the words typically retrieved is called *semantic anomia*
- Observe if the client gives some irrelevant responses; these, too may suggest word retrieval problems
- Observe whether the client can describe, gesture, write, and draw to suggest a word he or she cannot say, can correctly recognize the name when given; this suggests that the client has the word knowledge, but cannot retrieve the word during conversation or naming tasks

Hegde, M. N. (2006). *A coursebook on aphasia and other neurogenic language disorders* (3rd ed.). Clifton Park, NY: Thomson Delmar Learning.

Rosenbek, J. C., LaPointe, L. L., & Wertz, R. T. (1989). *Aphasia: A clinical approach.* Austin, TX: Pro-Ed.

**Aphasia.** Assessment of aphasia, which is a language disorder caused by recent brain injury (often a stroke), requires an understanding of neuropathologies, neurodiagnostic methods, and language impairments that are more striking than other impairments; in some forms of aphasia, neurological symptoms may be absent or mild; see the sources cited at the end of this main entry and the companion volume, *Hegde's PocketGuide to Communication Disorders* for epidemiology and ethnocultural factors, etiological factors, and symptomatology of aphasia.

### *Assessment Objectives/General Guidelines*

- To make a brief assessment of language skills in the early stages
- To make a more thorough assessment of communication skills including expressive, receptive, and gestural communication as the client's physical condition improves and stabilizes
- To diagnose aphasia and its type if feasible
- To help develop a treatment plan for the client and to help generate information useful for other professional members in the rehabilitation of the client
- To counsel the family members

## *Case History/Interview Focus*

- See **Case History** and **Interview** under Standard/Common Assessment Procedures
- Concentrate on the onset and recovery from stroke or other clinical conditions; review the client's medical records for the results of neurodiagnostic procedures (including brain scanning results)
- Obtain detailed biographic information including education, occupation, literacy, hobbies and interests, and premorbid intellectual and communication skills as well as current family communication patterns
- Obtain information on the family's affordability of treatment, resources for continued treatment, participation in treatment and rehabilitation programs, and the support systems needed

## *Ethnocultural Considerations*

- See the companion volume, *Hegde's PocketGuide to Communication Disorders,* for epidemiology and ethnocultural variables that differentially affect the prevalence of aphasia in different segments of the population
- See Ethnocultural Considerations in Assessment in this volume
- In taking the case history and during the interview of the family members, explore the family's cultural, linguistic, and ethnic factors that may influence the assessment and treatment of aphasia
- Select standardized tests that are relevant and appropriate for the ethnocultural background of the client; if such tests are not available, consider designing task-specific and client-specific assessment procedures
- If appropriate tests are not available for individual clients of a particular ethnocultural background, use a content-open, skill-oriented assessment outline of the kind given here; the outline specifies skills to be assessed and the clinician is free to select stimulus materials appropriate for the client; the responses also may be evaluated in a flexible manner
- If possible, consult with a speech-language pathologist who belongs to the client's ethnocultural background
- Get the help of a qualified interpreter in the case of bilingual clients

## *Assessment of Aphasia: General Considerations*

- Consider assessment of aphasia as a continuous process because the skill levels and the diagnosis of the specific type of aphasia may change over time
- Assess the most critical features of aphasia first; perhaps a quick assessment of naming will be more productive than a detailed auditory comprehension test with a client who is suspected to have (or has obvious signs of) Broca's aphasia
- Review previous assessment reports; judge whether the information on them is still applicable; if so, postpone the administration of certain procedures
- Based on your experience, use client-specific procedures that have yielded useful information; this may help avoid some lengthy procedures

## *Assessment of Communication Skills*

- Assess the most functional communication skills on a priority basis; both the client and the family members may be most concerned about one or a few especially troublesome problems ("I can't think of the words," or he or she "can say only one or two words")

- Obtain a language (discourse) sample
  - Tape record the entire conversation and assessment session
  - Ascertain information on the hearing status of the client; speak clearly or slightly loudly as the client's condition demands
  - Engage the client in conversation
  - Ask the client about his or her recent health problems, family, occupation and work experience, interests, hobbies, and so forth
  - Ask the client to narrate experiences
  - Ask the client to describe pictures
  - Do not ask questions that evoke yes/no answers unless the client's communicative skills are severely impaired
  - Make every attempt to evoke longer, grammatically more complete utterances by asking the client to "say more" or "say it in a sentence" and so forth
  - Use personally relevant questions that evoke better responses than neutral questions
  - Challenge the client whose auditory comprehension is mildly impaired with more complex sentences, stories, proverbs, logical-illogical statements, and narratives to detect subtle problems
- Assess auditory comprehension deficits
  - Consider administering one of the several auditory comprehension tests that are available; select from one of the following that are listed alphabetically:

| Auditory Comprehension Tests | Purpose |
|---|---|
| *Auditory Comprehension Test for Sentences* (C. M. Shewan) | To assess comprehension of vocabulary, sentence length, and syntactic complexity |
| *Discourse Comprehension Test* (R. H. Brookshire & L. E. Nicholas) | To assess comprehension of audio taped narrated stories |
| *Functional Auditory Comprehension Task* (L. L. LaPointe & J. Horner) | To assess comprehension of functional language at different levels of complexity |
| *Token Test* (E. DeRenzi & L. A. Vignolo) | To assess auditory comprehension by having the client touch requested token or tokens |

- Assess comprehension of commands
  - Use common commands first; use uncommon commands to challenge a mildly impaired client
  - Do not use gestures as you give your commands
  - Give direct commands; for example, ask "Point to the pen," not "Can you point to the pen?"
  - Give natural commands

    "Move your chair a bit closer"

    "Close your eyes"

    "Show me the door"

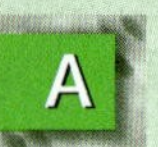



"Please turn off the lights"
"Please remove your glasses"

- Give multistep commands and note the number of steps completed
  "Pick up the pencil and the comb and place them in the box"
  "Fold this paper, put it in the envelope, and place the envelope on this book"

- Assess comprehension of single words; note that single words are not necessarily easy for aphasic clients; some clients benefit from the context that sentences may provide; write down the exact responses for analysis
- Assess first comprehension of category words; include objects, actions, numbers, colors, and letters
  "Point to books"
  "Point to colors"
  "Point to walking"
  "Point to letters"
  "Point to numbers"
- Assess comprehension of specific items within categories
  "Point to big book"
  "Point to blue"
  "Point to the man walking"
  "Point to the letter B"
  "Point to the number seven"
- Assess comprehension of single spoken sentences and connected speech
  - Take note of breakdowns in comprehension of sentences when you interview the client
  - Take note of breakdowns in comprehension of global discourse meaning
  - Make your sentences progressively longer or more complex
  - Use a variety of sentences (e.g., active, passive, question)
    "Point to the man who is walking"
    "Point to the woman who is wearing a red dress"
    "Point to the brown dog that is chasing a black cat"
- Assess comprehension of abstract and logical sentences
  "Will ice cubes melt in snow?"
  "Will a baby who can't swim drown in a pool?"
  "Can you drive a car with no gas?"
  "Why do you need a car?"
  "How would find someone's phone number?"
  "Can a thief arrest a policeman?"
- Assess comprehension of paragraph-length material
  - Tell a brief, unique, interesting story with some humor and emotionality in it; do not select a story that gives the client a special advantage
  - Ask yes/no questions about the story
  - Ask about the main ideas and specific details of the story
  - Ask about inferences one might make about the story
- Assess fluency
  - Use the conversational speech sample to evaluate fluency:
    - Observe and record the type and frequency of Dysfluencies

  - Observe and record the length of phrases measured in words
  - Observe and record the speech rate
  - Make notes about the rhythm and intonation of speech
  - Take note of the variety of grammatical structures used
  - Take notes about the ease with which the client produces sounds and words
- Assess repetition skills
  - Assess repetition of single words; model the words and ask the client to imitate (repeat)
    - Present a variety of single-syllable words with visible consonants that are commonly used (nouns, verbs, numbers, and letters; start with common words)

      Say "*bed*"
      Say "*pen*"
      Say "*men*"
      Say "*baking*"
      Say "*five*"
      Say "*B*"
    - Present blends and multisyllable words; present progressively longer and less familiar words until breakdowns occur

      Say "*basket*"
      Say "*bubble*"
      Say "*truck*"
      Say "*gingerbread*"
      Say "*fraternity*"
      Say "*refrigerator*"
      Say "*pediatrician*"
    - Write down the responses, including errors for later analysis
- Assess repetition of sentences
  - Present common, simple, short sentences and ask the client to imitate; present progressively longer and more complex sentences

    Say "*I like it*"
    Say "*He is here*"
    Say "*I am hungry*"
    Say "*It is getting dark*"
    Say "*Who did this?*"
    Say "*I can do it if you tell me*"
    Say "*Let us go out and have dinner tonight*"
    Say "*How do you do it, if you don't know anything about it*"
    Say "*The man who was watching the game was hit by the ball*"
- Assess word finding and naming skills
  - Assess responsive naming
    - Ask direct questions that give linguistic contexts for specific responses
    - Evoke nouns and verbs
    - Evaluate whether errors are due to auditory comprehension deficit or naming problems

      "What do you use to write?"

"What do you use to unlock a door?"
"What do you sleep on?"
"What color is snow?"
"What do you use to tell time?"
"What do you use when you can't see well?"
"What do you use to clean your body during a shower?"
"What do you use to brush your teeth?"
"What do you do with a knife?"
"What do you do with a pen?"
"What do you do when you are tired?"
"What do you do when you are hungry?"

- Assess confrontation naming
  - Show an item to be named and ask "What is this?"
  - Present both common and uncommon pictures or objects
  - Present objects, pictures of objects, letters, numbers, colors, body parts, and pictured actions
  - Record the stimulus presented and the actual responses for later analysis
  - Record your observations (e.g., *hesitant, self-correction*)
  - Show selected objects one at a time and ask "What is this?"
  - Show selected pictures one at a time and ask "What is this?"
  - Show pictures of various actions and ask the relevant question: "What is the woman doing?" or "What is the man doing?" or "What is the dog doing?"
  - Show selected colors and ask "What color is this?"
  - Show selected letters and ask "What letter is this?"
  - Show selected numbers and ask "What number is this?"
  - Show selected body parts on a picture and ask "What is this?"
- Assess categorical naming
  - Ask the client to name words belonging to different categories; allow 1 minute for each category
  - Use such common categories as animals, vegetables, fruits, furniture, and cities

    "Tell me the names of all the animals you can think of."
    "Tell me the names of all the vegetables you can think of."
    "Tell me the names of all the furniture items you can think of."
    "Tell me the names of all the fruits you can think of."
    "Tell me the names of all the cities in your state (specify)."
- Assess naming in the sentence completion context
  - Use the sentence completion procedure to assess naming
  - Ask the client to complete the sentence with one word
  - First present a trial sentence and you supply the answer

    "The sky is ____"
    "You drive this _____"
    "You can fly this _____"
    "When it is night, you turn on the _____"
    "When you are hungry, you want to _____"
    "When you are tired, you want to _____"

- Assess automatic serial naming
  - Ask the client to produce automatic, serial words and numbers
    "Name the days of the week"
    "Name the months of a year"
    "Please count to 20"
- Assess the client's production of grammatical structures
  - Assess the client's production of sentence structures and types; use the taped interview as well to analyze the language structures the client uses, misuses, and omits
    - Take an extended language sample; use pictures if necessary to stimulate connected speech
    - Tape record the sample
    - Analyze the average length of utterances and sentences measured in words; analyze the types and varieties of sentences the client correctly uses and those that the client misuses
  - Assess the client's production of morphologic features
    - Use the language sample to analyze the correct and incorrect use of Grammatical Morphemes of Language; take note of omissions and substitutions
    - To sample morphologic feature productions not found in the language sample, design a client-specific protocol to assess them; for instance, if irregular plural productions were not observed, ask questions that would evoke them or show pictures that would stimulate them
- Assess motor speech disorders
  - Because aphasia and motor speech disorders may coexist, assess apraxia and dysarthria in all clients with aphasia
    - Complete a thorough orofacial examination and analyze the conversational speech sample for evidence of apraxia of speech and dysarthria
    - Make a clinical judgment about the necessity and extent of additional evaluation of motor speech disorders
    - If additional and detailed assessment of motor speech disorders is warranted, use procedures described under Apraxia of Speech and Dysarthria.
- Assess understanding or expression of gestures
  - Assess understanding of gestures
    - Present a few common gestures (e.g., drinking from a glass, writing, looking at a distant object)
    - Ask the client to say what the gestures mean
  - Assess production of gestures
    - Take note of whether the client uses appropriate hand and facial gestures along with verbal expressions
    - Take note of whether the client can gesture the words he or she cannot say
    - Take note of whether the client has acquired any formal signs (such as those from the American Sign Language)

- Assess reading problems
  - Consider administering a comprehensive reading test to plan for intervention on reading problems; select one of the following:
    - *The Reading Comprehension Battery for Aphasia* by L. L. LaPointe and J. Horner; it is a comprehensive test for assessing reading skills in clients with aphasia
    - Because there are not many specialized reading tests for clients with aphasia, consider administering one of the commercially available standardized reading tests; commonly used tests include the *Gates-MacGinitie Reading Test* by W. H. Gates, R. K. MacGinitie, K. Maria, and associates; and *Nelson Reading Skills Test* by G. Hanna, L. M. Schell, and R. Shreiner; and the *Nelson-Denny Reading Skills Test* by J. I. Brown, V. V. Fischco, and G. Hanna
- Assess comprehension of silently read material
  - Select a prose passage that is appropriate to the client's age, education, interest, and cultural background
  - Ask the client to read the passage silently
  - Ask the client specific questions about the material to assess comprehension
- Assess errors in oral reading
  - To rule out peripheral visual problems, ask the client to match a few pictures with printed words and to match a few spoken words with printed words
  - Select a prose passage that is appropriate to the client's age, education, interest, and cultural background
  - Ask the client to read the passage
  - On a copy of the passage, mark the errors the client makes in reading (e.g., omission and substitution of sounds and words, misreading of words, self-corrections, and errors based on phonemic or semantic similarity)
  - Take note of the rate of reading and dysfluencies exhibited
  - To rule out visual neglect, note whether the client ignores the printed material on the left half the page
- Assess writing problems
  - Note that most aphasia test batteries contain writing subtests; administer one of those to assess writing skills; most clinicians do not administer special (dedicated) writing tests because very few are especially suitable for clients with aphasia; in addition to administering aphasia subtests on writing, assess writing skills with client-specific procedures
- Assess graphomotor skills (letter formation)
  - Find out the dominant hand the client used to write before the onset of aphasia
  - Note the hand the client uses to write (preferred but now weak right hand or nonpreferred left hand)
  - Ask the client to copy printed words, sentences, and a paragraph
  - Ask the client to spontaneously write about his or her family or work
  - Ask the client to write a description of a picture
  - Analyze the letter formation, upper- and lowercase letter usage, use of script or printed letters, overall quality of letter formation, legibility of letters, and letter formation errors

- Assess confrontation writing skills
    - Ask the client to write the names of pictures shown
    - Analyze the error patterns
    - Assess writing to dictation
    - Ask the client to write words and sentences you dictate
    - Analyze the error patterns
- Assess narrative writing with obtained writing samples; ask the client to bring a premorbid writing sample for later comparison
    - Analyze the error patterns
- Assess automatic or spontaneous writing
    - Ask the client to write his or her name and address
    - Ask the client to write the names of his family members
    - Ask the client to write the letters of the alphabet
    - Ask the client to fill out a check, a form, and to make a shopping list
    - Ask the client to write a brief message to a family member
    - Analyze the error pattern; be aware that automatic writing may be better preserved and may not be indicative of spontaneous and narrative writing problems
- Assess bilingual deficits
    - Find out the primary language the client used before the onset of aphasia
        - Assess the client in his or her primary language or the language of strong and frequent use before the onset
        - Refer the client to a clinician who can assess the client in primary language if you cannot do it
        - Obtain an interpreter who is trained in providing assistance in assessment of aphasia if you need to provide services
        - Assess the client in his or her second language if warranted
        - Compare the communication deficits in the primary and the secondary languages
        - Use culturally and linguistically appropriate assessment tools and materials
- Assess pragmatic communication problems
    - Make a discourse analysis
        - Use the conversational speech sample (discourse) to make an analysis of pragmatic problems
        - Tell a short story to the client and ask the client to narrate it back to you
        - Ask the client to narrate an experience or an event (e.g., the recent visit to hospital, the last vacation, a sports event of interest, or a hobby)
        - Take note of the event/temporal sequence and the details given or missed
        - Record the frequency with which the client correctly took turns during the interview and speech and language samples
        - Record the frequency with which the client initiated a new topic during conversation
        - Record the frequency with which the client abruptly switched from one topic to another
        - Make some ambiguous statements to see if the client asks for clarification (a conversational repair strategy)

- Frequently, ask for clarification (e.g., *I am not sure what you mean, Can you say it differently, I didn't get it,* and so forth) to see if the client would appropriately modify the statements (another conversational repair strategy)

## Aphasia Standardized Tests

- Select a test that is brief, but just as valid and reliable as a longer one
- Select a test that is ethnoculturally appropriate for the client
- There are several screening tests of aphasia, one of which may be initially administered before making a more thorough evaluation; consider the latest versions of one of the following or any other reliable and valid screening test:
    - *Acute Aphasia Screening Protocol* by M. A. Cray, N. J. Haak, & A. E. Malinsky
    - *Aphasia Language Performance Scales* by K. S. Keenan & E. G. Brassell
    - *Aphasia Screening Test* by R. M. Reitan
    - *Aphasia Screening Test* by R. Whurr
    - *Bedside Evaluation Screening Test* by J. Fitch-West, & E. S. Sands
    - *Boston Diagnostic Aphasia Examination—the short form* by H. Goodglass, E. Kaplan, & B. Barresi
- Administer one of the several diagnostic tests of aphasia that are available; administer the latest versions of selected test or tests; the following is an alphabetized list of some commonly used tests; consider one of these or any other reliable and valid test:

| Aphasia Diagnostic Test | Purpose |
|---|---|
| *Amsterdam-Nijemegen Everyday Language Test* (L. Blomert, C. Koster, H. van Mier, & M. L. Kean) | To assess pragmatic language skills; a functional assessment tool |
| *ASHA Functional Assessment of Communication Skills for Adults* (C. M. Frattali, C. K. Thompson, A. L. Holland, C. B. Whol, & M. M. Ferketic) | To assess functional communication skills in a variety of settings and environments |
| *Assessment of Nonverbal Communication (New England Pantomime Test)* (J. R. Duffy & J. R. Duffy) | To assess comprehension and expression of gestures through picture selection |
| *Auditory Comprehension Test for Sentences* (C. M. Shewan) | To assess comprehension of spoken sentences |
| *Boston Assessment of Severe Aphasia* (N. Helm-Estabrooks & associates) | To assess communication skills in severely aphasic clients |
| *Boston Diagnostic Aphasia Examination* (H. Goodglass & E. Kaplan) | To assess articulation, fluency, naming, repetition, serial speech, grammar, paraphasia, auditory comprehension, syntax, oral reading, and writing |

*(continues)*

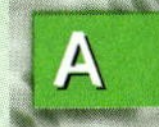



(continued)

| Aphasia Diagnostic Test | Purpose |
|---|---|
| *Boston Naming Test* (H. Goodglass, E. Kaplan, & S. Weintraub) | To assess naming skills through line drawings |
| *Communication Profile: A Functional Skills Survey* (J. C. Payne) | To assess functional communication skills, especially in ethnic minorities including African American, American Indian, and Asian American clients |
| *Communicative Abilities of Daily Living* (A. L. Holland) | To assess communication skills in daily living conditions; a functional assessment tool |
| Communicative Effectiveness Index (J. Lomas, L. Pickard, S. Bester, H. Elbard, A. Finlayson, & C. Zoghaib) | To assess pragmatic communication skills through a questionnaire filled out by a family member or a friend; a functional assessment tool |
| *Examining for Aphasia* (J. Eisenson) | To assess receptive and expressive language skills |
| *Functional Assessment of Communication Skills for Adults (ASHA FACS)* (C. Frattali, C. Thompson, A. Holland, C. Wohl, & M. Ferketi) | To rate functional communication skills including reading and writing; especially useful to evaluate a rehabilitation program's effectiveness |
| *Functional Auditory Comprehension Task* (L. L. LaPointe & J. Horner) | To assess functional auditory comprehension of spoken language |
| *Functional Communication Profile* (M. T. Sarno) | To assess various categories of communication; a functional assessment tool |
| *Multilingual Aphasia Examination—Third Edition* (A. L. Benton & Hamsher, K) | To assess oral expression, spelling, verbal understanding, reading, articulation, and writing in English, Spanish, French, or German |
| *Minnesota Test for Differential Diagnosis of Aphasia—Revised* (H. Schuell & H. Sefer) | To assess speech, language, auditory comprehension, reading, and writing skills |
| *Neurosensory Center Comprehensive Examination for Aphasia* (O. Spreen & A. L. Benton) | To assess language comprehension and production, memory, reading, and writing skills |
| *Porch Index of Communicative Ability* (B. E. Porch) | To assess auditory comprehension, reading, oral expressive language, pantomime, visual matching, writing, and copying |
| *Reading Comprehension Battery for Aphasia* (L. L. LaPointe & J. Horner) | To assess reading comprehension of words, sentences, and paragraphs; functional reading, synonyms, and morphosyntax |

(continues)

(continued)

| Aphasia Diagnostic Test | Purpose |
|---|---|
| *Revised Token Test* (M. M. McNeil &T. E. Prescott) | To assess auditory processing through token manipulation |
| *Western Aphasia Battery* (WAB) (A. Kertesz) | To assess speech content, fluency, auditory writing, comprehension, repetition,naming, reading, calculation, drawing, nonverbal thinking, and block design |

## Related/Medical Assessment Data

- Consider the results of medical neurodiagnostic techniques
- Consider the results of available psychological, cognitive, physical therapy, and related assessment information
- Consider the client's current medical condition and prognosis

## Standard/Common Assessment Procedures

- Complete the Standard/Common Assessment Procedures
- Pay special attention to orofacial examination to rule out peripheral neuromuscular involvement related to speech production

## Analysis of Assessment Results

- Analyze results of assessment to obtain both the strengths and limitations of the client
- Summarize the communication deficits in terms of:
  - Auditory comprehension deficits: levels of breakdown (e.g., intact comprehension of isolated sentences, but breakdown at paragraph level or in conversation)
  - The client's fluency skills and the types and number of dysfluencies
  - The client's repetition skills: describe the level of breakdown (e.g., can repeat words but not phrases)
  - Naming problems: describe the types of naming problems
  - Syntactic and morphologic problems: describe the sentence types produced and not produced, morphologic features used, not used, or misused
  - The client's limitations in understanding and using gestures
  - Reading and writing problems: describe the types of errors
  - The bilingual client's deficits in both the primary and secondary language
  - Pragmatic communication deficits: summarize problems in discourse
  - The results of standardized tests administered and integrate the results with client-specific procedures, observations, and the results of specific assessment procedures
  - Ratings of the severity of aphasia if appropriate
  - The type of aphasia if appropriate

## Diagnostic Criteria

- To diagnose aphasia, language disturbance should be due to recently acquired cerebral injury, except in some rare cases of gradual onset
- Language disturbances should outweigh any intellectual deficits observed
- Case history and available medical data (including neurological, radiological, and related data) should support the diagnosis of aphasia

- Pattern of deficits observed should help rule out related and similar disorders as specified under differential diagnosis

### *Differential Diagnosis*

- Distinguish aphasia from normal language with some aphasic-like characteristics, apraxia, dementia, dysarthria, language of confusion, schizophrenia, right hemisphere syndrome, and traumatic brain injury; use the following grids to make a differential diagnosis (adapted from Hegde, 2006):

#### Aphasia or Normal Language?

| Aphasia | Aphasic-like but Normal Language |
|---|---|
| Positive history of stroke, tumor, and other central neuropathology | Negative history of central neuropathology |
| Prior history of normal language; deterioration in language skills | Prior history of limited language; no evidence of deterioration in language skills |
| Lack of education does not explain the problems | Lack of education could explain the problems |
| Level of literacy does not explain the problem | Level of literacy could explain the problem |
| Current environment could not explain the problem | Current environment could explain the problem |
| Sudden onset | Lifelong problem |

#### Aphasia or Dementia?

| Aphasia | Dementia |
|---|---|
| Onset mostly is sudden | Onset mostly is slow |
| Damage in the left hemisphere | Bilateral brain damage |
| Focal brain lesions in most cases | Diffuse brain damage in most cases |
| Mood usually is appropriate, though depressed or frustrated at times | May be moody, withdrawn, and agitated |
| Impaired language, but generally intact cognition is mostly intact | Cognition is mildly or severely impaired, but better language skills until later stages |
| Memory typically is intact | Memory is impaired to various degrees, often severely |
| Behavior generally is relevant, socially appropriate, and organized | Behavior often is irrelevant, socially inappropriate, and disorganized |
| Mentally alert and oriented to time and space | Mentally confused and disoriented to time and space |
| No disorientation to self | Disorientation to self in later stages |
| Semantic, syntactic, and phonologic performance simultaneously impaired | Progression of deterioration from semantic to syntactic to phonologic performance |

*(continues)*

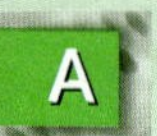



*(continued)*

| Aphasia | Dementia |
|---|---|
| Fluent or nonfluent | Fluent until dementia becomes worse |
| Relatively better performance on spatial and verbal recognition tasks | Relatively poor performance on spatial and verbal recognition tasks |
| Relatively better story retelling skills | Relatively poor story retelling skills |
| Relatively better description of common objects | Relatively poor description of common objects |
| Relatively better silent reading comprehension | Relatively poor silent reading comprehension |
| Relatively better pantomimic expression | Relatively poor pantomimic expression |
| Relatively better drawing skills | Relatively poor drawing skills |

*Caution: (1) Clients with fluent aphasia are more likely to be confused with dementia than are those with fluent aphasia; (2) aphasia and dementia may coexist; (3) an aphasic client may develop a neurological disease resulting in dementia (Alzheimer's disease); and (4) a client with dementia may suffer a stroke, resulting in aphasia.*

## Aphasia or the Language of Confusion?

| Aphasia | Confusion |
|---|---|
| Left hemisphere damage, focal | Bilateral damage, diffuse |
| Strokes are the most common cause | Traumatic brain injury and toxic and metabolic disturbances are the most common causes |
| Often relevant | Typically irrelevant |
| Attentional deficits are not the most striking | Attentional deficits are the most striking |
| Writing problems parallel speaking problems | Writing problems often greater than speaking problems |
| No confabulation | Confabulation |
| Syntactic difficulties | Little or no syntactic difficulties |
| Repetition skills often impaired | Repetition skills often intact |
| Significant word finding problems | No significant word finding problems |
| Varying degrees of auditory comprehension problems | Generally intact auditory comprehension problems |
| No disorientation except for the first few hours of stroke | Disoriented to time, place, and clients |
| History suggests stroke | History suggests brain trauma |
| No significant behavioral change | Significant behavioral change |
| More stable or slower change in symptoms | More rapid, positive changes in symptoms |

*Caution: Confusion may coexist with aphasia when a client with traumatic brain injury suffers focal left hemisphere damage.*

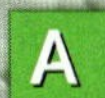




## Aphasia or Schizophrenia?

| Aphasia | Schizophrenia |
|---|---|
| Sudden onset | Gradual onset |
| Late onset (adult or old age) | Early onset (adolescent or early adulthood) |
| Not a psychotic disorder; no history of psychiatric disturbances | A psychotic disorder; a history of psychiatric disturbances |
| Due to a general medical condition (cerebral infarct) | Not due to a general medical condition |
| Left hemisphere damage | No evidence of left hemisphere damage |
| No thought disorders | Thought disorders including delusions |
| No such perceptual disorders as hallucinations | Perceptual disorders, especially auditory hallucinations |
| No confabulation, generally relevant | Confabulation, typically irrelevant |
| No evidence of disorganized speech | Disorganized speech |
| Deficits in auditory comprehension | No deficits in auditory comprehension (may be inattentive) |
| Reading and writing affected | Reading and writing may not be affected |
| Appropriate emotional responses | Lack of emotional expression and inappropriate or incongruent emotional responses |
| Social behavior, personal hygiene, and general behavior not affected or disorganized; any limitation due to motor problems | Social behavior, personal hygiene, and general behavior grossly disorganized; none due to physical limitations |
| Appropriate sexual behavior | Inappropriate sexual behavior |
| Absence of Catatonic Motor Behavior | Presence of Catatonic Motor Behavior |

*Caution: Aphasia and schizophrenia may coexist, especially when a client with schizophrenia suffers a stroke.*

## Aphasia or Right Hemisphere Syndrome?

| Aphasia | Right Hemisphere Syndrome |
|---|---|
| Significant or dominant problems in naming, fluency, auditory comprehension, reading, and writing | Only mild problems in naming, fluency, auditory comprehension, reading, and writing |
| No left-sided neglect | Left-sided neglect |
| No denial of illness | Denial of illness |
| Speech is generally relevant | Speech is often irrelevant, excessive, rambling |
| Generally normal affect | Often lack of affect |

*(continues)*

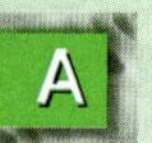



*(continued)*

| Aphasia | Right Hemisphere Syndrome |
|---|---|
| Intact recognition of familiar faces | Possible impaired recognition of familiar faces |
| Simplification of drawings | Rotation and left-sided neglect |
| No significant prosodic defect | Significant prosodic defect |
| Appropriate humor | Inappropriate humor |
| May retell the essence of a story | May retell only nonessential, isolated details (no integration) |
| May understand implied meanings | Understands only literal meanings |
| Pragmatic impairments less striking | Pragmatic impairments more striking (eye contact, topic maintenance, etc.) |
| Though limited in language skills, communication is often good | Though possessing good language skills, communication is very poor |
| Pure linguistic deficits are dominant | Pure linguistic deficits are not dominant |

*Note: Right hemisphere damage in those few individuals whose right hemisphere is dominant for language results in aphasia, and for the same etiologic factors.*

## Aphasia or Apraxia of Speech?

| Aphasia Without Apraxia of Speech | Apraxia of Speech Without Aphasia |
|---|---|
| Neurogenic language problem | Neurogenic speech problem |
| Trial and error, groping articulatory movements are not significant | Trial and error, groping articulatory movements are significant |
| Misarticulations less variable, more consistent | Misarticulations more variable, more inconsistent |
| Some impairment in auditory comprehension | Generally, no impairment in auditory comprehension |
| Prosodic problems not dominant | Prosodic problems dominant |
| Difficulty in initiating utterances is less obvious | Difficulty in initiating utterances is more obvious |
| Omission of function words | No significant tendency to omit function words |
| Word-finding problems | No word-finding problems |
| Limb or oral apraxia not dominant | Limb or oral apraxia or both may be dominant |

*Note: Apraxia of speech and Broca's aphasia often coexist. Pure apraxia is rare. It often is associated with Broca's aphasia.*

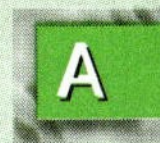



## Aphasia or Dysarthria?

| Aphasia Without Dysarthria | Dysarthria Without Aphasia |
|---|---|
| Neurogenic language problem | Neurogenic speech problem |
| The language problems are not due to muscle weakness | The speech problems are due to muscle weakness, spasticity, rigidity (except for ataxic dysarthria) |
| No consistent misarticulations | Consistent misarticulations |
| Intelligibility of speech not clearly related to the rate of speech | Intelligibility clearly related to the rate of speech |
| No respiratory problems associated with speech production | Respiratory problems associated with speech production |
| Phonatory problems not significant | Phonatory problems may be significant |
| Resonance disorders not significant | Resonance disorders may be significant |
| Prosodic disorders not as dominant | Prosodic disorders may be dominant |
| Abnormal voice quality not significant | Abnormal voice quality may be significant |
| Abnormal stress not significant | Abnormal stress may be significant |

*Note: Occasionally, aphasia and dysarthria may coexist. Subcortical lesions that produce aphasia are more likely to be associated with dysarthria.*

## Aphasia or Traumatic Brain Injury?

| Aphasia | Traumatic Brain Injury |
|---|---|
| Pure linguistic problems are dominant | Pure linguistic problems are not dominant |
| Significant grammatical errors | Grammatical errors not significant |
| Dysarthria not a part of the syndrome (although the two may coexist) | Dysarthria part of the syndrome |
| Language not confused | Initially, confused language |
| Slower improvement in language | Faster improvement in language |
| Less serious pragmatic problems | More serious pragmatic problems |
| Social interaction not as seriously impaired | Social interaction seriously impaired |
| Not disorganized or confused | Initially disorganized and confused |
| Not disoriented to time and space | Initially disoriented to time and space |
| Not inconsistent or irrelevant | May be inconsistent or irrelevant |
| Attentional problems not as serious | Serious attentional problems including distractibility, impulsivity, poor social judgment, and lack of insight |

*Note: Traumatic brain injury may cause aphasia as well.*

- Note that agrammatic writing suggests Broca's aphasia and helps rule out Wernicke's aphasia
- Note that severe writing skills suggest global aphasia

## Prognosis

- Evidence on such biographical variables as the age (at onset), gender, education, and occupational status is contradictory or ambiguous
- Aphasia resulting from traumatic brain injury may have better prognosis than that resulting from vascular pathology, which in turn may have better prognosis than that resulting from subcortical hemorrhage
- Larger lesions and bilateral lesions indicate less favorable prognosis than smaller and unilateral lesions
- More posterior lesions, especially in the temporoparietal regions, and deeper lesions suggest less favorable prognosis than more anterior and upper cortical lesions
- Better health and intact sensory modalities are associated with more favorable prognosis than poor health and sensory deficits
- More favorable prognosis for improved language without treatment during the first three to six months
- Less severe aphasia is associated with more favorable prognosis for higher level of language recovery than more severe aphasia, which may show greatest improvement yet stabilizing at a lower level of language

## Recommendations

- Recommend communication treatment for all clients with aphasia, at least on a trial basis
- Let the initial treatment outcome help make judgments about continued treatment
- See the companion volume, *Hegde's PocketGuide to Communication Disorders*, and the cited sources for additional information

Basso, A. (2003). *Aphasia and its therapy*. New York: Oxford University Press.

Benson, D. E., & Ardila, A. (1996). *Aphasia: A clinical perspective*. New York: Oxford University Press.

Brookshire, R. (2003). *An introduction to neurogenic communication disorders* (6th ed.). St. Louis, MO: Mosby Year Book.

Catani, M., & ffytche, D. (2005). The rises and falls of disconnection syndromes. *Brain, 128*(10), 2224–2239.

Chapey, R. (Ed.) (2001). *Language intervention strategies in adult aphasia* (4th. ed.) Baltimore, MD: Lippincott Williams & Wilkins.

Darley, F. (1982). *Aphasia*. Philadelphia, PA: W. B. Saunders.

Davis, G. A. (2000). *Aphasiology: Disorders and clinical practice*. Needham Heights, MA: Allyn and Bacon.

Demonte, J., Guillaume, T., & Cardebat, D. (2005). Renewal of the neurophysiology of language: Functional neuroimaging. *Physiological Review*, 85, 49–95.

Hegde, M. N. (2006). *A coursebook on aphasia and other neurogenic language disorders*. Clifton Park, NY: Thomson Delmar Learning.

Helm-Estabrooks, N., & Albert, M. L. (2004). *Manual of aphasia therapy* (2nd ed.). Austin, TX: Pro-Ed.

LaPointe, L. L. (Ed.) (2005). *Aphasia and related neurogenic language disorders* (2nd ed.). New York: Thieme Medical Publishers.

Nadeau, S. E., Gonzalez-Rothi, L., & Crosson, B. (2000). *Aphasia and language: Theory to practice*. New York: Guilford Press.

Payne, J. C. (1997). *Adult neurogenic language disorders: Assessment and treatment*. Clifton Park, NY: Thomson Delmar Learning.

Sarno, M. T. (Ed.) (1998). *Acquired aphasia* (3rd ed.). New York: Academic Press.

**Aphasia: Specific Types.** Assessment of variations in aphasia symptom complex is essential to make a typological classification in individual clients, although many clients cannot be classified into unambiguous types; most commonly described types include the following:

***Anomic Aphasia.*** The main assessment concern in this type of fluent aphasia is the persistent and severe naming problems; varied etiologic factors including closed head injury, focal lesions in the angular gyrus or second temporal gyrus, and Alzheimer's disease; pure anomic aphasia may be rare; chronic clients with a history of other kinds of aphasia may remain as anomic aphasic individuals; use the assessment procedures described under Aphasia and pay special attention to the distinguishing features of anomic aphasia

#### Diagnostic Criteria/Guidelines

- Persistent and significant naming problems that dominate the clinical picture are the hallmark of anomic aphasia
- Other language skills that are better preserved, even though paraphasic and empty speech due to persistent naming problems may be evident
- History and etiology consistent with anomic aphasia, although the cerebral lesion sites are ambiguous

#### Differential Diagnosis

- Relatively better auditory comprehension skills associated with anomic aphasia distinguish it from both Wernicke's aphasia and global aphasia, which are associated with poor auditory comprehension
- Good articulation and good grammatical structures associated with anomic aphasia distinguish it from Broca's aphasia, characterized by agrammatical speech and possible coexistence of dysarthria
- Better repetition skills associated with anomic aphasia distinguish it from conduction aphasia in which the repetition skills are impaired

#### Recommendations

- Aphasia treatment, with an emphasis on teaching naming skills

***Broca's Aphasia.*** The main assessment concern in this type of nonfluent aphasia with lesions in the third frontal convolution of the left or dominant hemisphere (Brodmann's area 44) is agrammatical, telegraphic, effortful, and nonfluent speech; a somewhat controversial diagnostic category because injury to Broca's area is neither necessary nor sufficient to produce aphasia;

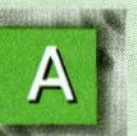



use the assessment procedures described under Aphasia and pay special attention to the following:

**Diagnostic Criteria/Guidelines**

- Dysfluent, effortful, agrammatical, slow speech with better receptive skills suggest Broca's aphasia
- History and etiology consistent with aphasia
- Obvious neurological symptoms including right-sided hemiparesis, paralysis, and initial confinement to a wheelchair
- Lesions in the frontal cortex, especially in and around Broca's area
- Potential association with apraxia and dysarthria

**Differential Diagnosis**

- Relatively better auditory comprehension skills distinguish Broca's aphasia from Wernicke's aphasia and global aphasia in which the auditory comprehension is poor
- Nonfluent speech, limited grammatical structures, and relative absence of paraphasia associated with Broca's aphasia distinguish it from Wernicke's aphasia, transcortical sensory aphasia, anomic aphasia, and conduction aphasia—all associated with fluent but paraphasic speech with good grammar
- Poor repetition skills associated with Broca's aphasia distinguish it from transcortical motor aphasia and transcortical sensory aphasia (better repetition skills)

**Recommendations**

- Aphasia treatment, with an emphasis on improving phrase length, fluency, and naming skills

***Conduction Aphasia.*** The main diagnostic feature of this rare type of fluent aphasia is impaired repetition skills in the context of normal auditory comprehension; sites of lesion include the supramarginal gyrus, the superior temporal lobe, and regions between Broca's and Wernicke's area; use the assessment procedures described under Aphasia and pay special attention to the following:

**Diagnostic Criteria/Guidelines**

- Markedly impaired repetition skills in the context of good to normal auditory comprehension are the main diagnostic features
- Other language skills are better preserved
- Some clients may present no neurological symptoms whereas others may present paresis of the right side of the face and right upper extremity
- History and etiology consistent with aphasia

**Differential Diagnosis**

- Severely impaired repetition skills associated with conduction aphasia distinguish it from anomic aphasia, transcortical motor aphasia, and transcortical sensory aphasia, which are associated with good repetition skills
- Relatively better auditory comprehension skills associated with conduction aphasia distinguish it from Wernicke's aphasia, transcortical sensory

aphasia, and global aphasia, which are all characterized by poor auditory comprehension
- Fluent speech, good articulation, and better grammatical structures associated with conduction aphasia distinguish it from Broca's aphasia, global aphasia, and transcortical motor aphasia, which are characterized by agrammatism, effortful articulation, and impaired fluency of speech

#### Recommendations

- Aphasia treatment, with an emphasis on teaching naming skills

*Crossed Aphasia.* Assessment of this atypical type of aphasia in right-handed clients, needs the documentation of right hemisphere injury; a somewhat rare occurrence; frequent causes include brain tumor or trauma (versus vascular pathology in the left-hemisphere injury); use the assessment procedures described under Aphasia and pay special attention to the following:

#### Diagnostic Criteria/Guidelines

- Right-hemisphere damage in right-handed individuals
- History and etiology consistent with aphasia; diagnosis of brain tumor or trauma in most cases

#### Differential Diagnosis

- Right-hemisphere damage in right-handed individuals distinguish crossed aphasia from other syndromes of aphasia caused by left hemisphere pathology
- High incidence of tumor and trauma causing right-hemisphere injury and aphasia distinguish it from left-hemisphere injury and aphasia that typically result from vascular pathology
  - Minimal problems in naming and auditory comprehension, combined with drawing problems and left-sided neglect, help distinguish crossed aphasia from aphasia resulting from left hemisphere pathology

#### Recommendations

- Aphasia treatment, with an emphasis on improving grammatical skills, fluency, left-sided neglect, and drawing skills

*Global Aphasia.* Assessment of this type of nonfluent aphasia takes into consideration the most severe deficits in both comprehension and production of language; all sensory modalities may be affected; due to extensive lesions in the frontal, temporal, and parietal lobes; lesions may extend to the white matter of the brain; Broca's and Wernicke's areas may both be involved; use the assessment procedures described under Aphasia and pay special attention to the following:

#### Diagnostic Criteria/Guidelines

- Severe deficits in all modalities of communication are essential for a diagnosis of global aphasia

#### Differential Diagnosis

- Extremely limited verbal expression distinguishes global aphasia from other nonfluent aphasias
- Extremely limited fluency, phrase length, grammatical skills, and prosodic features distinguish global aphasia from fluent aphasias

Recommendations

- Aphasia treatment, with an emphasis on basic and functional communication skills including the use of gestures, communication boards, simple writing, expression of basic words and phrases, and basic auditory comprehension

*Isolation Aphasia.* Assessment of this rare type of nonfluent aphasia is similar to the assessment of global aphasia; it is caused by lesions surrounding the perisylvian speech area, thus isolating language areas from other areas of the brain; resembles global aphasia; use the assessment procedures described under Aphasia and pay special attention to the following:

Diagnostic Criteria/Guidelines

- Symptoms similar to global aphasia except for the better preserved repetition skills
- Unique neuropathology

Differential Diagnosis

- All severely depressed language modalities except for repetition skills distinguish isolation aphasia from other types

Recommendations

- Aphasia treatment, with an emphasis on improved basic and functional communication skills

*Primary Progressive Aphasia.* Assessment of this atypical form of aphasia should document the progressive (versus the typical and stable) nature of aphasias that terminates in dementia; part of the frontotemporal Dementia; use the assessment procedures described under Aphasia as well as those described under Dementia and pay special attention to the following:

Diagnostic Criteria/Guidelines

- Initial symptoms of aphasia and subsequent symptoms of dementia characterize this special aphasic syndrome
- Documented frontotemporal neuropathology
- Possible diagnosis of Pick's disease (associated with frontotemporal dementia)

Differential Diagnosis

- Insidious onset, unlike most forms of aphasia that have an acute onset
- Initial aphasic symptoms; in some clients aphasia may be the nonfluent type, and in other cases it may be the fluent variety
- Muteness in the final stage, uncommon in most types of aphasia
- Dysarthria in a majority of clients, characteristic of the nonfluent variety
- Comprehension of the meaning of single words is more impaired in the fluent variety than in the nonfluent variety
- Eventually, emergence of symptoms of Dementia

Recommendations

- Aphasia and dementia treatment, with an emphasis on improved basic and functional communication skills, and checking deterioration in communication skills to the extent possible

*Subcortical Aphasia.* Assessment of several newer syndromes of aphasia that are due to damage to such left subcortical regions as internal capsule, putamen, and thalamus poses special challenges partly because of their controversial nature; cortical structures may still be affected, causing language dysfunctions; use the assessment procedures described under Aphasia and pay special attention to the following:

### Diagnostic Criteria/Guidelines

- Depends on the site of lesion
- Presence or absence of dysarthria and the presence or absence of auditory comprehension problems are helpful in diagnosis
- Neuropathology that contrasts with typical aphasia syndromes; evidence of subcortical damage on neurodiagnostic tests

### Differential Diagnosis

- Like clients with Broca's aphasia, those with lesions in the anterior limb of the internal capsule and putamen exhibit severe articulation problems and minimal auditory comprehension problems; unlike Broca's clients, they have good syntactic skills and fluency; right hemiplegia is common
- Clients with lesions in the posterior limb of the internal capsule and putamen resemble clients with Wernicke's aphasia, with severe auditory comprehension problems with only mild articulation problems except that they exhibit right hemiplegia (absent in Wernicke's clients)
- Clients with subcortical anterior and posterior lesions affecting internal capsule, putamen, and thalamus exhibit symptoms of global aphasia, with severe impairments in all speech-language skills
- Clients with left thalamic lesions exhibit symptoms of transcortical motor aphasia with difficulty initiating spontaneous speech and sparse, fluctuating, perseverative, neologistic, and echolalic speech

### Recommendations

- Aphasia treatment

*Transcortical Motor Aphasia.* Assessment of this type of nonfluent aphasia with intact repetition skills requires it to be differentiated from the similar Broca's aphasia; also to be distinguished from transcortical sensory aphasia, which resembles Wernicke's aphasia; use the assessment procedures described under Aphasia and pay special attention to the following:

### Diagnostic Criteria/Guidelines

- Intact repetition; can repeat long and complex sentences
- Lack of spontaneous speech; limited speech output only when strongly urged; limited syntax, short sentences; naming problems
- Agrammatical, paraphasic, telegraphic speech as in Broca's aphasia
- Generally fluent speech, good articulation
- Better auditory comprehension (may have mild to moderate deficits)
- History, etiology, and neuropathology consistent with transcortical variety of aphasia

### Differential Diagnosis

- General similarity to Broca's aphasia. Lack of spontaneous speech combined with limited word output in the absence of articulation problems contrasted with excellent repetition skills help distinguish transcortical motor aphasia from other types

### Recommendations

- Aphasia treatment, with an emphasis on improving spontaneous speech and phrase length

***Transcortical Sensory Aphasia.*** Assessment of this type of fluent aphasia is similar to the assessment of Wernicke's aphasia; the transcortical sensory aphasia is contrasted with transcortical motor aphasia; a form of aphasia commonly associated with Alzheimer's disease; use the assessment procedures described under Aphasia and pay special attention to the following:

### Diagnostic Criteria/Guidelines

- Symptoms of Wernicke's aphasia with intact repetition skills
- History and etiology consistent with aphasia

### Differential Diagnosis

- Intact and somewhat echolalic repetition skills distinguish transcortical sensory aphasia from Wernicke's aphasia
- Generally fluent but empty speech with severe to moderate auditory comprehension deficits distinguish transcortical sensory aphasia from transcortical motor aphasia with its nonfluent and limited spontaneous speech; intact repetition is a common feature of both types

### Recommendations

- Aphasia treatment, with an emphasis on improving naming skills

***Wernicke's Aphasia.*** Assessment of this type of fluent aphasia, which is less controversial than the nonfluent Broca's aphasia, requires an evaluation of fluent and paraphasic speech; use the assessment procedures described under Aphasia and pay special attention to the following:

### Diagnostic Criteria/Guidelines

- Fluent, paraphasic, and apparently grammatically correct speech with little meaning and severe auditory comprehension deficits
- History and etiology consistent with aphasia

### Differential Diagnosis

- Impaired repetition skills distinguish Wernicke's aphasia from transcortical sensory aphasia with its intact repetition skills
- Normal or excessive fluency; apparently normal grammar, articulation, and prosody; severe auditory comprehension deficits; and limited communication in spite of copious speech distinguish Wernicke's aphasia from Broca's aphasia
- Normal or excessive fluency and impaired repetition skills distinguish Wernicke's aphasia from transcortical motor aphasia with its dysfluent speech and intact repetition

### Recommendations

- Aphasia treatment
- For treatment of all types of aphasia, see the cited sources and *Hegde's PocketGuide to Treatment in Speech-Language Pathology* (3rd ed.)

Basso, A. (2003). *Aphasia and its therapy*. New York: Oxford University Press.

Benson, D. E., & Ardila, A. (1996). *Aphasia: A clinical perspective*. New York: Oxford University Press.

Brookshire, R. (2003). *An introduction to neurogenic communication disorders* (6th ed.). St. Louis, MO: Mosby Year Book.

Chapey, R. (Ed.) (2001). *Language intervention strategies in adult aphasia* (4th. ed.). Baltimore, MD: Lippincott Williams & Wilkins.

Davis, G. A. (2000). *Aphasiology: Disorders and clinical practice*. Needham Heights, MA: Allyn and Bacon.

Hegde, M. N. (2006). *A coursebook on aphasia and other neurogenic language disorders*. Clifton Park, NY: Thomson Delmar Learning.

Helm-Estabrooks, N., & Albert, M. L. (2004). *Manual of aphasia therapy* (2nd ed.). Austin, TX: Pro-Ed.

LaPointe, L. L. (Ed.) (2005). *Aphasia and related neurogenic language disorders* (2nd ed.). New York: Thieme Medical Publishers.

Nadeau, S. E., Gonzalez Rothi, L., & Crosson, B. (2000). *Aphasia and language: Theory to practice*. New York: Guilford Press.

Payne, J. C. (1997). *Adult neurogenic language disorders: Assessment and treatment.* Clifton Park, NY: Thomson Delmar Learning.

Sarno, M. T. (Ed.) (1998). *Acquired aphasia* (3rd ed.). New York: Academic Press.

**Aphonia.** To assess this phonatory disorder, which is a loss of voice, see Voice Disorders.

**Apraxia.** Assessment of disordered volitional movement in the absence of muscle weakness, paralysis, or fatigue is a concern in evaluating and diagnosing motor speech disorders, especially in those who have Apraxia of Speech in adults and Childhood Apraxia of Speech (see their main entries); the clinician may assess the following types of apraxia:

### *Assess Constructional Apraxia*

- Have the client draw simple and familiar pictures
  - Ask the client to draw a house, a human face, a clock, a chair, an apple, and so forth
- Have the client replicate three-dimensional designs or create them
  - Ask the client to copy block designs; use a block design subtest as a test of intelligence
  - Ask the client to construct stick designs you demonstrate
  - Ask the client to match any three-dimensional designs you show

### Assess Limb Apraxia

- Observe the client to see if the spontaneous movements are possible
  - Assess especially the intact spontaneous movement of the hands and legs
  - Give various commands to assess impaired volitional movements
- Have the client replicate three-dimensional designs or create them
  - Ask the client to wave good-bye
  - Ask the client to pick up an object on the floor
  - Ask the client to show how he or she would drink from a glass; then give a glass of water and ask the client to take a sip; performance may be better on the latter

### Assess Oral Apraxia (Nonverbal)

- Have the client perform various oral movements
  - Ask the client to lick lips, whistle, clear throat, smile, move the tongue around in the mouth or stick it out, puff the cheeks out, and so forth
  - Observe the same movements that are adequately performed spontaneously
  - Observe whether it co-occurs with apraxia of speech as it frequently does

**Apraxia of Speech (AOS) in Adults.** Assessment and differential diagnosis of this neurogenic motor speech disorder thought to be due to a motor programming problem in the absence of muscle weakness or neuromuscular slowness are essential to differentiate it from Aphasia or Dysarthria of the unilateral upper motor neuron type; AOS may be associated with nonverbal oral apraxia; language assessment is not critical in its pure form, but pure forms of apraxia of speech are rare.

### Assessment Objectives/General Guidelines

- To assess articulatory proficiency in volitional speech in the absence of muscle weakness
- To assess fluency and prosodic aspects of speech
- To assess other communication skills including auditory comprehension, oral language skills, and reading and writing skills
- To make a diagnosis or rule out general apraxia and to diagnose AOS
- To assess the role of sensory deficiencies as the cause or a contributing factor to apraxia or apraxic-like speech
- To distinguish AOS from other motor speech disorders including Dysarthrias, Neurogenic Fluency Disorders, Palilalia, and Aprosodia
- To distinguish AOS from neurogenic language disorders including Aphasia and Dementia
- To describe potential treatment targets and to assess prognosis
- To describe the client's strengths and intact skills
- To suggest potential neuropathology

### Case History/Interview Focus

- See **Case History** and **Interview** under Standard/Common Assessment Procedures
- Concentrate on orofacial examination to rule out orofacial muscle weakness or paralysis
- Concentrate on the client's detailed biographical data and medical data; pay special attention to family communication patterns

- Review the client's medical records to establish an etiologic factor associated with apraxia of speech (strokes, neurodegenerative diseases, trauma, and tumors, in that order of frequency)

### *Ethnocultural Considerations*

- See Ethnocultural Considerations in Assessment
- Select assessment procedures that are relevant to the client's ethnocultural and linguistic background
- Assess family resources, needed support systems, and access to medical and speech-language pathology services

### *Assessment of Apraxia of Speech*

- Note that assessment of apraxia of speech includes assessment of aphasia because these two conditions often coexist; pure apraxia of speech is rare
- Assess language to determine a coexisting aphasia
  - Obtain a language sample
  - Administer one or more standardized tests of Aphasia
  - Design client-specific procedures to assess specific language deficits (e.g., naming problems) associated with Aphasia
- Assess auditory comprehension deficits associated with aphasia
  - Make judgments during the interview of the client and throughout assessment
  - Administer a test of auditory comprehension of spoken speech; see Aphasia for a list of tests
  - Use the procedures described under Aphasia
- Assess reading and writing problems associated with aphasia
  - Have the client copy a written passage, spontaneously write a piece, or write to dictation
  - Use additional procedures described under Aphasia
- Assess speech production to diagnose AOS
  - Devise your own stimulus materials to assess speech production problems or use the following suggestions that are based on *Motor Speech Evaluation* described by Wertz, LaPointe, and Rosenbek (1991)[1]
  - Tape record the client's responses for later scoring, or score as you evoke the responses. Transcribe responses phonetically; take note of struggle, groping, self-correction, repetition, and other forms of dysfluencies; errors of articulation, delayed reaction, facial grimacing, and other behaviors that suggest apraxia
  - Evoke imitative production of a speech sound
    - Ask the client to say "/a/" as long and as evenly as you can; model the response for the client to imitate
  - Evoke the repetitive production of syllables; model all responses for the client to imitate
    - Ask the client to say "pʌ-pʌ-pʌ as long and as evenly as you can"
    - Ask the client to say "tʌ-tʌ-tʌ as long and as evenly as you can"
    - Ask the client to say "kʌ-kʌ-kʌ as long and as evenly as you can"

[1]Adapted from Wertz, R. T., LaPointe, L. L., & Rosenbek J. C. (1991). *Apraxia of speech in adults.* San Diego, CA: Singular Publishing Group. (1991) and used by permission.

- Evoke the repetitive production of multiple syllables
  - Ask the client to say "**pʌ-tʌ-kʌ**" as long and as evenly as you can
- Evoke imitative production of selected words; model the responses for the client
  - Say "*several*"
  - Say "*tornado*"
  - Say "*artillery*"
  - Say "*linoleum*"
  - Say "*snowman*"
  - Say "*television*"
  - Say "*catastrophe*"
  - Say "*gingerbread*"
  - Say "*probability*"
  - Say "*thermometer*"
  - Say "*refrigeration*"
  - Say "*responsibility*"
  - Say "*unequivocally*"
  - Say "*parliamentarian*"
  - Say "*statistical analysis*"
  - Say "*Encyclopedia Britannica*"
  - Say "*Boston, Massachusetts*"
  - Say "*Minneapolis, Minnesota*"
  - Say "*San Francisco, California*"
  - Say "*Nuclear Regulatory Commission*"
  - Say "*thick* "
  - Say "*thicken*"
  - Say "*thickening*"
  - Say "*love*"
  - Say "*loving*"
  - Say "*lovingly*"
  - Say "*please*"
  - Say "*pleasing*"
  - Say "*pleasingly*"
  - Say "*jab*"
  - Say "*jabber*"
  - Say "*jabbering*"
  - Say "*mom*"
  - Say "*judge*"
  - Say "*peep*"
  - Say "*bib*"
  - Say "*nine*"
  - Say "*tote*"
  - Say "*dad*"
  - Say "*coke*"
  - Say "*gag*"
  - Say "*fife*"

   - Say "*sis*"
   - Say "*zoos*"
   - Say "*church*"
   - Say "*churn*"
   - Say "*lull*"
   - Say "*shush*"
   - Say "*roar*"
- Evoke repeated, imitative production of words and phrases; score each production
   - Say "*artillery*" five times
   - Say "*impossibility*" five times
   - Say "*disenfranchised*" five times
   - Say "*catastrophically*" five times
   - Say "*barometric pressure*" five times
- Evoke the imitative production of sentences
   - Say "*The valuable watch was missing*"
   - Say "*In the summer they sell vegetables*"
   - Say "*The shipwreck washed up on the shore*"
   - Say "*Please put the groceries in the refrigerator*"
   - Say "*Please tell the gardner to fertilize the plants*"
- Evoke counting responses
  "Please count from 1 to 20"
  "Now please count backwards, from 20 down to 1"
- Evoke picture description that lasts at least 1 minute; use the "Cookie Thief" picture from the *Boston Diagnostic Aphasia Examination*
  "Tell me what is happening in this picture"
- Assess imitation of sentences the client produced during the examination; use any four sentences
   - Repeat [a sentence the client has produced]
   - Repeat [a second sentence the client has produced]
   - Repeat [a third sentence the client has produced]
   - Repeat [a fourth sentence the client has produced]
- Assess oral reading; use the *Grandfather* passage; take note of errors of significance
  "Please read this passage out loud"

• Assess prosodic features of speech
- Assess the speech rate in conversational speech
   - Ask the client to speak faster at times; the client typically fails
   - Note that, on occasion, the spontaneous speech may be faster than usual
- Assess continuity in speech
   - Take note of frequent pauses in between syllables and words
   - Assess the effects of such inappropriate pauses on the speech rate as well as the normal rhythm of speech
- Assess the durations of consonants and vowels
   - Take note of increased duration of speech sounds

    - Judge the effects of increased speech sound durations on the prosodic aspects of speech, including overall speech rate
  - Assess linguistic stress patterns
    - Judge the appropriateness of linguistic stress patterns in conversational speech
    - Take note of even stress on syllables and its effects on prosodic features, including the rhythm of speech
  - Judge variations in intonation
    - Make clinical judgments about patterns of intonation
    - Take note of relatively flat intonation and its effects on prosodic features of speech
  - Judge loudness and pitch variations
    - Make clinical judgment or an instrumental assessment of loudness and pitch variations
    - Assess the effects of lack of variations in loudness and pitch on the prosodic aspects of speech
  - Take note of any evidence of foreign accent syndrome
    - See Foreign Accent Syndrome
- Assess oral and nonverbal movement
  - To evaluate oral apraxia or a coexisting dysarthria in case of significant muscle weakness or paralysis, assess oral and nonverbal movement, conduct an Orofacial Examination described under Standard/Common Assessment Procedures
  - Conduct further evaluations by following suggestions from Wertz, LaPointe, and Rosenbek (1991)[2]
  - Assess isolated oral movements; ask the client to listen carefully and perform the action requested

    "Stick out your tongue"
    "Try to touch your nose with your tongue"
    "Try to touch your chin with your tongue"
    "Bite your lower lip"
    "Pucker your lips"
    "Puff out your cheeks"
    "Show me your teeth"
    "Click your teeth together"
    "Wag your tongue from side to side"
    "Clear your throat"
    "Cough"
    "Whistle"
    "Show that you're cold by making your teeth chatter"
    "Smile"
    "Show me how you would kiss a baby"
    "Lick your lips"

[2]Adapted from Wertz, R. T., LaPointe, L. L., & Rosenbek J. C. (1991). *Apraxia of speech in adults*. San Diego, CA: Singular Publishing Group. (1991) and used by permission.

- Assess oral motor sequencing; ask the client to watch you carefully and perform the actions you demonstrate
  - Touch the upper lip center with the tongue tip; lower and raise the jaw
  - Click teeth once; pucker lips
  - Lower and raise the jaw; bite lower lip with teeth; show teeth by stretching the lips
  - Touch the lower lip center with the tongue tip; bite the lower lip; lower and raise the jaw; lick the lips
  - Puff out the cheeks; pucker lips; lower and raise the jaw; lick the lips
  - Click teeth once; pucker lips; lower and raise the jaw; lick lips; bite the lower lip
  - Pucker lips; lick the lips; click teeth once; puff out the cheeks; touch the upper lip center with tongue tip
- Assess limb movements to evaluate limb apraxia
  - Use the following examples from Wertz, LaPointe, and Rosenbek (1991)[3] or use similar commands; ask the client to listen carefully and perform the following actions:
    - "Show how an accordion works"
    - "Show me how you salute"
    - "Wave good-bye"
    - "Threaten someone with your hand"
    - "Show that you are hungry"
    - "Thumb your nose at someone"
    - "Snap your fingers"
    - "Show how you would play a piano"
    - "Indicate that someone is crazy"
    - "Make the letter 'O' with your fingers"
- Take note of clients' personal variables
  - During the interview and assessment session, informally assess:
    - Awareness of problems
    - Motivation for treatment
    - Frustration and coping strategies
    - Response to instructions
    - Level of cooperation

***Standardized Tests.*** Very few standardized tests of AOS are commercially available; most procedures come from research clinicians who have described them in their writing. Administration of aphasia standardized tests, of which many are available, is typically a part of apraxia assessment

- Administer selected standardized tests listed under Aphasia
- Administer selected standardized tests listed under Articulation and Phonological Disorders
- Administer one of the following specialized tests of apraxia

[3]Adapted from Wertz, R. T., LaPointe, L. L., & Rosenbek J. C. (1991). *Apraxia of speech in adults*. San Diego, CA: Singular Publishing Group. (1991) and used by permission.

## Apraxia of Speech (AOS) in Adults

| Test | Purpose |
|---|---|
| *Apraxia Battery for Adults* (B. L. Dabul) | To measure the presence and severity of limb, oral, and speech apraxia and changes over time |
| *Comprehensive Apraxia Test* (F. G. DeSimoni) | To assess nonverbal and verbal apraxia |
| *Test of Oral and Limb Apraxia* (N. Helm-Estabrooks) | To assess oral and limb apraxia in developmental or acquired neurological disorders |

### *Related/Medical Assessment Data*

- Review medical records for evidence of strokes, neurodegenerative disorders, brain trauma, brain tumors, and other neurological diseases or disorders that may be of etiological significance
- Check neurodiagnostic test results for potential identification of lesion sites

### *Standard/Common Assessment Procedures*

- Complete the Standard/Common Assessment Procedures
- Pay special attention to orofacial examination to rule out peripheral neuromuscular problems

### *Analysis of Assessment Results*

- Analyze the language sample and the results of administered tests of aphasia to diagnose or rule out a possible, coexisting aphasia; follow the assessment procedures described under Aphasia
- Describe language formulation, expression, and comprehension problems associated with a coexisting aphasia
- Analyze the results of standardized articulation and phonological tests administered and describe and summarize the kinds of errors noted
- Analyze the speech sample and describe and summarize the kinds of articulatory and phonological errors noted
- Analyze and summarize the results of motor speech evaluation to diagnose AOS
- Analyze and summarize the results of orofacial examination, oral, nonverbal movement evaluation to identify paralysis, paresis, or oral apraxia
- Analyze and summarize the results of limb movement evaluation to assess limb apraxia
- Analyze and describe the reading and writing problems associated with aphasia as assessed by standardized aphasia tests or by client-specific procedures

### *Diagnostic Criteria*

- Evidence of pathology in the left hemisphere
- Evidence of vascular pathology typically involving the left middle cerebral artery
- Dominant symptoms of speech programming difficulties with inconsistent errors of articulation, groping and struggling, notable difficulties in volitional speech production, and prosodic problems

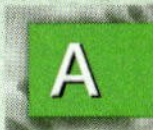




## Subtypes

- Controversial, but possibly based on site of lesion, patterns of articulatory errors, and prosodic problems
- One possible subtype associated with articulatory substitutions and transpositions coupled with less consistently abnormal prosodic features
- Another possible subtype associated with articulatory distortions and more consistently abnormal prosodic features

## Differential Diagnosis

- Distinguish apraxia from aphasia, dementia, language of confusion, dysarthrias, neurogenic stuttering, and palilalia
- Expect the greatest difficulty in distinguishing a coexisting AOS and aphasia in the same client; whereas aphasia often exists without AOS, AOS often exists with aphasia; aphasia associated with AOS often is the nonfluent variety
- Distinguish apraxia from other relevant disorders based on the characteristics listed in each of the 6 grids that follow (adapted from Hegde, 1994)

### Apraxia of Speech or Aphasia?

| Apraxia of Speech | Aphasia |
|---|---|
| Neurogenic speech problem | Neurogenic language problem |
| Without aphasia, more often or more strongly associated with posterior, frontal, or insular lesions | Without AOS, aphasia more often associated with temporal or temporoparietal lesions |
| Client complains of speech production problem (articulation) | Client complains of word retrieval and related language problem |
| Trial and error, groping articulatory movements are significant | Trial and error, groping articulatory movements are not significant |
| Misarticulations more variable, more inconsistent | Misarticulations less variable, more consistent |
| Generally, no impairment in auditory comprehension | Some impairment in auditory comprehension |
| Prosodic problems dominant | Prosodic problems not dominant, especially in fluent aphasias |
| Difficulty in initiating utterances is more obvious or due to difficulty in positioning the articulators | Difficulty in initiating utterances is less obvious or due to naming and language formulation problems |
| Attempts at self-correction | Lack of attempts at self-correction, especially by clients with fluent aphasia |
| Articulatory errors more frequent on initial sounds | Articulatory errors more frequent on final sounds |
| No significant tendency to omit function words | Omission of function words |

*(continues)*

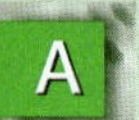



*(continued)*

| Apraxia of Speech | Aphasia |
|---|---|
| No word-finding problems | Word-finding problems |
| Limb or oral apraxia or both may be dominant | Limb or oral apraxia not dominant |
| No reading comprehension deficits | Reading comprehension deficits |
| AOS typically does not mask aphasia | If severe, aphasia can mask AOS |
| AOS with or without aphasia may be associated with unilateral upper motor neuron dysarthria | Aphasia without AOS is less likely to be associated with unilateral upper motor neuron dysarthria |
| Phonologic problems of AOS are predictable and approximations of the intended word | Phonologic problems of fluently aphasic clients are unpredictable, idiosyncratic, and off-target |

*Note: AOS and aphasia share similar neuropathology (vascular etiology and gross neuropathology); AOS in its pure form is uncommon; AOS and Broca's aphasia often coexist, but not AOS and fluent aphasias; phonologic problems associated with AOS may be confused with similar problems found in fluent aphasias.*

### Apraxia of Speech or Dementia?

| Apraxia of Speech | Dementia |
|---|---|
| Sudden onset | Slow onset in many cases |
| Unilateral brain damage | Bilateral brain damage |
| CVA, trauma, or surgery more typical causes | Degenerative neurological diseases more typical causes |
| More localized brain damage | Diffuse brain damage in most cases |
| Intact language and mental functions | Impaired language and mental functions |
| Relatively intact intellectual functions | Progressively deteriorating intellectual functions |
| More errors of fluency and syntax | Fewer errors of fluency and syntax |
| Better preserved reading comprehension | Disturbed reading comprehension |
| Intact semantic and syntactic skills | Semantic and syntactic errors in the initial stages |
| Predominant errors of articulation | Errors of articulation not predominant; such errors appear only in later stages |
| Moodiness, withdrawal, and agitation not a frequent characteristic | May be moody, withdrawn, and agitated |
| Cognition better preserved | Cognition is mildly or severely impaired, but better language skills until later stages |
| General behavior is relevant, socially appropriate, and organized | Behavior often is irrelevant, socially inappropriate, and disorganized |
| Except for the initial acute stage, mentally alert and oriented to time and space | Mentally confused and disoriented to time and space |

*(continues)*

*(continued)*

| Apraxia of Speech | Dementia |
|---|---|
| Well-oriented to self | Disorientation to self in later stages |
| Often less fluent, especially when Broca's aphasia coexists | Fluent until dementia becomes worse |

*Caution: Note that degenerative CNS pathology may cause AOS in about 16% of cases. In such cases, dementia and AOS may coexist.*

## Apraxia of Speech or the Language of Confusion?

| Apraxia of Speech | Language of Confusion |
|---|---|
| Unilateral, focal damage | Bilateral, diffuse damage |
| Vascular pathology and neurosurgical trauma in most cases | Traumatic brain injury and toxic and metabolic disturbances in most cases |
| Speech is relevant | Typically irrelevant |
| Attention deficits are not characteristics | Attention deficits are the most striking |
| Symptoms relatively persistent | Symptoms are more transient |
| Dominant fluency problems | Relatively intact fluency |
| Dominant errors of articulation | Few errors of articulation |
| More syntactic errors | Fewer errors of syntax |
| Fewer writing problems than speech production problems | Writing problems often greater than speaking problems |
| No confabulation | Confabulation |
| No disorientation | Disoriented to time, place, and clients |
| No significant behavioral change | Significant behavioral change |

## Apraxia of Speech or Dysarthria?

| Apraxia of Speech | Dysarthrias |
|---|---|
| The cause is motor programming deficit, not muscle weakness | The cause is muscle weakness |
| Lesions often in the Supratentorial Level of the brain | Lesions in supratentorial and other areas (including posterior fossa, spinal structures, or peripheral nerves) |
| Supratentorial lesions producing apraxia tend to be cortical | Supratentorial lesions producing dysarthria tend to be subcortical |
| Huntington's chorea, parkinsonism, Pick's disease, and ALS are *not* associated with apraxia | Huntington's chorea, parkinsonism, Pick's disease, and ALS *are* associated with dysarthrias |

*(continues)*

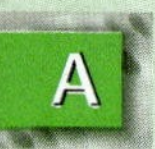



*(continued)*

| Apraxia of Speech | Dysarthrias |
|---|---|
| Can be associated with normal orofacial mechanism and function (except for NVOA) | Often associated with abnormalities of orofacial mechanism and function |
| NVOA may be associated with AOS | NVOA not typically associated with dysarthrias |
| Absence of dysphagia | Presence of dysphagia (but usually not in ataxic dysarthria) |
| Variable misarticulations | Consistent misarticulations (except for ataxic dysarthria which shows irregular articulatory breakdowns) |
| Better production of automatic utterances than propositional productions | The same problems with automatic and propositional productions |
| Word length, meaningfulness, frequency of occurrence are significant variables | Word length (with a possible exception of ataxic dysarthria), meaningfulness, frequency of occurrence are *not* significant variables |
| Besides distortions, complications of speech gestures may be noticeable | Distortions and simplification of speech gestures are dominant |
| More frequent and variable dysfluencies | Less frequent and less variable dysfluencies |
| Frequent articulatory groping | Articulatory groping not characteristic |
| Many attempts at self-correction | Few, if any, attempts at self-correction |
| Respiratory, phonatory, and resonance problems *not* as significant as articulatory and prosodic problems | Respiratory, phonatory, and resonance problems as significant as articulatory and prosodic problems |
| Frequently associated with aphasia | Infrequently associated with aphasia |

*Note: Both AOS and dysarthrias are neurogenic speech disorders. The two are not confused in most cases. Some symptoms are common to AOS and spastic, hyperkinetic, and ataxic dysarthrias; however, it is more difficult to distinguish AOS from ataxic dysarthria. See Dysarthrias for differential diagnosis between AOS and specific types of dysarthrias.*

## Apraxia of Speech or Neurogenic Stuttering?

| Apraxia of Speech | Neurogenic Stuttering |
|---|---|
| Lesions typically in the left hemisphere | Varied site of lesion including brainstem, basal ganglia, cerebellum, all cortical lobes except for the occipital lobe |
| Generally, dysfluencies due to articulatory groping, attempts at self-correction, articulatory revision, and searching | Generally, dysfluencies unrelated to articulatory problems found in AOS |
| Dysfluencies on the off-target sounds or in an effort to revise them | Repetitions and prolongations of target sounds |

## Apraxia of Speech or Palilalia?

| Apraxia of Speech | Palilalia |
|---|---|
| Lesions typically in the left hemisphere | Bilateral lesions typically in the basal ganglia |
| Mechanism of dysfluencies not clear | Mechanism of dysfluencies is neuromuscular problems |
| Sound, syllable, and word repetitions; sound prolongations | Mostly word and phrase repetitions |
| Less commonly associated with hypokinetic dysarthria | More commonly associated with hypokinetic dysarthria |
| Progressive increase in speech rate not evident | The speech rate may increase progressively |
| Slower speech rate | Not necessarily slower speech rate |
| Dysfluencies may be accompanied by effort and groping | Easy and effortless repetition of word and phrase |

## Apraxic Muteness or Muteness of Other Kinds?

| Apraxic Muteness | Muteness of Other Kinds |
|---|---|
| Normal oral mechanism or slight weakness that cannot explain muteness; normal crying, yawning, smiling | Impaired neuromuscular control, paresis or paralysis of orofacial muscles in anarthric mutism |
| Clients with apraxic muteness try to speak and are frustrated at their inability | Muteness due to other reasons (e.g., abulia) are totally disinterested in talking |
| Apraxic mutism may be persistent | Mutism in aphasia may be transient, present often only in the acute stage |
| Apraxic mutism is not drug-induced | Mutism in some cases is due to documented drug use or abuse |
| Apraxic mutism is not a psychiatric disorder | Mutism in some cases may be associated with such psychiatric disorders as schizophrenia and depression; in some cases, mutism is thought to be a conversion reaction |

### *Prognosis*

Clinically proven, strong, and generally applicable and universally agreed-upon variables that clearly predict prognosis are few or nonexistent; however, clinical experience suggests the following:

- Good prognosis for improvement in speech with systematic treatment
- In a few cases, complete or nearly complete recovery in a matter of a few days
- Less favorable prognosis for severe, persistent AOS
- More favorable prognosis with better physical health and lack of sensory deficits
- Less favorable prognosis with larger lesions

- More favorable prognosis with a single, small lesion confined to Broca's area
- Less favorable prognosis with multiple strokes
- More favorable prognosis if treatment is initiated within a month postonset than if the treatment is much delayed
- More favorable prognosis in the absence of serious nonverbal, oral apraxia
- More favorable prognosis with coexisting aphasia that is less severe

### *Recommendations*

- Treatment to improve communication
- See the cited sources and the two companion volumes: *Hegde's PocketGuide to Communication Disorders* and *Hegde's PocketGuide to Treatment in Speech-Language Pathology* (3rd ed.) for details

Bhatnagar, S. C. (2002). *Neuroscience for the study of communication disorders* (2nd ed.). Baltimore, MD: Williams & Wilkins.

Brookshire, R. H. (2003). *An introduction to neurogenic communication disorders* (6th ed.). St. Louis, MO: Mosby Year Book.

Croot, K. (2002). Diagnosis of AOS: Definition and criteria. *Seminars in Speech and Language, 23*(4), 267–279.

Darley, F. L., Aronson, A. E., & Brown, J. R. (1975). *Motor speech disorders.* Philadelphia, PA: W. H. Saunders.

Deger, K., & Wolfram, Z. (2002). Speech motor programming in apraxia of speech. *Journal of Phonetics, 30,* 321–335.

Duffy, J. R. (2005). *Motor speech disorders: Substrates, differential diagnosis, and management* (2nd ed.). St. Louis, MO: Elsevier Mosby.

Love, R. J., & Webb, W. G. (2001). *Neurology for the speech-language pathologist* (4th ed.). Boston, MA: Butterworth-Heinemann.

McClain, M., & Foundas, A. (2004). Apraxia. *Current Neurology and Neuroscience Reports, 4*(6), 471–476.

McNeil, M. R., Doyle, P. J., & Wambaugh, J. (2000). Apraxia of speech: A treatable disorder of motor planning and programming. In S. E. Nadeau, L. J. Gonzalez-Rothi, & B. Crosson (Eds.), *Aphasia and language: Theory to practice* (pp. 221–265) New York: Guilford.

Ogar, J., Slama, H., Dronkers, N., Amici, S., Gorno-Tempini, M. L. (2005). Apraxia of speech: An overview. *Neurocase: Case Studies in Neuropsychology, Neuropsychiatry, and Behavioral Neurology, 11*(6), 427–432.

Ogar, J., Willock, S., Baldo, J., Wilkins, D., Ludy, C., & Donkers, N. (2006). Clinical and anatomical correlates of apraxia of speech. *Brain and Language, 87,* 343–350.

Wertz, R. T., LaPointe, L. L., & Rosenbek, J. C. (1991). *Apraxia of speech.* San Diego, CA: Singular Publishing Group.

**Aprosodia and Dysprosody.** Assessment of prosodic disturbances of speech is important in several disorders of communication, including Apraxia of Speech, Dysarthria, and Right Hemisphere Syndrome; people who have been treated for stuttering with slow speech with the syllable prolongation technique also exhibit dysprosody; technically, *aprosodia* is lack of prosodic features in speech whereas *dysprosody* means impaired prosody of speech; assess prosodic features in any client whose speech sounds unnatural; to assess prosodic problems, see Apraxia of Speech.

**Articulation and Phonological Disorders.** Assessment of speech disorders characterized by difficulty in correctly producing speech sounds is a major responsibility of speech-language pathologists; assessment of omissions, distortions, or substitutions of sounds should lead to a differential diagnosis of an articulation disorder versus a phonological disorder; absence or presence of phonological patterns or presumed rule governance of errors helps make this distinction; assessment procedures described in this section are pertinent to younger and older children who may be classified as having a *functional articulation disorder* with no significant or convincing evidence of organic deficits; to assess articulation problems as a part of Dysarthria in children with neuromuscular disorders, see Cerebral Palsy; to assess speech production problems in children with apraxia of speech with presumed motor planning or programming deficits in the absence of neuromuscular impairments, see Childhood Apraxia of Speech.

### Assessment Objectives/General Guidelines

- To assess the articulatory performance of the client in single word positions and in conversational speech
- To assess the presence of phonological processes that may help establish patterns in misarticulations
- To evaluate a child's performance in light of developmental norms
- To evaluate stimulability of speech sounds that are misarticulated
- To identify potential treatment targets
- To evaluate treatment effects by repeated measurement

### Case History/Interview Focus

- See **Case History** and **Interview** under Standard/Common Assessment Procedures
- Pay special attention to articulation disorders as described by the parents; seek information on speech and language acquisition
- Take note of such other clinical conditions as hearing loss, intellectual disabilities, cleft palate and other craniofacial anomalies, and neuromuscular problems the child may exhibit
- Depending on the age and judged sophistication, talk to the child about his or her speech problem to assess awareness of the speech problems, personal reactions to the problem, reactions from the peers and teachers, difficulties the child experiences in social and academic contexts, and so forth

### Ethnocultural Considerations

- See Ethnocultural Considerations in Assessment
- Pay special attention to the client's bilingual/multilingual status; be aware that there can be substantial variations within one language (e.g., Puerto Rican vs. Mexican vs. Cuban Spanish) and that Asian Americans are a linguistically heterogeneous group with varied language families and numerous dialectal variations of each language

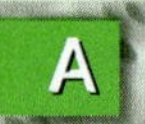



- Consider the dialectal variations of the client and do not diagnose an articulation or phonological disorder solely on the basis of a dialect; see Articulation and Phonological Disorders in African American Children, Articulation and Phonological Disorders in Bilingual Children, and Articulation and Phonological Disorders in Native American Children
- Consider using standardized tests in the client's first language (e.g., a Spanish test of articulation for a child whose primary language is Spanish)
- Consider working with an interpreter who speaks a bilingual child's primary language

### Screening Articulation Skills

- When an articulation disorder is not obvious, screen articulation to determine whether a more detailed assessment is needed
  - Evoke a brief conversation from the child and take note of articulatory errors
  - Ask a few questions about the child, names of family members, friends and their names, interests, hobbies, school activities, favorite television shows, teachers, sport activities, recent vacations, and so forth; ask the child to count to 20, recite days of the week, months of the year, and so forth
  - Take a brief conversational speech sample from an adult and evaluate speech sound productions
  - Have an adult read the *Rainbow* passage or the *Grandfather* passage to screen errors in speech sound productions

### Use Standardized Screening Instruments

- Administer one of the following standardized screening tests or measures

| Test | Purpose |
|---|---|
| *Denver Articulation Screening Test* (A. F. Drumright) | To screen production of 30 sounds in initial and final word positions |
| *Fluharty Speech and Language Screening Test for Preschool Children* (N. B. Fluharty) (administer the speech screening portion) | To screen production of speech sounds with object stimuli |
| *McDonald Screening Deep Test* (E. T. McDonald) | To screen production of frequently misarticulated sounds in 10 coarticulatory contexts |
| *Joliet 3-Minute Speech and Language Screen* (Revised) | A quick screening instrument for children 2.6 to 4.6 years of age |
| *Predictive Screening Test* (C. Van Riper & R. L. Erickson) | To screen production of sounds to predict articulatory skills by the end of second grade |
| *Preschool Language Scale* (Zimmerman, Steiner, & Pond) | To screen production of 18 individual sounds and one cluster |
| *Quick Screen of Phonology* (N. W. Bankson & J. E. Bernthal) | To screen 10 phonological processes |

(continues)

*(continued)*

| Test | Purpose |
|---|---|
| *Templin-Darley Screening Test* (M. C. Templin & F. L. Darley) | To screen production of sounds with color and black and white pictures |
| *Test of Minimal Articulation Competence* (W. Secord) | To screen speech sound production in 3 to 5 minutes; also includes the Rapid Screening Test |

## Assessment of Articulation and Phonological Disorders

- Take a representative sample of connected speech
  - Use the general procedures of obtaining a speech and language sample described under Standard/Common Assessment Procedures
  - In the case of younger children, have the mother and child interact with each other; let them interact in their usual manner; supply toys and picture books the mother and the child prefer; tape record the interactions; observe and take notes
  - Engage the child in conversational speech
  - Use a quiet room and avoid noisy stimulus materials; use a tablecloth or any soft material to dampen noise; sit on carpeted floor
  - Use large pictures, storybooks, and soft toys; consider the child's interests and ethnocultural background in selecting stimulus materials
  - Tape record the entire speech sample for later analysis
  - Record in stereo for a more dynamic range
  - When possible, transcribe on the spot
  - Talk less, do not interrupt the child, and listen carefully
  - Echo what you think the child said when you are not sure what the child said
  - Do not ask yes/no questions; ask open-ended questions
  - Use the following to evoke conversation; modify them as necessary to make them appropriate for individual child; use the questions/suggestions within the parentheses for follow-up:
    - "Tell me about your favorite TV show"
    - "Tell me about the shows you watch on Saturday mornings (tell me what happens in ______ show or ______ show?)"
    - "Tell me about your favorite video game (tell me how to play it; what are some of your other favorite video games?)"
    - "What did you do last weekend? (what do you plan to do next weekend?)"
    - "Tell me about your favorite vacation (tell me about your other vacations)"
    - "Tell me the story of Cinderella (did you see the movie? did you like it?)"
    - "Tell me the story of [a recent children's movie] (did you see the movie? did you like it?)"
    - "Tell me the story of the *Three Little Pigs* should only be"
    - "Tell me the names of your friends (describe them for me; how much time do you spend with them?; do you play with them on weekends?; what do you play with them?)"
    - "Who is your best friend (why?)"

    - "Tell me about your favorite babysitter (why is she your favorite?)"
    - "Tell me how to make popcorn"
    - "Tell me how to make hot dogs"
    - "Tell me how your mom makes cookies (do you help mom when she bakes cookies? how do you help her?)"
    - "Pretend I have never had pizza before and describe it to me (have you ever helped your mom make pizza at home? how did you help her?)"
    - "Who is your favorite teacher (and why?)"
    - "What subjects do you like the most (and why?)"
  - Show large picture cards that depict a variety of activities and ask the child to tell a story; when the response is sparse, ask such follow-up questions as the following while you point to different aspects of the picture:
    - "What about this?"
    - "What about that?"
    - "What is going on here?"
    - "What is he doing here?"
    - "Why is she doing that?"
    - "What is she (he, they) doing over there?"
    - "What is happening here? why?"
  - Show funny and incongruous pictures and ask such questions as the following:
    - "What is funny about this?"
    - "What is wrong here?"
  - Ask the child to narrate a story; prompt the child to say more; direct the child's attention to aspects of the story he or she ignores
  - Tell a story and ask the child to retell it; prompt the child about details not given
  - Tell a story about a picture and then ask the child to retell it as he or she looks at the picture
  - Pretend to go on a shopping trip to a store; have a toy cash register, plastic food items, and some play money; let the child do the shopping and talking
  - Use hand puppets to carry on a conversation and to tell stories to each other
  - Misname objects, toys, or pictures and let the child correct you
  - Show the child only parts of a disassembled toy (such as Mr. Potato Head); let the child ask for missing parts
  - Role play daily activities (cooking, shopping, planning a picnic)
  - Create a play or toy farm and ask questions about the animals and farm activities
  - Use a dollhouse to engage the child in conversation and description of stimuli
  - Ask the child to explain a game (e.g., hide-and-seek)
  - Have the child play teacher and talk to the kids or teach words to the kids
  - Obtain a sample of oral reading from children who can read; but note that fewer errors are revealed in reading tasks than in connected speech tasks
- Take a sample of single word productions
  - Use a standardized test that samples single word productions

- Make your own stimulus material to test sounds in the initial, medial, and final positions; minimally, include the most frequently misarticulated speech sounds: /s, z, θ, ð, ʃ, ʧ, ʤ, v, r/
- Select attractive and unambiguous pictures to evoke single word responses
- Use a combination of pictures and objects (especially toys with young children) to introduce variety
- Ask the child to name the picture
- Record the response for later analysis; preferably, write down the response in the phonetic alphabet
- If the child does not seem to know the name of a picture or object, name it and move on to the next stimulus
- After a while, re-present the stimulus you had named earlier
- With a client-specific procedure (not a standardized test), ask for repetition of any unclear response that is difficult to score (note that standardized tests may not allow this)
- Ask the child to repeat given responses if it appears that oral-motor problems are creating inconsistent responses
- Note that articulatory performance in single word productions may not totally reflect the problems the child may have in connected speech; however, by using single word production tasks you can make sure of sampling all sounds in all positions; do not use single word performance data exclusively unless the child's connected speech is extremely limited or unintelligible
- Compare single word performance data with connected speech performance data; the two sets of data may diverge, especially in the case of oral-motor problems

### *Assess Stimulability of Misarticulated Sounds*

- Select the sounds the child misarticulates and assess their stimulability
  - Ask the child to watch, listen carefully, and say what you say; do not give special instructions on the correct production (e.g., about the placement of the articulators or voicing)
  - Model the production of selected phonemes and ask the child to imitate
  - Model them initially in isolated sound levels
  - Model the sounds in words
  - Take note of the percent success rate to determine the stimulability for each sound
  - Note the limitations of stimulability tests; though popular, their value in predicting improvement either with or without therapy is questionable; lack of stimulability does not suggest poor prognosis for treatment; treatment is recommended regardless of stimulability scores; poor stimulability should discourage neither the clinician nor the client

### *Make a Structured Contextual Assessment*

- Administer a deep test of articulation
  - Deep testing helps assess the production of sounds in different phonetic contexts; note that although conversational speech provides contextual

information, structured assessment of contextual influence is valuable in identifying contexts in which a misarticulated sound is correctly produced; such contexts may be used in treatment; structured assessment allows for systematic alterations in the phonetic context in ways that may not naturally occur in conversational speech

- Assess consistency of misarticulations by sampling speech in varied phonetic contexts
  - Analyze phonetic contexts of conversational speech in which each of the misarticulated phonemes is produced correctly
  - Compare the results with those of a deep test of articulation

### *Standardized Tests of Articulation*

- Select tests of known reliability and validity
- Evaluate each test for its appropriateness for a child with a varied ethno-cultural background
- Administer one or more of the following standardized tests; always use the current edition of the test listed:

| Test | Purpose |
|---|---|
| *Arizona Articulation Proficiency Scale* (J. B. Fudala & W. B. Reynolds) | To assess primarily single phoneme productions with black and white picture stimuli; a few sentences |
| *Clinical Probes of Articulation Consistency (C-PAC)* (W. Secord) | To assess sound productions in varied phonetic contexts including pre- and postvocalic positions. |
| *Fisher-Logemann Test of Articulation Competence* (H. Fisher & J. Logemann) | To assess single phonemes with color pictures and sentence productions; includes a screening component |
| *Goldman-Fristoe Test of Articulation* (R. Goldman & M. Fristoe) | To assess single phonemes with color pictures and sentence productions |
| *Iowa Pressure Test* (H. L. Morris, D. D. Spriestersbach, & F. L. Darley) | To assess mostly fricatives and plosives and indirectly assess the adequacy of velopharyngeal closure; items from the *Templin-Darley Test of Articulation* |
| *McDonald Deep Test of Articulation* (E. T. McDonald) | To assess contextual production of phonemes (two-word combinations and in sentences) |
| *Photo Articulation Test* (K. Pendergast, S. F. Dickey, J. W. Selmar, & A. L. Soder) | To assess single phoneme productions with color pictures of objects |
| *Templin-Darley Test of Articulation* (M. C. Templin & F. L. Darley) | To assess sound production in words, sentences, and in sentence completion formats |
| *Test of Minimal Articulation Competence (T-MAC)* (W. Secord) | To assess speech sound production with a picture confrontation format |

## Measures of Phonological Processes

- Use one of the following tests to make a phonological analysis of misarticulations; always use the current edition of the instrument listed:

| Test | Purpose |
|---|---|
| *Assessment of Link Between Phonology and Articulation—Revised* (R. J. Lowe) | To assess 15 phonological processes through short sentences and with picture stimuli |
| *Assessment of Phonological Processes—Revised* (B. W. Hodson) | To assess 40 phonological processes in seven categories with objects, pictures, and body parts |
| *Bankson-Bernthal Test of Phonology* (N. W. Bankson & J. E. Bernthal) | To assess consonant productions, phonological error patterns, and intelligibility |
| *Compton-Hutton Phonological Assessment* (A. J. Compton & J. S. Hutton) | To assess sound productions in initial and final word positions to identify phonological error patterns |
| *Computerized Articulation and Phonology Evaluation System* (J. Masterson & B. Bernhardt, 2001) | To assess phonological processes through color photographs |
| *Computerized Profiling* (S. Long & M. Fey) | To assess phonological processes with an IBM-compatible or Macintosh computer |
| *Hodson Assessment of Phonological Processes* (B. Hodson) | To identify priorities in the treatment of unintelligible children; not a traditional test of phonological processes |
| *Khan-Lewis Phonological Analysis* (L. Khan & N. Lewis) | To assess 15 phonological processes with 44 words from the *Goldman-Fristoe Test of Articulation* |
| *Macintosh Interactive System for Phonological Analysis* (J. Masterson & F. Pagan) | To assess 27 phonological processes or rules with a Macintosh computer |
| *Natural Process Analysis* (L. Shriberg & J. Kwiatkowski) | To assess 8 natural phonological processes with a 90-word spontaneous speech sample |
| *Phonological Process Analysis* (F. Weiner) | To assess 16 phonological processes with 136 picture stimuli |

## Related Assessment Data

- Obtain results of intellectual and behavioral assessment in cases of children with intellectual disabilities and behavioral disorders
- Obtain information on academic and language performance with school-age children

- Obtain information on physical or neurological disabilities and dental abnormalities
- Obtain information on such developmental disorders as Asperger syndrome and autism, if relevant
- Obtain information on audiological assessment, if relevant
- Obtain information on other sensory impairments, if relevant

### *Standard/Common Assessment Procedures*

- Complete the Standard/Common Assessment Procedures
- Conduct a thorough orofacial examination
- Rule out or describe craniofacial anomalies that may be contributing to the client's speech production problems

### *Scoring and Analysis of Assessment Data*

- Transcribe the speech sample to determine the errors of articulation
- Use the International Phonetic Alphabet to transcribe the speech of the child
- If practical, use diacritics to make a narrower transcription (close transcription system) to obtain a more specific and detailed description of errors especially for children with cleft palate or bilingual backgrounds
- Take note of the consistency with which errors are produced; calculate the percentage of misarticulation for each phoneme in error (e.g., /s/ misarticulated in 100% of the sampled contexts; /p/ misarticulated in 70% of the sampled contexts); calculate the percentage of misarticulation of each phoneme in the initial and final position of words
- List the phonetic contexts in which any of the misarticulated sounds were correctly produced
- Calculate the percent correct production of misarticulated sounds that the child correctly imitated on stimulability trials
- Analyze the results of standardized tests according to the test manuals
- Make a phonological analysis if the child has multiple misarticulations and it appears that a pattern analysis will be worthwhile
- Analyze the results of phonological assessment instruments according to the prescribed procedures
- Make a phonetic inventory analysis; count sounds that occur at least three times in a speech sample versus those that occur just one or two times; this analysis reveals the size of the child's phonetic inventory; a child's phonetic inventory may be limited to only a few sounds (many errors or error patterns) or may contain many sounds (few errors)
- Integrate information from different sources (case history, speech samples, standardized tests, phonological assessment instruments, reports from other specialists that bear upon the diagnosis, etc.)
- List the sounds in error; classify them according to an acceptable format (e.g., omissions, substitutions, and distortions; errors in the initial, medial, and final positions); compare the child's performance to Developmental Norms for Phonemes
- List the Phonological Processes that were identified in your phonological analysis

- List the child's phonological processes in the order of early disappearing to late disappearing processes; use the following guidelines given by Stoel-Gammon and Dunn (1985) to evaluate the processes that should have disappeared in the assessed child

| Processes Disappearing by Age 3 Years | Processes Persisting After Age 3 Years |
|---|---|
| Unstressed syllable deletion | Cluster reduction |
| Final consonant deletion | Epenthesis |
| Consonant assimilation | Gliding |
| Reduplication | Vocalization |
| Velar fronting | Stopping |
| Diminutization | Depalatalization |
| Prevocalic voicing | Final devoicing |

- Take note that processes that may persist the longest include gliding of liquids, stopping, cluster simplification, vocalization, and final consonant deletion; significant decrease in the use of processes between the ages of 2.5 and 4 years (Peña-Brooks & Hegde, 2007)
- If preferred, list the Distinctive Features that are missed or misused; organize the errors according to the missing distinctive features
- Calculate the percent intelligibility based on the number of words or utterances understood with or without the knowledge of context; if preferred, rate severity on a 3- or 5-point rating scale

### Diagnostic Criteria

- Errors of speech sound production when the child is expected to be producing them correctly
- Multiple errors that fall into patterns that suggest one or more phonological processes
- Evidence of phonological processes beyond the expected age at which such processes should no longer be observed
- Clinically significant problem of unintelligible speech
- The number of phonemes in error that is above the cutoff score for offering treatment services as established in given clinical service settings (e.g., public schools)
- Clinically and socially significant problem regardless of the number of sounds in error; family concern and need for services

### Differential Diagnosis

- Distinguish an articulation disorder in the child assessed from a phonological disorder
- Diagnose an articulation disorder if the errors are few and cannot be organized on the basis of place-manner-voice, phonological, or distinctive feature analysis

- Diagnose a phonological disorder in a child when the child's multiple errors can be grouped according to a pattern or linguistic rule; most often, clinicians analyze errors in terms of phonological processes to make this diagnosis, although grouping errors on the basis of distinctive features or the place-manner-voice analysis also will help identify patterns in multiple errors
- Distinguish articulation and phonological disorders from Childhood Apraxia of Speech (CAS); the characteristics of oral apraxia, motor incoordination, poor imitative skills for articulation, inconsistent and variable errors, groping and silent articulatory postures, and speech sound sequencing problems distinguish CAS by their presence, and articulation and phonological disorders by their absence
- Distinguish articulation and phonological disorders from Dysarthria associated with Cerebral Palsy; the characteristics of a history of cerebral damage to the immature nervous system, obvious neuromuscular problems, and associated respiratory, resonance, phonatory, and prosodic problems distinguish cerebral palsy by their presence, and articulation and phonological disorders by their absence
- Distinguish functional articulation and phonological disorders from those associated with hearing impairment; a confirmed audiological diagnosis of hearing impairment, and characteristics of hypo- and hypernasality, reduced rate of speech, pauses, slower articulatory transitions, disturbed stress patterns, disorders of vocal pitch (too high or too low), disturbed prosodic features, hoarse or breathy voice quality, predominance of voiced-voiceless and oral-nasal confusion, and imprecise or distorted vowel production distinguish hearing impairment by their presence, and articulation and phonological disorders by their absence
- Distinguish an articulation disorder in the assessed child from a dialectal difference; if the "errors" (variations from standard English productions) are a part of the child's first language phonological features, do not diagnose a disorder; if the variations are due to a different dialect of the same language (e.g., African American English or one of the other English dialects), then do not diagnose a disorder
- Describe such associated conditions as emotional disorders, Asperger syndrome, or autism, and suggest additional or more intensive evaluation when needed

### *Prognosis*

- Generally good for children with articulation and phonological disorders; most children's articulation skills improve with systematic treatment
- The presence of such additional variables as hearing impairment, intellectual disabilities, physical disabilities, negative environmental factors, and sensory deficits may affect the rate of improvement and the final outcome; nonetheless, these variables are not a basis to withhold treatment

### *Recommendations*

- Detailed assessment for the client who has failed the screening evaluation
- Treatment for the client who is diagnosed to have an articulation and phonological disorder

- See the cited sources and the two companion volumes: *Hegde's PocketGuide to Communication Disorders* and *Hegde's PocketGuide to Treatment in Speech-Language Pathology* (3rd ed.)

Bernthal, J. E., & Bankson, N. W. (2004). *Articulation and phonological disorders* (5th ed.). Boston, MA: Allyn and Bacon.

Lowe, R. J. (1994). *Phonology: Assessment and intervention applications in speech pathology*. Baltimore, MD: Williams & Wilkins.

Peña-Brooks, A., & Hegde, M. N. (2007). *Assessment and treatment of articulation and phonological disorders in children* (2nd ed.). Austin, TX: Pro-Ed.

Smit, A. B. (2004). *Articulation and phonology: Resource guide for school-age children and adults*. Clifton Park, NY: Thomson Delmar Learning.

Stoel-Gammon, C., & Dunn, C. (1985). *Normal and disordered phonology in children*. Austin, TX: Pro-Ed.

Williams, A. L. (2003). *Speech disorders: Resource guide for preschool children*. Clifton Park, NY: Thomson Delmar Learning.

## Articulation and Phonological Disorders in African American Children.

Assessment of disorders of speech sound production in children who speak African American English (AAE) and a variety of Standard American English (SAE) require a thorough knowledge of the phonological, grammatical, and pragmatic aspects of African American English along with the African American culture; an important assessment objective is to distinguish a (normal) dialectal difference from a disorder of speech production; many African American children who speak AAE also speak SAE competently; assessment presents challenges to clinicians who do not know the phonological properties of AAE; in assessing children who speak both the AAE and SAE, the clinician should not (1) mistakenly diagnose an articulation disorder in SAE when the sound productions simply reflect the influence of AAE, and (2) overdiagnose or underdiagnose an articulation disorder in AAE; both can be avoided with (1) a good knowledge of the phonological system of AAE, and (2) a general understanding that AAE is a product of unique historical and cultural forces, and that it is a recognized form of English with its own phonological, syntactic, semantic, and pragmatic rules and conventions; see Ethnocultural Considerations in Assessment for general guidelines, Articulation and Phonological Disorders for a general description that applies to most children who misarticulate speech sounds, and *Hegde's PocketGuide to Communication Disorders* and other sources cited at the end of this entry to understand articulation and phonological disorders in African American children

### *Assessment Objectives/General Guidelines*

- To diagnose an articulation or phonological process disorder in AAE and SAE if a child speaks both forms; note that this requires knowledge of the phonological characteristics of AAE
- To diagnose an articulation or phonological disorder if African American child speaks only SAE; still, a general knowledge of the AAE and family communication patterns are essential to make this diagnosis

- To analyze errors in SAE that are not due to the influence of AAE in a child who speaks both dialects of English; note that such errors do constitute a true articulation disorder; note, too, that this task requires knowledge of the phonological system of AAE
- To analyze patterns of SAE speech sound productions that vary from those of SAE, but are a function of AAE patterns; note that such variations are not a basis to diagnose an articulation disorder; this analysis is done to achieve a comprehensive understanding of child's phonological skills; however, elective treatment may be offered if the child, the family, or both, wish to minimize variations in SAE articulation
- To identify potential treatment targets that are ethnoculturally appropriate for the child and consistent with the wishes and needs of the child, the educational demands faced by the child, and the desires of the child's parents or other caretakers

### *Case History/Interview Focus*

- See **Case History** and **Interview** under Standard/Common Assessment Procedures
- In addition to completing the standard case history and related procedures, concentrate on the child's unique cultural and linguistic background; ask questions designed to obtain information on the family communication patterns; for instance:
  - Do the family members speak only AAE at home?
  - Do the family members also speak SAE at home?
  - How is the talking time roughly distributed across the two forms of English?
  - What is the level of SAE proficiency of the family members?
  - What is the level of AAE proficiency of the family members?
  - Do they all effectively code-switch depending on communicative situations?
  - What are the parents' expectations regarding clinical services? Are they concerned about proficiency in SAE and SAE phonological patterns?
  - What kinds of educational demands are made on the child?
  - Does the child's classroom teacher accept AAE?
  - How is the child doing in the classroom?
  - Is there an indication of poor performance due to limited SAE proficiency, limited AAE proficiency, or both?
  - Are there any associated clinical conditions that might affect treatment prognosis (e.g., developmental disabilities, hearing loss, neurological impairment, genetic syndromes)?
  - What are the recommendations of the child's teachers?
  - What are the educational and career goals of the client or as envisioned by the parents?

### *Assessment of Articulation and Phonological Disorders in African American Children*

- Note that there are very few satisfactorily standardized tests to evaluate articulatory proficiency in African American children; currently, use of nonstandardized, systematic, client-specific procedures with a good background in AAE is the best diagnostic approach

- Note that most standardized tests of articulation and phonology may not have adequately sampled African American children in their standardization process; many test developers have made and are still making efforts to improve the sampling of minority children, including African American children in their re-standardization of popular tests of speech and language; keep track of newer editions of older tests that may be more suitable to assess articulation (and language) skills in minority children
- Note that SAE speech sound errors need to be assessed even if no diagnosis of a disorder is made solely on this basis; because the parents and the child may opt for articulation treatment geared toward standard English productions, it is essential to make a thorough analysis of errors in both forms of English
- Use the procedures described under Articulation and Phonological Disorders to structure and evoke speech from the child; however, in selecting stimulus materials to evoke speech, consider the child's family and cultural background; let the parents guide the selection of materials that are familiar to their child
- Let the parents interact with the child as you tape record the conversational interaction; assist the parents in manipulating the stimulus materials to evoke a variety of speech productions to sample all speech sounds; let the parents guide the selection of materials that are familiar to their child; some parents may bring material to the assessment session if prior arrangements are made
- Take a sample of single word productions; use the procedures described in Articulation and Phonological Disorders

### *Assessment of Stimulability of Misarticulated Sounds*

- Select the sounds the child misarticulates in both forms of English and assess their stimulability
- Use procedures described under Articulation and Phonological Disorders

### *Related Assessment Data*

- Obtain results of intellectual and behavioral assessment of children if warranted
- Obtain information on academic and language performance with school-age children
- Obtain information on physical or neurological disabilities and craniofacial abnormalities including malocclusions, dental abnormalities, cleft palate, and weakness or paralysis of facial muscles
- Obtain information on audiological assessment
- Obtain information on other sensory impairments

### *Standard/Common Assessment Procedures*

- Complete the Standard/Common Assessment Procedures with an emphasis on the orofacial examination

### *Scoring and Analysis of Assessment Data*

- Use the procedures described under Articulation and Phonological Disorders
- Take the help of an African American speech-language pathologist (SLP) or one with a good knowledge of AAE

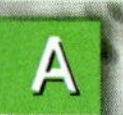



- Analyze errors in AAE in light of the AAE phonological patterns; only those productions that are inconsistent with AAE phonological patterns are a basis to diagnose an articulation disorder in AAE
- Analyze variations in SAE phoneme productions that may be a function of the phonological patterns of AAE; these variations are not a basis to diagnose an articulation disorder
- Analyze errors in SAE that are independent of the phonological patterns of AAE; these errors are a basis to diagnose an articulation disorder in SAE

## Diagnostic Criteria

- Note that the phoneme inventory of children speaking AAE will match that of SAE; a majority of phonemes are used in the same way in both AAE and SAE; only some phonemes will be used differently, substituted for other phonemes, or omitted in certain contexts
- Assess which AAE phonemic usages that differ from those of SAE are indeed characteristics of AAE; in making this assessment, consider the following phonological patterns that are accepted in AAE and hence are not a basis to diagnose an articulation disorder:
    - /l/ lessening or omission (e.g., *too'* for *tool*; *a'ways* for *always*)
    - /r/ lessening or omission (e.g., *doah* for *door*; *mudah* for *mother*)
    - /θ/ substitution for /f/ in word final or medial positions (e.g., *teef* for *teeth*, *nofin'* for *nothing*)
    - /t/ substitution for /θ/ in word initial positions (e.g., *tink* for *think*)
    - /d/ substitution for /ð/ in word initial and medial positions (e.g., *dis* for *this* and *broder* for *brother*)
    - /v/ substitution for /ð/ in word final positions (e.g., *smoov* for *smooth*)
    - omission of consonants in clusters in word initial and final positions (e.g., *thow* for *throw* and *des'* for *desk*)
    - Consonant substitutions within clusters (e.g., *skrike* for *strike*)
    - Unique syllable stress patterns (e.g., ***gui*** *tar* for *guitar* and ***Ju*** *ly* for *July*)
    - Modification of verbs ending in /k/ (e.g., *li-id* for *liked* and *wah-tid* for *walked*)
    - Metathetic productions (e.g., *aks* for *ask*)
    - Devoicing of final voiced consonants (e.g., *bet* for *bed* and *ruk* for *rug*)
    - Deletion of final consonants (e.g., *ba'* for *bad* and *goo'* for *good*)
    - /i/ substitution for /e/ (e.g., *pin* for *pen* and *tin* for *ten*)
    - /b/ substitution for /v/ (e.g., *balentine* for *valentine* and *bes'* or *vest*)
    - Diphthong reduction or ungliding (e.g., *fahnd* for *find* and *ol* for *oil*)
    - /n/ substitution for /g/ (e.g., *walkin'* for *walking* and *thin'* for *thing*)
    - Unstressed syllable deletion (e.g., *bout* for *about* and *member* for *remember*)
- Note that a diagnosable articulation disorder for a child who speaks AAE is a disorder in the context of AAE (and SAE), not in the sole context of SAE

## Differential Diagnosis

- Use all the guidelines for differential diagnosis summarized under Articulation and Phonological Disorders

- Note that the most critical task of differential diagnosis is to separate articulatory errors in AAE and those in SAE that are not a function of AAE phonological patterns; take note of all variations in SAE that may be a basis for treatment request from the parents, child, or both; however, diagnose a disorder in SAE only if the errors are not due to the phonological patterns of SAE
- Diagnose articulatory errors in AAE only when they are inconsistent with AAE phonological patterns

### *Prognosis*

- No systematic evidence suggests that prognosis for improved articulation in African American children is any different from that in other children
- When systematic and effective treatment is offered, African American children will improve in their articulation skills like any other children
- The presence of such additional variables as developmental disabilities, genetic syndromes, and sensory disabilities (e.g., hearing loss) may affect the rate of improvement as they do in any other children with articulation and phonological disorders

### *Recommendations*

- Recommend treatment for articulation disorders in AAE; recommend treatment targets that are consistent with AAE
- Recommend treatment for articulatory variations in SAE only if the client or the family members request such treatment because of the advantage standard English offers in educational, social, and occupational settings
- Recommend treatment on a priority basis for errors in phonemes that are common to AAE and SAE

Battle, D. E. (2002). *Communication disorders in multicultural populations* (3rd ed.). Boston, MA: Butterworth-Heinemann.

Genesee, F., Paradis, J., & Crago, M. B. (2004). *Dual language development and disorders.* Baltimore, MD: Paul H. Brookes.

Goldstein, B. A. (2004). *Bilingual language development and disorders in Spanish-English speakers.* Baltimore, MD: Paul H. Brookes.

Kamhi, A. G., Pollack, K. E., & Harris, J. L. (1996). *Communication development and disorders in African American children.* Baltimore, MD: Paul H. Brookes.

Kayser, H. (1995). *Bilingual speech-language pathology: An Hispanic focus.* San Diego, CA: Singular Publishing Group.

Peña-Brooks, A., & Hegde, M. N. (2007). *Assessment and treatment of articulation and phonological disorders in children* (3rd ed.). Austin, TX: Pro-Ed.

Roseberry-McKibbin, C. (2002). *Multicultural students with special language needs* (2nd ed.). Oceanside, CA: Academic Communication Associates.

**Articulation and Phonological Disorders in Bilingual Children.** Assessment of disorders of speech sound production in children who speak two (or more) languages can be challenging because it requires the knowledge of the languages involved in an individual case; the disorder may be evident in one or both of the languages spoken by a large and varied group of children in the United States; present assessment challenges because of the variety of primary languages that influence the secondary English spoken in the United States; see Ethnocultural Considerations in Assessment for general guidelines; see also Articulation and Phonological Disorders for a general description that apply to most children who misarticulate speech sounds.

### *Assessment Objectives/General Guidelines*

- To analyze errors of speech sound production and phonological processes evident in the primary language of the child; note that this requires knowledge of the primary language's phonological characteristics; in the absence of such knowledge, refer the child to an SLP who has the knowledge; or, use a qualified interpreter
- To analyze errors in English that are not due to the influence of the primary language; note that this task, too, requires knowledge of a bilingual child's primary language
- To analyze English sound productions that vary from those in standard or a regional American English; such an analysis need not result in a diagnosis of an articulation disorder and a recommendation for treatment; this analysis is done to achieve a comprehensive understanding of the child's phonological skills; however, treatment may be offered if the child, the family, or both, wish to minimize the English articulatory variations
- To identify potential treatment targets that are ethnoculturally appropriate for the child and consistent with the wishes and needs of the child and his or her family

### *Case History/Interview Focus*

- See **Case History** and **Interview** under Standard/Common Assessment Procedures
- In addition to completing the standard case history and related procedures, concentrate on the child's unique cultural and linguistic background; ask questions designed to obtain information on the family communication patterns; for instance:
  - What percentage of the time do the family members speak the primary language such as Spanish or Hmong at home?
  - What is the level of English proficiency of the family members?
  - What is the level of primary language proficiency of the family members?
  - What is the specific variety of the primary language spoken at home (e.g., Mexican Spanish or Puerto Rican Spanish)?
  - Do they speak English and, if so, what percentage of the time, or in what kinds of communicative situations?
  - Is one or the other language dominant in certain speaking situations?
  - What are the parents' expectations regarding clinical services? Are they concerned about proficiency in SAE and English speech sound production?
  - What kinds of educational demands are made on the child? Is the child in a regular classroom or in a special bilingual program?
  - How is the child doing in the classroom? Is there an indication of poor performance due to English language deficiency, primary language

deficiency, or deficiency in both the languages?
  - Are there any associated clinical conditions that might affect prognosis (e.g., developmental disabilities, hearing loss, neurological impairment, genetic syndromes)?
  - What are the recommendations of the child's teachers?
  - What are the educational and career goals of the client or as envisioned by the parents?

### *Assessment of Articulation and Phonological Disorders in Bilingual Children*

- Note that there are very few satisfactorily standardized tests to evaluate articulatory proficiency in bilingual children; a few tests of Spanish language may be available, but for bilingual children who speak an Asian language, standardized tests are even more limited or nonexistent
- Make sure that an available Spanish test of articulation samples the specific variety of Spanish (e.g., Mexican Spanish or Cuban Spanish) the child and the family members speak; very few standardized tests are available that are suitable to all varieties of Spanish spoken in the United States
- Note that English speech sound errors need to be assessed even if no diagnosis of a disorder is made solely on this basis; because the parents and the child may opt for articulation treatment geared toward standard English productions, it is essential to make a thorough analysis of errors in both the languages
- Take extended, representative samples of connected speech in both English and the primary language of a bilingual child; use the general procedures of obtaining a speech and language sample described under Standard/Common Assessment Procedures; note that when one language is more dominant than the other, the samples will differ in their extent
- Use the procedures described under Articulation and Phonological Disorders to structure and evoke speech from the child; however, in selecting stimulus materials to evoke speech, consider the child's family and cultural background; let the parents guide the selection of materials that are familiar to their child; some parents may bring material to the assessment session if prior arrangements are made
- Let the parents interact with the child as you tape record the conversational interaction; assist the parents in manipulating the stimulus materials to evoke a variety of speech productions to sample all speech sounds
- Take a sample of single word productions; use the procedures described under Articulation and Phonological Disorders

### *Assessment of Stimulability of Misarticulated Sounds*

- Select the sounds the child misarticulates in both languages and assess their stimulability
- Use procedures described under Articulation and Phonological Disorders

### *Related Assessment Data*

- Obtain results of intellectual and behavioral assessment if relevant
- Obtain information on academic and language performance and academic demands made on the child

- Obtain information on physical, medical, neurological, and craniofacial abnormalities including cleft palate, malocclusions, and dental deviations
- Obtain information on audiological assessment
- Obtain information on other sensory impairments, if relevant

### *Standard/Common Assessment Procedures*

- Complete the Standard/Common Assessment Procedures with an emphasis on the orofacial examination

### *Scoring and Analysis of Assessment Data*

- Use the procedures described under Articulation and Phonological Disorders
- Take the help of a bilingual speech-language pathologist who knows the child's primary language
- Analyze errors separately in the primary language and the secondary English
- Analyze errors in English that may be a function of the primary language; in this case, the errors are variations and not a basis to diagnose an articulation disorder

### *Diagnostic Criteria*

- Use the following characteristics of Spanish-influenced English in diagnosing articulation and phonological disorders in a child whose primary language is Spanish; note that these characteristics, when they influence the production of English as second language, are not the bases to diagnose an articulation and phonological disorder in English:
  - Unlike English, which has 15, Spanish has only 5 vowels: /i/, /e/, /u/, /o/, and /a/; therefore, a Spanish speaking child may produce the other English vowels in a somewhat variable manner
  - The English consonants /v/, /θ/, /ð/, /z/, /ʤ/, and /ʒ/ are not in Spanish; the nasal /ŋ/ and the liquid /j/ also are absent in Spanish; while speaking English as a second language, some Spanish speaking children may produce those consonants as allophonic variations of phonemes present in Spanish; such productions are not disorders
  - Some Spanish consonants, though similar to certain consonants in English, may be produced differently; for example, the Spanish /s/ may be produced more frontally, giving the impression of a lisp; but this is not to be diagnosed as a disorder
  - Spanish has only a few consonants in word final positions (only /s/, /n/, /r/, /l/, and /d/); consequently, other English consonants in final word positions may be omitted
  - Spanish consonantal clusters are fewer and simpler; the /s/ cluster, most common in English, does not occur in Spanish; final clusters are rare in Spanish; therefore, a Spanish speaking child's English may not contain some of the clusters
  - English /t/, /d/, and /n/ tend to be dentalized, also as an influence of the Spanish language
  - Final consonants may be devoiced (e.g, *dose* for *doze*) as a consequence of the Spanish influence

- /b/ may be substituted for /v/ (e.g., *bery* for *very*)
- Weak or deaspirated stops may give the impression of omission of stop sounds
- /ʧ/ may be substituted for /ʃ/ (e.g., *Chirley* for *Shirley*)
- /d/ or /z/ may be substituted for /ð/, which does not exist in Spanish (e.g., *dis* for *this* or *zat* for *that*)
- Schwa may be inserted before word-initial consonant clusters (*eskate* for *skate* or *espend* for *spend*)
- /r/ may be trapped (as in the English word *butter*) or *trilled*
- Word-initial /h/ may be silent (e.g., *old* for *hold* or *it* for *hit*)
- /y/ may be substituted for /ʤ/, an absent sound in Spanish (e.g., *yulie* for *Julie*)

- In diagnosing articulation and phonological disorders in children whose primary language is an Asian language
  - Use the general guidelines already specified for assessing bilingual children
  - Note that because of the diversity of Asian languages—they belong to different language families with diverse phonological properties—a general description of phonological characteristics is neither practical nor meaningful
  - Note that many descriptions in the literature under the heading of *Asian* children or speakers apply only to Chinese, not to other Asian languages
  - Develop a database of Asian languages spoken in your service area and prepare lists of their phonological characteristics of the kind provided for Spanish in this section
  - Make a diagnosis of articulation and phonological disorders based on such characteristics
- In diagnosing articulation and phonological disorders in children whose primary language is a Native American language
  - Use the general guidelines already specified for assessing bilingual children; ethnocultural considerations in assessment may be less critical in the case of a Native American child who is a monolingual English speaker than in the case of a child whose primary language is a Native American language and English is the second language; still, the ethnocultural variables cannot be ignored in offering clinical services because the family and the immediate social structure and values have to be taken into consideration
  - Ethnocultural variables are important for all these reasons if a Native American child speaks English as a second language and the primary language is one of the Native American languages
  - Regardless of the language status of the child, the parents of a Native American child may want the child assessed for an articulation disorder in standard English; the clinician would then assess only English speech productions if the child is a monolingual English speaker or assess both English and the Native American speech sound productions if the child is a bilingual
  - Note that because of the diversity of Native American languages—they belong to different language families with diverse phonological

properties—a general description of phonological characteristics is neither practical nor meaningful; develop resources on the Native American languages spoken in your service area; local experts, speakers of Native American languages, and various web sites will be helpful

  - Determine first if a Native American child is a bilingual speaker; then follow the guidelines offered in this section; if the child is a monolingual English speaker, especially living in the mainstream society, still pay attention to cultural and family communication patterns but generally follow procedures described under Articulation and Phonological Disorders.

## *Differential Diagnosis*

- Use all the guidelines for differential diagnosis summarized under Articulation and Phonological Disorders
- Note that the most critical task of differential diagnosis is to separate articulatory errors in English from articulatory variations that are caused by the child's primary language; take note of all variations in English; however, diagnose a disorder only if the errors are not due to the phonological patterns of the child's first language
- Differentiate articulatory errors in the primary language in light of the phonological characteristics of that language
- Diagnose articulation errors in English as you typically would if the child is a monolingual English speaker; still consider the family cultural and communication patterns and their purpose in seeking services

## *Prognosis*

- No systematic evidence suggests that prognosis for improved articulation in bilingual children is any different from that in monolingual children
- With systematic and effective treatment, bilingual children with articulation disorders will improve like any other children
- The presence of such additional variables as developmental disabilities, genetic syndromes, and sensory disabilities (e.g., hearing loss) may affect the rate of improvement as they do in any other children

## *Recommendations*

- Recommend treatment for articulation disorders in the first language that are consistent with the phonological patterns of that language
- Recommend treatment for articulatory variations in standard English only if the client or family members request such treatment because of the advantage standard English offers in educational, social, and occupational settings
- Recommend treatment for errors in phonemes that are common to the child's primary language and the secondary standard English on a priority basis
- Refer the child to a bilingual clinician who knows the child's primary language
- See the sources cited at the end of this entry and the two companion volumes: *Hegde's PocketGuide to Communication Disorders* and *Hegde's PocketGuide to Treatment in Speech-Language Pathology* (3rd ed.)

Battle, D. E. (2002). *Communication disorders in multicultural populations* (3rd ed.). Boston, MA: Butterworth-Heinemann.

Genesee, F., Paradis, J., & Crago, M. B. (2004). *Dual language development and disorders*. Baltimore, MD: Paul H. Brookes.

Goldstein, B. A. (2004). *Bilingual language development and disorders in Spanish-English speakers*. Baltimore, MD: Paul H. Brookes.

Kamhi, A. G., Pollack, K. E., & Harris, J. L. (1996). *Communication development and disorders in African American children*. Baltimore, MD: Paul H. Brookes.

Kayser, H. (1995). *Bilingual speech-language pathology: An Hispanic focus*. San Diego, CA: Singular Publishing Group.

Peña-Brooks, A., & Hegde, M. N. (2007). *Assessment and treatment of articulation and phonological disorders in children* (3rd ed.). Austin, TX: Pro-Ed.

Roseberry-McKibbin, C. (2002). *Multicultural students with special language needs* (2nd ed.). Oceanside, CA: Academic Communication Associates.

**Assimilation Processes.** To assess this phonological process, which may be a part of phonological disorders in children, see Articulation and Phonological Disorders.

**Ataxic Dysarthria.** To assess this type of motor speech disorder, see Dysarthria: Specific Types.

**Auditory Agnosia.** To assess difficulty recognizing auditory stimuli, in spite of normal peripheral hearing, see Aphasia with which it is often associated.

**Augmentative and Alternative Communication (AAC).** Assessment of a need for nonverbal modes of communication that either augment limited verbal skills of individuals, or for the most part replace verbal skills, is essential in the case of individuals who have severe oral communication disorders; also to be assessed for AAC potential are the individuals who have an extremely limited capacity to develop and sustain functional oral language skills; modes of augmented or alternative communication may be aided with an external device (e.g., pointing to drawings, or drawing by hand) or unaided, in which the client may communicate without the assistance of external means but may maximize the use of gestures and facial expression; see the sources cited at the end of this entry and the two companion volumes: *Hegde's PocketGuide to Communication Disorders* (for an overview of AAC systems and terms), and *Hegde's PocketGuide to Treatment in Speech-Language Pathology* (3rd ed.) (for intervention approaches).

### *Assessment Objectives/General Guidelines*

- To assess the existing oral speech and language skills and comprehension of spoken language; even in severely impaired individuals who are being considered for an AAC system, an assessment of language production and comprehension skills is essential because the nonverbal means of communication builds on the existing language skills
- To assess whether an individual's oral communication skills are so limited as to require an augmentative or alternative communication system,

whether for a short duration or for an indefinite duration; it is inappropriate to exclude candidacy for AAC because the client is "not ready" for whatever the reason (e.g., a preschool child) or does not need because the handicapping condition may dissipate in a short duration (e.g., as severe form of aphasia)

- To assess the communication needs of the potential AAC user; a need-based assessment tends not to exclude people who were traditionally excluded from AAC services (e.g., people with severe forms of aphasia or apraxia, intellectual impairment, or preschool children)
- To assess what sorts of communication needs are met by the individual's existing communication skills (oral plus nonoral forms) and what communication needs are not met by those existing skills
- To assess what kinds of AAC systems will help meet the unmet communication needs of an individual
- To assess the degree to which an individual with limited oral communication skills participates in communication situations; this *participation model of assessment* includes the following components:
  - An analysis of the degree to which the peers of the student or colleagues of an adult can participate and thus help the individual who uses an AAC system; the peers or colleagues of an AAC system user may themselves need training and support and without their participation, AAC user's efforts to communicate may be unproductive
  - An analysis of the barriers the individual with an AAC system faces that prevent full or possibly maximal participation; barriers may be due to institutional policies (e.g., a school district's policy to exclude children with severe disabilities from regular classrooms); hospital policies may exclude the use of electronic devices that interfere with sensitive medical equipment
  - An analysis of knowledge and skill barriers on the part of individuals who interact with the client who uses an AAC device; lack of technical knowledge and skill in using devices on the part of those who interact with the AAC user will limit participation in communication situations
  - An analysis of dispositions of people who interact with the AAC user; negative dispositions or beliefs on the part of family members, teachers, or health care workers that individuals with severe limitations cannot be effective communicators may be a significant barrier to effective participation
- To assess the educational or occupational demands made on the potential AAC user; whether the child is in a regular or special education class, the structure and support available in the classroom, technical assistance offered, and so forth; whether an adult in an occupational setting is supported by his or her colleagues and supervisors, and the kinds of barriers faced in communication as well as the effective discharge of duties
- To assess the physical capabilities of the potential AAC user; this part of the assessment will include such considerations as limited motoric skills, paresis or paralysis of the limbs, such movement disorders as chorea and tics, and so forth

- To obtain information on the cognitive level of the potential AAC user; this part of the assessment will include obtaining the results of tests of intelligence, assessment of memory, alertness, willingness to learn a new system of communication, and so forth
- To assess the kinds of environmental modifications that have been made and those that still need to be made to better promote full participation of the AAC user in activities and communication situations; modifications may be simple or inexpensive (e.g., a desk at the height of a wheelchair) or may be complex or expensive (remodeling a house or a bathroom for wheelchair access)
- To assess the family constellation and its communication strengths and limitations; this part of the assessment will concentrate on the dispositions of different family members toward the client who uses or needs an AAC system, their support to participate in communication with the individual, the amount of time they spend communicating with the individual, and so forth
- To assess the client's sensory capabilities; this assessment includes an analysis of such limitations as hearing loss, blindness, agnosias, and other sensory deficits that may have an effect on the potential selection of an AAC system
- To assess the overall strengths and limitations of the potential AAC user; this analysis will take into consideration the results of all the previous assessment components, including the unmet communication needs, barriers to participation, cognitive and neuromotor limitations, judged motivation to learn new systems of communication, family and teacher support, support from colleagues and supervisors in occupation settings, and so forth
- To assess candidacy for a particular type of AAC and to assess the cost of AAC device options that may be appropriate for a client; once a particular type of an AAC device has been selected for the individual, the cost of the device needs further assessment; devices can be as inexpensive as a notebook and a pencil that the individual uses regularly or as expensive as a speech synthesizing computer; the goal of assessment is to select the one that is most affordable to the parties involved and yet is capable of meeting the communication needs and promoting optimal participation
- To suggest a particular type of AAC for a client and to make the final recommendation or a set of recommendations

## *Case History/Interview Focus*

- See **Case History** and **Interview** under Standard/Common Assessment Procedures
- Pay special attention to the clients' motor and sensory capabilities that may be needed to use AAC
- During the interview, assess the parents' views about AAC systems, their level of knowledge and acceptance of nonverbal means of communication, family resources to gain access to a system that may be expensive, their

motivation of level of interest in learning to use the system and in supporting the child

### *Ethnocultural Considerations*

- See Ethnocultural Considerations in Assessment
- Consider the special challenges bilingual (e.g., Spanish-English speaking children), bidialectal (Standard American English and African American English), or monolingual non-English speaking children face in using an AAC system
- Assess bilingual children in both languages; this is essential because an assessment for AAC includes an evaluation of existing spoken language skills and comprehension of spoken language; similarly, assessment of bidialectal children should include both variations of English (e.g., mainstream English and African American English)
- Select an appropriate AAC system that contains both languages or dialectal variations, while allowing for code switching
- Assess family communication patterns, literacy, and competence in native language and English or the two dialects of English, beliefs, and values related to communication and augmented or alternative communication; assess the suitability of a potential AAC system in promoting communication between the child and the family members
- Assess family resources and needed support system because the AAC-based rehabilitation can be expensive and tax the family's resources
- Supplement standard assessment with a culturally sensitive assessment tool (e.g., M. B. Huer's the Protocol for Culturally Inclusive Assessment of AAC)

### *Typical AAC Target Population*

- Note that in most diagnostic categories that follow, individuals who are the most severely affected have the greatest need for an AAC system; in some cases, an AAC device may be helpful in the acute stage of the disorder
  - Individuals with aphasia, especially global aphasia and primary progressive aphasia, need an AAC system; some clients in their acute phase of aphasia may use an AAC device until they regain some of their communication skills
  - Adults and children with severe apraxia of speech
  - Individuals with Amyotrophic Lateral Sclerosis; these individuals exhibit Dysarthria, and may be unable to talk (anarthric) in the late stage of the disease and can benefit from an AAC device
  - Clients with Multiple Sclerosis; only a small percentage of people with multiple sclerosis and the resulting dysarthria may need an AAC device
  - Individuals of all ages with autism spectrum disorders
  - Clients with Guillain-Barŕe syndrome who have a depletion of the myelin sheath of the peripheral nerves resulting in paralysis; most of the them recover from their symptoms, but they may benefit from an AAC system while the recovery is in progress; a few who do not recover may need an AAC system on a more permanent basis
  - Some individuals with Parkinson's disease may need a system that augments their natural speech

- Individuals with brainstem stroke that is associated with a severe form of Dysarthria and Anarthria often need an AAC system
- People with the locked-in syndrome, who are fully conscious but are quadriplegic and have no movements except for eye movements need an AAC system
- Children and adults with cerebral palsy, especially those with more severe neuromotor control problems, may benefit from an AAC system
- Individuals who have severe hearing impairment with extremely limited oral speech may opt to use an AAC system, although most deaf adults are competent sign language users who may need oral interpreters only while interacting with hearing people who do not know the sign language
- People with neurodegenerative diseases that result in dementia may need an AAC device and may be able to use one until the final stages of the disease
- Clients who have undergone intubation for various reasons may be unable to orally communicate for a certain duration during which an AAC system will be beneficial; for example, clients who have had an endotracheal tube inserted through the mouth and into the trachea (to sustain air supply to the lungs) may be unable to phonate and articulate speech
- People who have had such surgical procedures as laryngectomy and glossectomy also need an AAC system to communicate
- Individuals who sustained various kinds of orofacial injuries and spinal cord injuries may need an AAC system temporarily or permanently, depending on the degree of recovery from their injuries
- Individuals with tracheostomy, a surgical procedure in which an opening is created in the front part of the neck and into the trachea to sustain air supply to the lungs, cannot speak because the air will not pass through the vocal folds; such individuals will need an AAC system
- Most people with traumatic brain injury, especially if it is severe, may benefit from an AAC, particularly in the initial stage of recovery from the trauma; others with more lasting effects may use a system on a long-term basis or even permanently
- Individuals with intellectual deficits (mental retardation), especially when combined with severe physical disabilities that makes natural speech difficult to produce, need an AAC system

### *Assessment: General Strategies*

- Assess the current communication skills of the client (speech, writing, typing, gestures, any special skills such as sign language); take a speech-language sample and design client-specific procedures (have the client type a passage, use sign language, take a writing sample)
- Assess the current communication demands the client faces; describe all daily communicative activities of the client; document activities in home, school, occupational settings, social settings, and so forth
- Assess how others (family members, teachers, peers, colleagues, supervisors) react with the client: gestures, signs, writing, words, connected speech, a combination of several means

- Assess what problems or barriers that limit interaction between the client and his or her communication partners seem to exist (e.g., poor gesturing or signing skills in family members; poor motor control in the client); assess the client's participation in a variety of communication contexts or situations
- Assess dispositions of significant clients toward communication, the individual with communication disabilities, and new methods that may be appropriate (e.g., family members' negative disposition toward sign language or mechanical instruments; supervisors' negative dispositions toward individuals who need to communicate in unusual ways)
- Assess dispositions of the client to various forms of AAC (e.g., rejection of artificial larynx by a laryngectomy or synthesized speech by a neurologically impaired client); find out the reasons for such dispositions (e.g., a physician's negative comments about electronic larynx)
- Evaluate how well the client and his or her communication partners can learn a new system of communication: their general level of education, sophistication, expressed willingness and enthusiasm, ease with which they understand the information offered, and willingness to put efforts into the venture to make it work
- Evaluate funding sources because those AAC methods involving instruments can be expensive (e.g., personal sources, health insurance, community organizations, government agencies)
- Determine, to the extent possible, the current or maintaining causes of the limited communication skills; take note of the reasons for expressive problems (e.g., paralysis of facial muscles; neurological diseases; laryngectomy; intellectual disabilities, hearing loss, visual problems)
- Assess whether the clinical condition creating the problems is progressive, stable, or temporary
- If and when appropriate, assess Articulation and Phonological Disorders, Language Disorders in Children, Voice Disorders, and Fluency Disorders; assess receptive communication skills; recognize that most of the communication skills will be at the basic level in a potential candidate for AAC
- Note that the final selection of an AAC method or device is a team decision involving the client, family members or other caregivers, educators, physical therapists, psychologists, medical specialists, and social workers
- In consultation with the clients involved, make a preliminary judgment about one or two potential AAC methods or devices that might be useful to the client

### *Use an Assistive Technology—AAC Assessment Tool*

- Several AAC assessment tools, a part of the broader category called assistive technology tools, are available to obtain information during assessment; these tools include questionnaires, printed profiles, software programs, protocols for culturally sensitive assessment, and so forth; one or more of these assessment tools may help complete a comprehensive assessment efficiently; the following alphabetized list samples a few more commonly available tools; use the latest versions of each instrument and find others that may be just as useful; given in parentheses are sources from which the tool may be obtained by visiting their web sites:

- AAC Feature Match (Doug Dodgen and Associates): A computer software program designed to help match the communication needs of school-age to adult AAC users with specific features of systems that may be selected for them
- AAT Assessment Tool (Doug Dodgen and Associates): A computer software program that helps assess the communication needs and strengths, including sensory and motor capabilities of school-age children and adults in need of an adaptive or assistive system
- Assistive Technology Assessment Questionnaire (Tech Connections, Atlanta, GA): Includes printed forms to systematically gather information about a client's AAC needs and strengths; designed to assess adults
- Assistive Technology Predisposition Assessment (Institute for Matching Person and Technology, Inc): A comprehensive assessment battery that includes separate tools to assess consumers' experiences and expectations, help select the right kind of AAC for an individual, relate educational goals and AAC systems, identify workplace variables that are barriers to an AAC system use, and to evaluate barriers to using health care technologies; may be used with adolescents and adults
- Assistive Technology Screener (Technology and Inclusion, Austin, TX): Printed forms that help evaluate the AAC needs of school-age children
- Augmentative Communication Assessment Profile (Speechmark Publishing): To assess the usefulness of a low-technology AAC system that may include manual signs and pointing items on a display system; especially designed for children ages 3–11 who have an autism spectrum disorder
- EvaluWare (Assistive Technology Inc): A computer software program designed to assess the AAC needs, computer-related skills, and the most efficient method of computer access (e.g., the use of a touch screen or keyboard) school-age children can use
- Matching Assistive Technology and Child (Institute for Matching Person and Technology, Inc): To assess the AAC needs of infants and young children and their families; helps identify training needs
- Medicare Funding of AAC Technology Assessment/Application Protocol (posted on the Communication Enhancement Website): To assess the AAC needs of an adult with an acquired communication disorder and to document them to justify Medicare funding
- Needs First (Computer Options for the Exceptional, Inc): A computer software program designed to match school-age children's AAC needs with an AAC device after an assessment has been made through other means
- Protocol for Culturally Inclusive Assessment of AAC (M. B. Huer, in *Journal of Children's Communication Development*, *19*, 1997, 23–34): To assess the AAC needs and use of technological devices by children and families from diverse ethnocultural backgrounds; includes a self-assessment of skills and knowledge of professionals for making a culturally sensitive assessment

## *Assess the Client's Motor Skills*

- Note that the level of motor skills plays the most important role in the use of AAC; hence their assessment is important
- Assess the mobility and dexterity of the hands first because they are the most important for AAC
- Assess the functional integrity of the muscles of the neck and face next
- Assess the functional integrity of the legs and feet last because they are important only when the mobility and dexterity of the hands, neck, and face are extremely limited
- Assess motor skills in a hierarchical fashion: If the client exhibits a higher skill, there is no need to assess lower skills
- Assess movements of the elbow, hand, wrist, fingers, shoulders, head, and neck; assess movements of the jaw, forehead muscles, cheek muscles, eyebrow muscles; assess blinking, eye closing and opening; assess movements of thigh, legs, and feet
- Assess motor skills necessary to gain direct access to an AAC instrument, device, or method: Assess whether the client can operate various kinds of switches, including cursor movements in a hierarchical fashion (e.g., if not with hands, may be with head movement or leg or foot movement); assess skills in pressing, holding, and releasing switches; assess whether the client can wait, can minimize errors, and can be prompt in operating switches
- Assess hand and finger mobility and fine motor skills if a sign language system is being considered
- Take note of difficulties in understanding instructions, need to repeat instructions and suggestions, client's attention span, and apparent speed of learning
- Assess the client's current level of symbolic communication: Select 10 to 15 objects or concepts with which the client is familiar; find a variety of symbols (pictures, photographs, line drawings) that represent them; assess the client's understanding of the symbol (e.g., ask the client to point to a particular symbol or give the symbol to you); ask the client to match the object and its symbol; ask the client to sort symbols (all symbols of houses in one pile and those of dogs in another pile)
- Assess word and letter recognition; present a set of simple printed words that are relevant to the client
- Assess paragraph reading comprehension; use a passage relevant to the client
- Assess spelling skills; use a set of simple words relevant to the client

## *Considerations in Selecting an Unaided (Gestural) AAC System*

- Hand movement flexibility allows for one of the sign languages (ASL or AMER-IND); the family and other regular communication partners need to learn the system; most efficient nonverbal communication; AMER-IND is easier for others to understand
- Movement flexibility of both hands allows for most gestural systems

- Movement flexibility in one hand allows for somewhat limited gestural systems (e.g., Manual Shorthand)
- Some facial and hand movement flexibility will allow for mimes and other organized gestural systems
- Only eyeblink or eyebrow movement capability will allow for eyeblink encoding and/or gestural Morse code; limited communication potential

### *Considerations in Selecting an Aided (Gestural-Assisted) AAC System*

- Pointing gesture capability allows for any symbol set usage, including the use of communication boards
- Limited cognitive functions require concrete symbol sets
- Inability to read or spell requires a system such as Blissymbolics, photographs, and other symbol sets
- Potential for learning to read or the presence of reading skills allows for a combination of printed words and symbol sets
- Limited vision will allow the use of plastic symbols or Braille
- Hand dexterity allows for written communication
- Simplicity, ease of learning to use, and cost to obtain and to run will determine the selection of a switching mechanism
- Portability, editing capability, and need for a printer will determine the selection of an electronic-assisted display device

### *Considerations in Selecting a Neuro-Assisted (Aided) AAC*

- Extremely limited movement capability of extremities dictates the use of neuro-assisted devices
- Slight movement capability of a muscle or muscle group allows for the use of neuro-assisted devices (e.g., eye blink, eyebrow movement, facial muscle movement)

### *Related/Medical Assessment Data*

- Obtain available medical and related reports from the client's physician, orthopedic surgeon, neurologist, and physical therapist, to evaluate the general medical and physical capabilities and limitations of the client
- Obtain psychological assessment reports that indicate the intellectual and cognitive levels of the client, although intellectual levels should not be a basis to exclude children or adults from AAC devices and services
- Obtain educational assessment reports that suggest the strengths, limitations, and needs of the child and the demands the child faces in his or her academic setting
- Obtain information from the occupational settings to understand the strengths, limitations, and needs of the client and the demands the client faces
- Obtain audiologic and ophthalmologic information on the client's hearing and vision

### *Standard/Common Assessment Procedures*

- Complete the Standard/Common Assessment Procedures
- During the interview, gather information on the family's communication patterns, views, and knowledge of AAC devices, disposition to having their

family member use a device, willingness to acquire the skills in using a device, and financial or professional support the family may need

- Examine the case history form closely to gather as specific information as possible on the child's physical and behavioral status, conditions that now warrant the use of an AAC device (e.g., cerebral palsy, intellectual or physical impairments, autism and other serious pervasive developmental disorders, brain injury, neurodegenerative diseases)

### *Analysis of Results and Preliminary Selection of AAC*

- Integrate information obtained from different sources with your data on assessment of the client's AAC needs
- In consultation with the client, the family members, educational specialists, and work setting supervisors, select a form of AAC that best suits the client; the selected AAC system should meet the communication needs and enhance social, academic, and family communication participation
- Finalize the selection only through a period of intervention; note that the initial selection may not work for the client; initial intervention may suggest modifications in the selected strategy or a different strategy
- Get the client, the family, teachers, supervisors, and other relevant persons involved in making modifications or selecting a new device

### *Prognosis*

- Highly variable because the population for which AAC is appropriate is extremely heterogeneous
- Clients usually benefit from a method that has been carefully selected based on a comprehensive assessment of the needs and strengths of both the user and the family; benefits enhanced and sustained with continuous professional support for the user and the family

### *Recommendations*

- A form of AAC that will help meet the communication needs of the client, the family, educational personnel, and people in the work setting; a system that increases communication participation
- Training the client, the family members, educators, peers, or coworkers in making good use of the selected method and in maintaining the instrument selected
- Periodic assessment to ensure continued success or to suggest a different form of AAC
- See the cited sources and the two companion volumes: *Hegde's PocketGuide to Communication Disorders* and *Hegde's PocketGuide to Treatment in Speech-Language Pathology* (3rd ed.)

Beukelman, D. R., & Mirenda, P. (2005). *Augmentative and alternative communication: Supporting children and adults with complex communication needs*. Baltimore, MD: Paul H. Brookes Publishing.

Light, J. C., Beukelman, D. R., & Reichle, J. (2003). *Communicative competence for individuals who use AAC*. Baltimore, MD: Paul H. Brookes.

Silverman, F. H. (1995). *Communication for the speechless* (3rd ed.). Boston, MA: Allyn and Bacon.

**Autism Spectrum Disorders.** Assessment of communication disorders associated with autism spectrum disorders requires an understanding of a multitude of unusual behavioral symptoms that characterize a group of disorders including Asperger's syndrome, autism, Rett syndrome, and childhood degenerative disorder; all these disorders within the spectrum begin in childhood and persist into adulthood; speech-language pathologists are now increasingly called upon to assess and treat children who have autism and Asperger syndrome—the two dominant disorders within the spectrum; generally, procedures used to assess Language Disorders in Children and Articulation and Phonological Disorders are appropriate, but all need to be modified in light of the unique characteristics of the disorders within the spectrum; see the sources cited at the end of this main entry and the two companion volumes: *Hegde's PocketGuide to Communication Disorders* and *Hegde's PocketGuide to Treatment in Speech-Language Pathology* (3rd ed.)

***Asperger's Syndrome (Disorder).*** Assessment of individuals with Asperger's disorder is similar to that of individuals with autism; diagnostic distinctions between the two include language and intellectual skills; individuals with autism have significant impairment in language, but those with Asperger's disorder have good language skills but poor sense of social appropriateness and tact; those with autism may have IQs below normal, whereas those with Asperger's disorder may have near normal or even superior IQs; generally, use the assessment procedures given in greater detail for autism, with the following special considerations:

#### Assessment Objectives/General Guidelines

- To assess communication and behavioral characteristics of individuals with Asperger's syndrome
- To make a differential diagnosis between Asperger's syndrome and autism
- To evaluate the strengths and limitations of the individual with a view to develop a treatment plan for the client and family
- To work with an interdisciplinary team of specialists and contribute to the assessment and treatment of individuals with the disorder

#### Case History/Interview Focus

- Note that unlike children with other genetic syndromes or even some children with autism, those with Asperger's disorder may have no distinguishing physical characteristics
- Ask parents about language acquisition, intellectual skills, and developmental milestones; note that these may be normal
- Interview parents about the early signs of repetitive and stereotyped behaviors, odd social behaviors, and an inability to appreciate the thoughts and feelings of others, in spite of being intellectually capable
- Ascertain whether the child has an intense interest in specific topics (e.g., snakes or train schedules)
- Seek information on the child's interest in social contacts or making friends; note that unlike children with autism, those with Asperger's disorder may try to make friends, but may get rebuffed because of their awkward social behavior

- Ask parents about independent living skills that individuals with Asperger's disorder may attain (in contrast to those with autism)

### Ethnocultural Considerations

- See Ethnocultural Considerations in Assessment
- Use the guidelines offered under Autism, the next subentry

Assessment of Communication Disorders

- Use the additional procedural details given under Autism
- Take a language sample for analysis of phonological, semantic, syntactic, and pragmatic language skills
- During the interview and throughout the assessment period, take note of adequate or superior vocabulary, grammar, and production of varied syntactic structures
- Take note of the most significant diagnostic feature of the disorder: socially inappropriate or completely tactless verbal behavior (e.g., to a clinician's question, "What will you like to be doing when you are a grown-up man?," a child is reported to have replied, "I don't know, but you will be dead then!")
- Ask the individual to talk about his or her special interests; note that the child is eager to talk, but it is not a conversation with you; note that the child talks endlessly and passionately, but it may be a lecture or monologue
- As the individual is speaking on his or her favorite topic, interrupt with your questions, pretend that you don't understand; note that the individual is unlikely to respond appropriately to your questions or requests for clarification
- Give nonverbal cues to indicate that it is time to stop, or that you are bored with the topic; note that the individual is unlikely to respond to such cues
- As the individual is talking, try to interject comments and note that the person is unlikely to yield the floor
- Assess the possibility of a more impaired language in older students and adults with Asperger's disorder
- See Autism for differential diagnosis

*Autism.* Assessment of individuals with autism may be more or less challenging depending on the severity of the disorder; the more severely impaired children show such obvious signs of inappropriate and stereotypic behaviors that the diagnosis is not especially difficult; however, milder forms of autism may be difficult to diagnose and distinguish from children with intellectual disabilities; careful observation and assessment of behavioral and communicative symptoms will reveal important differences; in addition to using relevant procedures described under Language Disorders in Children and Articulation and Phonological Disorders, consider the following in assessing and diagnosing autism.

### Assessment Objectives/General Guidelines

- To assess communication disorders associated with autism and to support a diagnosis of autism with known patterns of communication deficits

- To assess the strengths and limitations of the child because many children with autism may have an uneven profile of deficits and strengths
- To assess the family constellation and support for communication intervention; because the disorder affects every member of the family, it is important to include family members, and their concerns and expectations, in assessing the child
- To suggest components of a treatment or rehabilitation plan that may be integrated into the child's educational and social program or into an adult individual's social and occupational rehabilitation program

## Case History/Interview Focus

- See **Case History** and **Interview** under Standard/Common Assessment Procedures
- During the parent interview, seek information on the early signs of autism; question the parents about lack of interest in the mother's voice, lack of mutual gaze or joint attention, reluctance to be held and cuddled, interest in objects rather than people, and so forth
- Seek information on early signs of intellectual disabilities and delayed attainments of developmental milestones
- Get detailed information on the child's speech and language development; seek information on the onset of speech and language; progression in learning words, phrases, and sentences; appropriateness of the child's language productions; pay special attention to any evidence of echolalia
- Ask the parents to describe the child's play activities; take note of a lack of play activities or bizarre or unusual play activities
- Question the parents about early signs of stereotypic body movements (persistent rocking, fixating on their own bizarre hand movements); excessive preoccupation with a few objects, mechanical noises, and so forth
- Ask the parents whether the child prefers the same physical arrangements in their home and especially in his or her room
- Find out if the parents have observed any self-injurious behaviors
- Ask the parents to describe any special talents and strengths the child may have; seek information on exceptional musical, mathematical, or writing skills in spite of limited language skills or intellectual disabilities
- Find out whether the parents have observed extreme sensitivity to certain kinds of noise or visual stimuli

## Ethnocultural Considerations

- See Ethnocultural Considerations in Assessment
- Seek information from the parents and other family members about their knowledge of autism, and educational and clinical resources available to children with autism and their families
- Gauge the family's strengths and limitations in managing a child whose problem may demand much time, effort, attention, supervision, and cost of rehabilitation
- Informally assess the family's disposition toward the child and the diagnosis and their willingness to seek clinical and educational services

- Select books, toys, and other stimulus materials the child is familiar with and those that are ethnoculturally appropriate

## Assessment of Communication Disorders

- Assess communication disorders
  - Take a Speech and Language Sample (see Standard/Common Assessment Procedures)
  - Use the procedures described under Speech and Language Sample and Language Disorders in Children; however, take note that depending on the severity of autism, the child may not interact verbally; observation of the child's interaction with a parent or family member may yield diagnostic information
  - Assess phonological skills; note that a child with autism is likely to exhibit the same kinds of articulation disorders as the one without autism:
    - During language sampling, take note of the kinds of phonological errors the child produces
    - Record the sample for later analysis
    - Administer a standardized test of articulation
  - Assess semantic difficulties; assess word knowledge and meaning:
    - Assess whether the child has an exceptionally good vocabulary related to a particular topic; ask the child to talk about the topic to make an analysis
    - Do not neglect to give simple commands to see if the child can perform simple and relatively complex actions; even the child with an impressive vocabulary in an area of interest may fail to perform such simple commands as "Stand up" or "Point to the cup;" give progressively complex commands
    - Ask the child to label a set of concrete objects (or pictures of such concrete objects); also ask the child to name relatively abstract pictures (geometric shapes, "good guys" and "bad guys") to assess the relatively better understanding of concrete words; be aware that a few autistic children's specialized vocabulary may be abstract words rather than concrete words
    - Assess whether the child can generalize simple word meanings: see if the child would name vehicles of different shape, size, and color as cars or trucks; see if different toys would all be named as such; see if books of different shape, size, and color would all be named books
    - Assess whether the child would associate words that typically go together to evaluate an understanding of relational meaning; ask the child to match pictures that go together (e.g., pictures of a chair and table, paper and pencil, knife and fork)
    - Assess comprehension of selected proverbs, slang, idioms, and such other abstract forms of language; ask the child to tell what the presented abstract statements mean

- Assess syntactic and morphologic skills
  - Note that some children, especially with higher near-normal intellectual levels, may have few syntactic or morphologic errors; in such cases, more than deficiencies, peculiar usage (idiosyncratic productions) may be the main characteristic
  - Assess deficient syntactic or morphologic skills like you would in any child with language disorders
  - Take note of phrase productions or short, simple sentences that affect prosody and flow of speech
  - Assess word order in sentences and take note of unusual or incorrect word order
  - Take note of pronoun reversal while recording a conversational speech sample; ask the child questions to which the child will have to answer with the pronoun "you" or "your"; (e.g., *I am a teacher; who am I? My name is Maria; what is my name?*); ask questions to which the child will have to answer with "I" or "me"; (e.g., *What are you doing now? If you want this, what do you ask?*); take note of whether the child's echolalia seems to account for pronoun reversals
  - Take written notes on missing grammatical morphemes because the child talks or describes pictures
- Assess pragmatic communication skills
  - Expect to find significant deficits in pragmatic language skills as the impaired social communication and interaction are diagnostic of autism
  - Take note of absent or fleeting eye gaze during conversation
  - Assess the number of times the child initiated a new topic of conversation; the number may be zero or close to it
  - Introduce three or more topics for conversation (e.g., by saying *now let us talk about this here* . . .) and measure the duration for which the child maintained conversation on each of the topics introduced; take note of irrelevant comments, abrupt termination of conversation, introduction of inappropriate topics, and such other disorders of social interaction
  - Assess turn-taking skills during conversation; take note of a failure to take turns when indicated or interrupting to take an inappropriate turn
  - Assess conversational repair skills; make such ambiguous or unclear requests as "Show me the car" when you display two or more toy cars of different colors or, "Point to the man" when you display the pictures of several men, each in a different colored shirt; note the number of times the child asked for clarification; frequently request for clarification with such statements as "What did you say?" "What was that?" "I am not sure of what you just said" and so forth; count the number of times the child modified his or her statements to promote better comprehension

    - Assess social appropriateness of the child's speech, comments, and answers to questions and requests; this is a matter of clinical judgment, but count the number of inappropriate, irrelevant, or offensive comments the child made during the assessment sessions
  - Throughout the assessment period observe and document certain general communication characteristics that are unique to children with autism:
    - Pay special attention to echolalia; observe whether the child echoes your instructions, requests, questions, or picture descriptions; note that some of the echolalic responses may be delayed
    - Document a general lack of interest in communication; note whether child gets engrossed in stimulus materials, toys and other objects, repetitive motor behaviors, and so forth
    - Take note of a lack of interest in any kind of reciprocal interaction including such nonverbal interactions as pat-a-cake
  - Take note of high-pitched and monotonous speech; or a sing-song prosodic feature
  - Judge whether the child speaks with an abnormal pattern of inflections (rising or falling inflection that suggests different kinds of meaning)
- Observe and record nonverbal communication patterns
  - Observe such nonverbal or maladaptive behaviors that may be a means of communication in children with autism
    - Temper tantrums during assessment; ask the child to put together a difficult puzzle to see if the child requests help or throws temper tantrums instead
    - Take note of instances where the child took your hand and led you to the desired objects in the room
    - Assess the frequency of crying, fussing, grunting, and so forth that may indicated that the child needed something
    - Find out whether the child grabs something instead of requesting it
    - Take note of any attempts at kicking, pinching, spitting, biting, and so forth
    - Take note of such destructive actions as throwing things, breaking materials, hitting objects, and so forth
    - Keep an eye on many such maladaptive behaviors, some of which may have a communicative effect
- Observe and record associated problems
  - Although the speech-language pathologist is most concerned with communication deficits and deviations associated with autism, it would be negligent not to observe and record general behavioral characteristics that suggest a diagnosis of autism
  - Take note of any self-injurious behaviors the child may exhibit during the interview (e.g., poking into eyes, biting one's own fingers, hitting his or her head against an object)
  - Observe reluctance to be touched or held; note how the child reacts when you manually guide the child's hand to point to a stimulus picture

  - Record any tendency toward abnormal, stereotypic, and obsessive play; for example, the child may be fixated with a single toy although several are available for play
  - Document stereotypic body movements such as endless rocking
  - Observe perseverative movements, postures, and other motor behaviors

### Standardized Tests

- Consider one of the tests of language listed under Language Disorders in Children
- Consider one of the tests of articulation described under Articulation and Phonological Disorders

### Related/Medical Assessment Data

- Obtain medical reports of relevance, especially a neurological report
- Obtain psychological reports, to rule out significant intellectual impairments that need to be considered in treatment planning
- Obtain audiological reports to rule out hearing impairment that needs to be considered in communication treatment planning
- Obtain reports from teachers and special educators for the results of their assessment and recommendations

### Standard/Common Assessment Procedures

- Complete the Standard/Common Assessment Procedures
- Conduct a thorough orofacial examination to rule out potential craniofacial anomalies

### Analysis of Results

- Make an analysis of the speech and language sample as described under Language Disorders in Children and Articulation and Phonological Disorders
- Analyze the unique features of autism noted during the assessment and as evidenced in the speech and language sample
- Integrate the information from different sources
- Relate communication disorders that suggest autism with the behavioral analysis and diagnosis
- Summarize the observed speech and language characteristics that might support the diagnosis of autism

### Diagnostic Criteria

- An independent diagnosis of autism supported by behavioral assessment or psychiatric evaluation is important
- A pattern of communication disorders that is supportive of the diagnosis
- Early signs of autistic behaviors as revealed by the case history and parent interview
- Significant disinterest in people and communication and a preoccupation with objects and stereotypical behaviors

### Differential Diagnosis

- Differentiate autism from intellectual disabilities, even such disabilities that may be found in several children with autism: the unique characteristics of autism that distinguish it from intellectual disabilities (mental retardation) include a lack of interest in people, feelings, affection, and communication; preoccupation with routines; interest in objects versus people; and some unusual language including pronoun reversal, wrong word order, and echolalia—all uncharacteristic of children with intellectual disabilities

- Differentiate autism from Asperger's Syndrome; children with Asperger's syndrome often have better language skills and normal or even superior intellectual levels compared to those with autism; their main characteristic is tactless social behavior, but children with Asperger's syndrome are eager to talk, talk a lot on a topic of their interest, and are unaware of listener's indifference or lack of interest in what they say
- Differentiate autism from hearing impairment: children with hearing impairment do not exhibit unusual and stereotypic verbal or nonverbal behaviors; clients with hearing impairment have an independent audiological diagnosis; speech and voice characteristics associated with hearing impairment also help distinguish the two types of disorders
- Differentiate children with autism from those with brain injury: children with brain injury may occasionally make inappropriate statements; may have difficulty concentrating on the task at hand, may be mute or severely impaired in their expressive speech; but a clear history and medical evidence of recent brain injury will be absent in children with autism; other physical evidence of paralysis or paresis, altered states of consciousness, and neurological signs of brain injury also may be absent in children with autism

### Prognosis

- Variable depending on the severity of autistic behaviors; children without severe intellectual disabilities who receive early and intensive behavioral treatment are known to improve enough to be mainstreamed in schools
- Most, if not all, children benefit from behavioral and communication intervention; but the intervention needs to be intensive and long-term

### Recommendations

- Early intervention for communication deficits
- Coordination of treatment with general behavioral intervention
- Family counseling and training for home treatment
- Coordination of treatment with academic programs in the case of school-age children
- See the cited sources and the two companion volumes: *Hegde's Pocket-Guide to Communication Disorders* and *Hegde's PocketGuide to Treatment in Speech-Language Pathology* (3rd ed.)

***Childhood Disintegrative Disorder (CDD).*** Assessment and diagnosis of this variety of pervasive developmental disorder depend on the observation of at least 2 years of normal development that precedes its onset; assessment concern is to document a significant regression in behavior of a child who was developing normally; regression should be evident after age 2 and before age

10 to diagnose this disorder; use the general procedures described under Autism, Language Disorders in Children, and Articulation and Phonological Disorders to make a complete analysis of communication deficits associated with CDD; take note of the following special features:

### Assessment Objectives/General Guidelines

- To document regression in behavior after age 2 and before age 10
- To assess communication skills and behavior characteristics and to take note of physical characteristics of the disorder
- To work with an interdisciplinary team to make a thorough assessment that will help generate a treatment and rehabilitation plan for the child and the family
- To make a differential diagnosis of the disorder

#### *Case History/Interview Focus*

- Take a detailed case history from the parents to document a relatively abrupt or insidious loss of skills, loss of voluntary hand skills, impaired gait or trunk movements, often occurring between the age of 5 and 30 months, and seizure disorders
- Ask parents about and observe stereotyped hand movements (e.g., hand-wringing and hand washing)
- Notice a loss of interest in social interactions as you interview the child and seek information from the parents on the child's social development and loss of play activities
- Seek information on the child's stereotypical and restricted activities, interests, and movements
- Ask the parents about the child's loss of bowel or bladder control

#### *Assessment of Communication and Behavior Deficits*

- Observe and record poor motor coordination and lack of interest in play materials as you show such materials to the child
- Take a speech and language sample to assess oral communication skills and note severe speech and language impairments
- Assess both language production and comprehension; note that both may be severely affected
- Obtain a psychologist's report on intellectual deficits and relate language disorders to such deficits
- Document, through case history and interview, improvement in skills as the child grows older, but none remarkable
- Conduct repeated assessments to record progressive deterioration, especially if a neurological disorder is also present
- Assess similarities between the established total symptom complex associated with CDD and that of autism; note that the two may be indistinguishable

#### *Differential Diagnosis*

- To differentially diagnose CDD, document normal development during the early childhood years, up to age 2
- Document deterioration in skills after age 2 and before age 10
- See Autism and Rett Syndrome for additional diagnostic information

***Rett Syndrome (Disorder).*** Assessment of this progressive neurodevelopmental disorder, considered a part of autism spectrum disorder or pervasive developmental disorder, requires the assessment of intellectual functions because the disorder is a common cause of profound intellectual disabilities in girls; development is typically normal until the age of 6 to 18 months; affected children begin to show speech impairment and the inability to purposefully use their hands; other symptoms soon follow; see also Asperger's Syndrome, Autism, and Childhood Disintegrative Disorder, all considered pervasive developmental disorders.

### Assessment Objectives/General Guidelines

- To assess autistic-like behaviors in the early stage of the disorder and the more prominent physical symptoms in older individuals
- To help make a differential diagnosis of Rett disorder, autism, or Asperger's disorder
- To work with the interdisciplinary team to make a comprehensive assessment that will help generate a treatment and rehabilitation plan for the individual and a support plan for the family

### Case History/Interview Focus

- Interview the parents about the physical growth of the child; question about decelerated head growth, resulting in microcephaly; observe and record this craniofacial anomaly
- Ask the parents about neuromotor disturbances including reduced muscle tone, gait disturbances, ataxia, spasticity, seizure disorders, and tremors and dystonia; observe and record these impairments during assessment
- Ask the parents to describe unusual behaviors of the child; these may include wringing hand movements, clapping, and mouthing; observe and record these behaviors during assessment
- Seek information on early language development; find out the time when they noticed arrested development
- Obtain information on such breathing abnormalities as hyperventilation and apnea

### Assessment of Communication Disorders

- Generally, follow the procedures described under Autism
- Assess or ascertain through the parental interview an initial lack of interest in social interactions (similar to children with autism)
- Seek evidence of regression of language skills
- Obtain reports from a psychologist to document intellectual disabilities

### Differential Diagnosis

- Differentiate the childhood disintegrative disorder from Rett syndrome and autism
- Distinguish childhood disintegrative disorder by its absence in boys, initial normal development but regression in skills after the onset of the disorder, and characteristic neuromotor problems
- See Autism and Rett Syndrome for additional information

American Psychiatric Association. (1994). *Diagnostic and statistical manual of mental disorders* (4th ed.). Washington, DC: Author.

Hegde, M. N., & Maul, C. A. (2006). *Language disorders in children: An evidence-based approach to assessment and treatment.* Boston, MA: Allyn and Bacon.

Neisworth, J. T., & Wolfe, P. S. (2004). *The autism encyclopedia.* Baltimore, MD: Paul H. Brookes.

Nelson, N. W. (1998). *Childhood language disorders in context* (2nd ed.). New York: Macmillan.

Paul, R. (2001). *Language disorders from infancy through adolescence: Assessment and intervention* (2nd ed.). St. Louis, MO: Mosby.

Reed, V. (2005). *An introduction to children with language disorders* (3rd ed.). Boston, MA: Allyn and Bacon.

Weatherby, A. M., & Prizant, B. M. (2000). *Autism spectrum disorders.* Baltimore, MD: Paul H. Brookes.

# B

**B-Mode Carotid Imaging.** A noninvasive neurodiagnostic method to assess the health of the superficial arteries, especially those of the neck; also known as *echo arteriogram*; similar to ultrasound imaging of the fetus; in this procedure:
- A high frequency sound generator is placed over the neck
- A computer analyzes the sound deflected by the arteries and reconstructs the images of the arteries
- Such arterial diseases as stenosis or ulceration may be revealed

**Bardet-Biedl Syndrome.** To assess this syndrome, also known as the Laurence-Moon syndrome, see Syndromes Associated With Communication Disorders.

**Binswanger Disease.** To assess this neurodegenerative disease associated with a form of dementia, see Vascular Dementia.

**Bound Morphemes.** Assessment of grammatical morphemes is essential to diagnose language delay or disorder in younger or older children; impaired production of grammatical morphemes that do not convey much meaning by themselves and are usually combined with other morphemes (hence the term "bound morphemes") is an essential diagnostic feature of language disorders; bound morphemes are not whole words, but elements that are inflected with words; clients with aphasia also may omit bound morphemes, resulting in telegraphic speech; to assess the common bound morphemes:
- Tape record an extended language sample
- Manipulate the stimulus items during language sampling to give the child opportunities to produce the bound morphemes; for instance:
  - Show single and multiple objects and ask such questions as "What do you see?' or "What are these?" to evoke the regular plural inflections (s, z, əz)
  - Show pictures that depict actions and ask the child such questions as "What is he doing? or "What is she doing" to evoke the present progressive *ing*
  - Show pictures that depict actions or perform an action (e.g., touch your nose, open a book) and ask the child either what had happened in the picture or what you just did to evoke past tense inflections (*t*, as in *walked*, *d* as in *opened*, *ted* as in *painted*, and *ded* as in *loaded*)
  - Show pictures of people who possess objects and ask such questions as "Whose hat is it?" or "Whose toy is it?" to evoke the production of the possessive morpheme; sample all allomorphic variations (possessive *s*, as in *cat's*, *z* as in *boy's*, and *əz* as in *mouse's*)
- Use the sentence completion format as an alternative to asking questions to evoke bound morphemes; for instance, say, "He painted yesterday. What did he do yesterday? Yesterday he . . ." and let the child finish the sentence
- Evoke the production of each morpheme multiple times to calculate the percent correct production of each bound morpheme

**Brachman-de Lange Syndrome.** To assess this syndrome, also known as the Cornelia de Lange syndrome, see Syndromes Associated With Communication Disorders.

**Broca's Aphasia.** To assess this variety of nonfluent aphasia due to damage to Broca's area or surrounding areas, see Aphasia and Aphasia: Specific Types.

C

C

**Carotid Phonoangiography.** A noninvasive neurodiagnostic method to assess the health of the blood vessels by recording and analyzing the sound of blood flow; in this procedure:

- A scanning machine picks up and amplifies the sound of the blood gushing through the arteries
- The machine analyzes the properties of sounds it records to help diagnose arterial stenosis, which creates turbulence as the blood moves through a constricted artery.

**Case History.** A standard assessment procedure; includes chronological information on the onset, development, and progression of a disease; also includes information on the client's general health, development, and academic or occupational information; see Standard/Common Assessment Procedures for obtaining a detailed case history before making an assessment; see specific disorders for unique features that must be considered in taking case histories.

**Cerebellar Mutism.** To assess this form of transient mutism, often found in children who have had their posterior fossa tumors removed surgically, see Mutism.

**Cerebral Angiography.** An invasive, radiographic diagnostic procedure to evaluate the health of the vascular system, often that of the carotid artery; in this procedure:

- A catheter is inserted into a femoral artery in the groin, moving it upward into the selected artery (often, the ceratoid or vertebral artery)
- A radio-opaque contrast material is injected through the catheter
- A rapid series of X-rays is then taken of the artery or arteries to reveal variations in blood flow that might suggest vascular occlusions.

**Cerebral Palsy (CP).** Assessment of a group of congenital and nonprogressive neuromotor disorders found in children and older individuals requires an understanding of neurological impairments and their consequences for speech production; the disorder is the result of damage to a child's brain before, during, or shortly after the birth. See the companion volume, *Hegde's PocketGuide to Communication Disorders*, for details on epidemiology, symptoms, and etiological factors.

### *Assessment Objectives/General Guidelines*

- To assess the communication deficits associated with CP
- To note neuromotor problems associated with the communication disorders during assessment
- To assess the strengths of the child and the educational demands made on the child
- To assess the occupational consequences of dysarthria associated with CP in adolescents and adults
- To work closely with other professionals involved in the rehabilitation of the child with CP, because the assessment (and treatment) of children with CP is a team effort involving special education specialists, educational psychologists, and medical and related specialists (e.g., pediatrician, orthopedic surgeon, neurologist, physical therapist, occupational therapist)

- To help develop a rehabilitation program for the child and to identify family support needs
- To help coordinate the services of many professionals whose expertise is needed to help children and adults with CP
- To plan a schedule of periodic assessment of the child with CP, as most children will need long-term care
- To adapt testing and assessment procedures when necessary to suit the child's needs and physical limitations (e.g., let the child look at a stimulus instead of pointing to it; nod or shake the head instead of a verbal response; let the child tap the table instead of clapping hands)

### *Case History/Interview Focus*

- See **Case History** and **Interview** under Standard/Common Assessment Procedures
- Obtain detailed information on prenatal, perinatal, and postnatal conditions that are associated with CP in children
- Seek information on early feeding and swallowing difficulties and any history of nonoral feeding that may have been necessary
- Seek details on the child's physical development, social behavior, and speech-language development; obtain information on the degree of independence or dependence in self-care
- Ask questions about the child's academic performance, difficulties the child may have in the classroom
- Let the parents list skills the child performs well or adequately
- Explore the family's strengths and needs in meeting the child's long-term and often expensive needs related to special educational and medical rehabilitation

### *Ethnocultural Considerations*

- See Ethnocultural Considerations in Assessment
- With families that belong to ethnocultural minorities, explore the need for resources and support systems
- Assess the family members' disposition toward physical limitations and rehabilitation efforts

### *Assessment*

- Observe and obtain information on neuromotor functions
  - Obtain reports from the child's physician or neurologist on the child's physical and neuromuscular status
  - Take note of the neuromuscular disorders you observe during assessment, especially the more common plasticity and rigidity of muscles; observe any sign of athetosis (slow, involuntary, writhing movements); symptoms of ataxia (impaired balance); tremors (involuntary, repetitive, rapid, and rhythmic movements); and paralysis of one or more limbs
- Observe and obtain information on motor development
  - Use a developmental scale or checklist to assess the child's motor and general behavioral development
  - Obtain systematic information from the parents

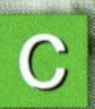


- Obtain information on the child's intellectual and academic status
    - Obtain information or assessment results from educational psychologists
    - Get reports from special education specialists
    - Make clinical judgments based on your assessment of speech and language development
- Assess speech disorders and speech intelligibility
    - Take an extended Speech and Language Sample (see Standard/Common Assessment Procedures)
    - Obtain a speech sample involving the child and the parent or another family member
    - Make clinical judgments about speech intelligibility for single words and sentences and with and without contextual cues; make a more detailed analysis of articulation skills when intelligibility is reduced
    - Take into consideration any oral structural deviations (e.g., tongue weakness, asymmetries in the tongue and soft palate, abnormalities of the jaw, unusually high palate, malocclusions)
    - Take into consideration functional oral-motor problems (e.g., oral apraxia, lateral tongue deviations, sluggish movement of the tongue; uncontrolled movements of facial muscles, chewing, sucking, and swallowing problems)
    - Analyze the speech samples for individual sound errors and for patterns of errors suggesting phonological processes (e.g., final consonant deletion, cluster reduction, fronting); use procedures described under Articulation and Phonological Disorders; pay special attention to dysarthric speech characteristics associated with CP
        - Take note of possibly greater articulatory breakdowns on longer words or words with phonetically more complex sequences
        - Compare the accuracy levels of labial versus glottal sounds; nasals versus fricatives; voiced sounds versus voiceless sounds
        - Take note of articulatory movement disorders associated with dysarthric speech (e.g., deviations in tongue and jaw movements; reduced range of articulatory movements; jerky, effortful, and labored movements)
        - Observe irregular articulatory breakdowns, prolonged sound productions, and inappropriate periods of silence during continuous speech
- Assess language disorders
    - Use the recorded speech and language sample to analyze the child's language skills
    - Take note of the language structures the child produces and those the child does not
    - Use the procedures described under Language Disorders in Children
    - Analyze the language problems in light of other complicating problems that may be present, including hearing impairment and intellectual disabilities
    - Take note of syntactic, morphological, and pragmatic deficiencies; these deficiencies are likely to be similar to those found in other children with language disorders
- Assess fluency problems
    - Use the recorded speech and language sample to make a clinical judgment about the presence or absence of a fluency disorder

- If warranted, make a more detailed analysis of the types and frequency of dysfluencies
- Use the procedures described under Stuttering for procedures, analysis, and diagnostic criteria

- Assess prosodic problems
  - Take note of misplaced stress patterns, lack of intonation, irregular rate of speech, and inappropriate pauses during speech
  - Assess the length of utterances to document short phrases
  - Make clinical judgments about overall prosodic features
- Assess voice and respiratory problems
  - Make clinical judgments about vocal loudness and pitch and their social adequacy and appropriateness for age and gender of the client; judge whether the voice is weak and soft
  - Judge whether variations in loudness and pitch are smooth and normal or jerky and abnormal; take note of any irregular bursts in loudness
  - Take note of voice quality (harshness, hoarseness, breathiness, strained-strangled voice)
  - Take note of any difficulty in voicing that may be due to vocal folds that are either too tightly adducted or remain abducted for too long; document brief periods of aphonia, breathiness, and delayed voice onset
  - Judge the adequacy of breath support for speech
  - Take note of the listed breathing abnormalities; see Make an Aerodynamic Evaluation under Voice Disorders for additional procedures used in assessing respiratory functions
  - Use the assessment procedures described under Voice Disorders including the use of instrumental assessment of voice characteristics
- Assess resonance problems
  - Observe the presence of hypernasality, hyponasality, generally reduced oral resonance, and nasal emission
  - Consider the resonance data along with information on velopharyngeal functioning
  - Use the assessment procedures described under Voice Disorders including the use of instrumental assessment of nasal resonance
- Assess oromotor dysfunctions
  - Complete a detailed orofacial examination; see Standard/Common Assessment Procedures
  - Pay special attention to orofacial muscle weakness or paralysis
- Assess swallowing disorders
  - Take note of early feeding, sucking, and swallowing disorders and current drooling
  - If a swallowing disorder is present according to the parental reports, assess swallowing problems or make a referral to a speech-language pathologist who is a specialist in pediatric swallowing disorders
- Assess the need for augmentative and alternative methods of communication
  - Assess the child's oral communication potential; if low, assess potential for a variety of alternative and augmentative communication devices the child might use

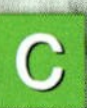

  - See Augmentative and Alternative Communication (AAC) for assessment methods and selection of an appropriate means of communication
- Observe and obtain information on other areas
  - Observe perceptual and attentional problems; obtain the psychological report
  - Observe the child's emotional responses during assessment; obtain parent's report on the child's emotional stability and reactivity
  - Obtain information from teachers and parents on the child's educational performance and problems
  - Screen hearing; refer the child to an audiologist when warranted; if already assessed, get an audiological report
  - Obtain information on the child's visual problems
  - Obtain information from the child's physical therapist

### Related/Medical Assessment Data

- Obtain reports from other specialists as indicated in earlier sections
- Integrate your assessment data with those offered in the various reports obtained

### Standard/Common Assessment Procedures

- Complete the Standard/Common Assessment Procedures
- Pay special attention to the orofacial examination

### Analysis of Assessment Data

- Analyze the speech and language sample as needed to identify language and speech disorders; use the procedures described under Language Disorders in Children and Articulation and Phonological Disorders; list language and speech disorders of the child including the characteristics of dysarthria found in the child
- Analyze data relative to voice, resonance, and breathing abnormalities and list the disorders or deviations
- Analyze data relative to fluency and prosody and summarize the problems noted; calculate the percent dysfluency rate; see Stuttering for procedures
- Integrate data from other professional sources and summarize the overall strengths and weaknesses

### Diagnostic Criteria

- History consistent with damage to a developing brain
- Neuromotor symptoms, behavioral patterns, and communication problems (especially dysarthria) consistent with damage to a developing brain

### Prognosis

- The typical course of CP is highly variable depending on the severity of neuromotor involvement and associated sensory, perceptual, and intellectual deficits
- Typically, children with CP improve because it is not a degenerative disorder
- Generally, prognosis for improved functioning with systematic and comprehensive rehabilitation is good for most if not all children with CP
- Prognosis for improved oral or augmentative and alternative communication is favorable for most if not all children with CP

### *Recommendations*

- Communication treatment as a part of a comprehensive rehabilitation program
- See the cited sources and the two companion volumes, *Hegde's Pocket-Guide to Communication Disorders* and *Hegde's PocketGuide to Treatment in Speech-Language Pathology* (3rd ed.)

Hardy, J. C. (1983). *Cerebral palsy*. Englewood Cliffs, NJ: Prentice Hall.

Love, R. J. (2000). *Childhood motor disability* (2nd ed.). New York: Macmillan.

Mecham, M. J. (1996). *Cerebral palsy* (2nd ed.). Austin, TX: Pro-Ed.

Yorkston, K. M., Beukelman, D. R., & Bell, K. R. (1999). *Management of motor speech disorders in children and adults* (2nd ed.). Austin, TX: Pro-Ed.

**Cerebrovascular Accidents (Strokes).** To assess the interruption of blood supply to a part of the brain or bleeding in the brain that causes neurological and communication problems, see Aphasia.

**Childhood Apraxia of Speech (CAS).** Assessment of childhood apraxia of speech requires an understanding of motor planning and programming concepts; also known as developmental *apraxia of speech* or *developmental verbal apraxia; childhood apraxia of speech*, the term that is gaining currency, is difficulty in positioning and sequentially moving muscles for the volitional production of speech in the absence of muscle weakness or paralysis; may be severe in some cases, resulting in unintelligible speech; presumed to be a disorder of motor programming for speech; unlike in Apraxia of Speech (AOS) in Adults, there usually is no demonstrated neuropathology, hence controversial; see the cited sources at the end of this entry and *Hegde's PocketGuide to Communication Disorders* for details on epidemiology, etiology, and symptomatology.

### *Assessment Objectives/General Guidelines*

- To assess the child's speech production skills
- To evaluate or rate the child's speech intelligibility
- To assess other aspects of communication, including prosodic features, language skills, voice characteristics, and fluency
- To assess oral apraxia (independent of speech)
- To describe the nature of a child's speech production problems
- To make a diagnosis of CAS
- To rate or evaluate the severity of CAS
- To identify the child's strengths and limitations
- To assess prognosis for improvement with speech treatment or rehabilitation with augmentative or alternative means of rehabilitation
- To help develop a treatment plan for the child, including any augmentative and alternative forms of communication if the severity of apraxia warrants
- To identify initial treatment targets

### *Case History/Interview Focus*

- See **Case History** and **Interview** under Standard/Common Assessment Procedures

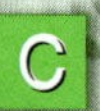


- Make a thorough orofacial examination to rule out the presence of any neuromuscular weakness or paralysis of any speech muscles that would also rule out apraxia; the problem may be one of dysarthria
- During the interview, concentrate on any potential factors that may be related to brain injury in the child
- Obtain detailed information on the academic consequences of apraxia, especially a severe one
- Ask the parents about any familial incidence of apraxia of speech in children or adults because the familial incidence is higher than that in the general population; in case of children with apraxia of speech, the mother is more likely to be affected than the father

### Ethnocultural Considerations

- See Ethnocultural Considerations in Assessment
- Although ethnocultural information specific to childhood apraxia of speech is limited, question parents about familial incidence
- Pay attention to the family's resources and support the family may need because treatment in cases of severe apraxia of speech is long term and expensive

### Assessment

- Assess nonimitative speech production skills
  - Obtain a speech and language sample of 75 to 100 utterances; see Speech and Language Sampling under Standard/Common Assessment Procedures
  - Record nonimitative (evoked) production of a set of single words that sample all phonemes; a standardized test of articulation may be appropriate
  - Use object or picture naming and description tasks to evoke nonimitative productions; select age-appropriate and ethnoculturally meaningful stimulus materials; during this part of the assessment:
    - Initially evoke productions of shorter words
    - Ask the child to produce progressively longer words (e.g., *love, loving, lovingly*)
    - Ask the child to describe the pictures; instruct the child to "Say more," "Say it in a sentence," or "Say it in a real long sentence"
  - Observe and record signs of speech motor programming problems
    - Take note of articulatory groping in an effort to produce the target sounds or words
    - Record the frequency of silent articulatory postures
    - Take note of dysfluencies as the child makes frequent attempts to produce the target sound or the word
  - Observe and record speech production problems as the length of words increases; take notes during assessment
  - Use stimulus materials described under the main entry, Apraxia of Speech (AOS) in Adults; modify the materials to suit the child or use parallel stimulus items selected from the child's vocabulary
  - Phonetically transcribe the utterances and speech sound errors

- Assess imitative speech production skills
  - Assess the accuracy with which the child can produce imitative speech:
    - Model individual sounds and syllables and ask the child to imitate their productions
    - Initially, hide your oral movements to see whether the visual cues are essential or not for correct or attempted imitation
    - If the child cannot imitate, show the normal articulatory movements
    - Model a series of shorter and longer words and ask the child to imitate
    - Model shorter and longer sentences and ask the child to imitate
- Assess consistency and variability of articulatory errors
  - Sample speech productions in varied phonetic contexts
  - Sample speech production at different complexity levels
  - Sample speech production in imitative and spontaneous modes
  - Sample production of the same phoneme (in the same word) in multiple trials
- Assess any unusual errors of articulation
  - Note that such unusual errors of articulation help distinguish childhood apraxia of speech from articulation and phonological errors without a suspected motor planning and programming deficit
    - Assess metathetic errors, which are the transposition of sounds or reversal of phoneme sequences (e.g., *maks* for *masks* or *soun* for *snow*); uncommon in children without apraxia of speech
    - Assess phonemic additions (e.g., *applesacks* for *applesauce* or *clat* for *cat*)
    - Prolongation of speech sounds
    - Repetition of even the final sounds and syllables in words
    - Nonphonemic productions that cannot be transcribed
- Assess other kinds of articulation errors
  - Note that to some extent these errors also may be found in children with articulation and phonological disorders with no evidence of motor control problems
    - Omissions and distortions of speech sounds that may be more frequent than other kinds of articulation errors
    - Distortions that are more frequent than other kinds of errors in a few older students
    - Varied patterns of simplification of consonantal blends (e.g., omission of a sound or a substitution of a sound)
    - Errors of voicing unvoiced sounds and unvoicing voiced sounds
    - Distorted vowels and reduction of diphthongs
- Assess intelligibility of speech
  - Assess intelligibility with already collected assessment data
    - Assess intelligibility at different topographic levels including syllables, words, phrases, and sentences
    - Rate intelligibility on a 5- or 7-point rating scale if desired
    - Note that severity of CAS may range from mild to severe; such judgments are often subjective, even with rating scales

- Assess language production and comprehension skills
  - Use the recorded conversational speech sample to diagnose a language disorder in addition to the speech disorder; if there is a language disorder, the characteristics are likely to be similar to such a disorder in other children with no apraxic features; see Language Disorder in Children for assessment procedures
  - Ascertain from the case history whether the child's language development has been delayed, as it is in some children with apraxia of speech
  - In the case of very young children, estimate the size of the vocabulary from parental reports
  - Assess language comprehension by giving increasingly complex verbal commands to be followed by the child; note the number of correct and incorrect responses given to commands
  - Ask the child to narrate a story; record the child's narration
  - Tell a story and ask the child to retell it; record the child story retelling
- Assess resonance problems
  - Assess hypernasality, hyponasality, and nasal emission by clinical judgment
  - Use a nasal mirror to judge nasal emission in the production of nonnasal sounds
  - Visually inspect the velopharyngeal mechanism as a part of the orofacial examination
  - When found necessary or feasible, use mechanical instruments to diagnose resonance problems (see Instruments for Resonance Assessment)
- Assess prosodic problems
  - Prosodic problems may be significant in children with apraxia of speech; such problems may help distinguish children with usual articulation and phonological disorders
    - Take note of any flat speech prosody (monotonous speech quality)
    - Evaluate the appropriateness of pitch and loudness variations; they may be unpredictable
    - Clinically evaluate the linguistic stress patterns that may be abnormal
- Assess fluency and dysfluencies
  - Count the frequency of each dysfluency type exhibited in the speech sample
  - Count the frequency of each dysfluency type exhibited in an oral reading sample
- Assess literacy skills
  - Tape-record a reading sample
  - Obtain a handwriting sample to assess general handwriting skills
  - Give a brief and simple spelling test to assess the spelling errors
  - Test printing and alphabet recognition in the case of preschoolers to assess preliteracy skills
- Observe any associated conditions that the child may exhibit
  - Screen hearing and make a referral to an audiologists if the screening results warrant it
  - Observe any signs of intellectual impairment
  - Observe and record any signs of ataxic CP and generalized hypotonia
  - Note any signs of attention deficit disorders or hyperactivity

## Standardized Tests

- Administer selected tests of articulation described under Articulation and Phonological Disorders to sample speech sound productions
- Consider administering the most recent edition of one of the specialized tests for childhood apraxia of speech or general measures of apraxia
  - *The Apraxia Profile* by L. Hickman
  - *The Kaufman Speech Praxis Test for Children* by N. Kaufman
  - *The Screening Test for Developmental Apraxia for Speech* by R. Blakely
  - *The Test of Oral and Limb Apraxia* by N. Helm-Estabrooks

## Medical, Psychological, and Educational Assessment Data

- Obtain any available medical data including the results of brain imaging techniques or neurological examinations
- Obtain psychological data including the results of intelligence testing and cognitive functioning
- Obtain data on the child's educational achievement and assessment that might suggest learning disabilities

## Standard/Common Assessment Procedures

- Complete the Standard/Common Assessment Procedures
- Pay special attention to the orofacial examination to rule out muscle weakness or paralysis and to find any evidence of nonoral apraxia

## Analysis of Assessment Data

- Analyze the assessment data
- Analyze the language samples and summarize the morphological, semantic, syntactic, and pragmatic problems noted
- Analyze and summarize the reading, writing, and other literacy skill levels
- Summarize the orofacial examination data
- Calculate the percent dysfluency rate based on the number of words spoken or read orally
- Describe groping, struggle, and related articulatory problems
- Analyze the phonetically transcribed nonimitative word productions and describe the kinds of articulatory and sequencing errors exhibited; identify the locus of breakdown (e.g., syllables, monosyllabic words, and multisyllabic words)
- Analyze and summarize the kinds of errors noted on imitative speech tasks
- Analyze and summarize consistency and variability in error patterns
- Calculate the percentage of spoken or orally read words that are intelligible
- Determine the presence or absence of resonance problems
- Analyze and summarize the noted prosodic problems
- Take into account medical, psychological, and educational assessment data
- Make a summary statement

## Diagnostic Criteria

- Deficiency in sequenced speech movements that are not attributable to other factors, especially to peripheral neuromuscular disorders or deficiencies
- Demonstrated problems of speech intelligibility associated with articulatory breakdowns are essential to diagnosing childhood apraxia of speech

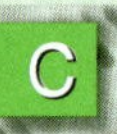

- Prosodic problems that distinguish articulatory breakdowns also are diagnostic features of childhood apraxia of speech versus articulation disorders not associated with presumed motor planning and programming deficits
- Articulatory groping and other characteristics of disordered speech motor control also are essential diagnostic features

## *Differential Diagnosis*

- Distinguish CAS from functional articulation disorder by applying the diagnostic criteria
- Rule out paralysis, paresis, and weakness of the speech production mechanism
- When such other problems as sensory or intellectual impairments are documented in children who otherwise qualify for the diagnosis of apraxia of speech, consider them as coexisting problems

## *Prognosis*

- Generally, more treatment time and effort are needed to produce significant changes; several years of treatment may be needed in many cases
- In cases of severe apraxia of speech, some errors may persist in spite of best clinical efforts
- Intensive and competent treatment can produce functionally adequate speech in many children; expectation of normal speech may be unrealistic in children with severe apraxia of speech
- Augmentative and alternative communication may be needed in cases of children with extremely severe apraxia of speech who have received competent oral communication treatment with no significant benefits

## *Recommendations*

- Intensive and prolonged treatment is recommended for most children with apraxia of speech
- Counseling the family about the need for such treatment is essential because the treatment regimen is likely to be long, and family participation in treatment and home management is essential for success
- Augmentative or alternative communication may be recommended when found necessary and appropriate
- See the cited sources and the two companion volumes, *Hegde's PocketGuide to Communication Disorders* and *Hegde's PocketGuide to Treatment in Speech-Language Pathology* (3rd ed.)

Forrest, K. (2003). Diagnostic criteria of developmental apraxia of speech used by clinical speech-language pathologists. *American Journal of Speech-Language Pathology, 12,* 376–380.

Hall, P. K., Jordan, L. S., & Robin, D. A. (1993). *Developmental apraxia of speech: Theory and clinical practice*. Austin, TX: Pro-Ed.

Hayden, D. A. (1994). Differential diagnosis of motor speech dysfunction in children. *Clinics in Communication Disorders, 4*(2), 119–141.

Hodge, M. M. (1994). Assessment of children with developmental apraxia of speech: A rationale. *Clinics in Communication Disorders, 4*(2), 91–101.

Hodge, M. M., & Hancock, H. R. (1994). Assessment of children with developmental apraxia of speech: A procedure. *Clinics in Communication Disorders*, *4*(2), 102–118.

Lewis, B. A., Freebairn, L. A., Hansen, A. J., Iyengar, S. K., & Taylor, H. G. (2004). School-age follow-up of children with childhood apraxia of speech. *Language, Speech, and Hearing Services in Schools, 35*, 122–140.

Love, R. J. (2000). *Childhood motor speech disability* (2nd ed.). Boston: Allyn and Bacon.

Peña-Brooks, A., & Hegde, M. N. (2007). *Assessment and treatment of articulation and phonological disorders in children* (2nd ed.). Austin, TX: Pro-Ed.

**Cleft Lip.** Assessment of communication disorders associated with facial clefts is a significant responsibility of speech-language pathologists; cleft lips are congenital malformations that result in an opening in the lip, usually the upper lip and very rarely the lower lip; often associated with cleft of the palate, although clefts of the palate are often not associated with cleft lip; the clefts of the lip alone may not cause serious speech problems; because a combination of cleft palate and cleft lip are common and produce speech production problems, an understanding of cleft lips is essential; see Cleft Palate for assessment procedures.

**Cleft Palate.** Assessment of children with clefts of the palate and clefts of the palate and lips requires a good knowledge of the oral, pharyngeal, and especially the velopharyngeal structures and functions; early assessment is essential to design a treatment program that might help minimize speech errors and compensatory patterns of articulation that result from the clefts; in most cases, a thorough assessment of the velopharyngeal mechanism and its inadequacies is an important aspect of assessing children with clefts; see the cited sources at the end of this main entry and *Hegde's PocketGuide to Communication Disorders* for details on epidemiology, symptomatology, and etiology of clefts.

### *Assessment Objectives/General Guidelines*

- To determine communication disorders associated with the clefts in a child
- To make periodic assessments of communication and its potential to generate information that might help plan surgical intervention
- To suggest communication treatment targets
- To suggest prosthetic and other rehabilitation procedures when warranted

### *Case History/Interview Focus*

- See **Case History** and **Interview** under Standard/Common Assessment Procedures
- Concentrate on the medical and surgical history related to the child's cleft
- Take detailed information on speech and language development of the child
- Obtain information on any middle ear infection and conductive hearing loss that are frequently observed in children with palatal clefts
- Ask questions about any feeding or swallowing difficulties in the child
- Ask questions about how the parents perceive the speech in their child; concentrate not only on articulation problems but also on nasal emission and hypernasality

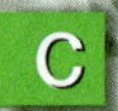

- Be aware of the different kinds of clefts that are likely to be found in male and female children
- Seek information on the familial history of clefts
- See *Hegde's PocketGuide to Communication Disorders* for a summary

## Ethnocultural Considerations

- See Ethnocultural Considerations in Assessment
- Clefts are distributed differently in different ethnocultural groups; be aware of the differential prevalence rates across groups
- Be aware that different types of clefts may predominate in different ethnocultural groups; also be aware that paternal and maternal ethnocultural backgrounds influence the types of clefts in children; see *Hegde's PocketGuide to Communication Disorders* for a summary

## Assessment

- Assessment of velopharyngeal dysfunction
  - Note that clinical judgments about hypernasality and hyponasality described under Assessment of Resonance Disorders later in this section yield indirect information about the velopharyngeal mechanism
  - Note that besides posterior and superior movement of the soft palate, lateral movement of the pharyngeal wall is necessary for adequate velopharyngeal closure
  - Note that different individuals show different patterns of velopharyngeal closures; all or only some of the involved structures may move or move more notably (e.g., primary lateral movement of the pharyngeal walls; primary movement of the soft palate; movements of the soft palate and lateral pharyngeal walls but little or no movement of the posterior pharyngeal wall; and all structures moving to achieve a sphincteric action)
    - Make an objective assessment of the velopharyngeal mechanism
    - Make an endoscopic examination of the velopharyngeal mechanism (nasopharyngoscopy); see Endoscopy; follow the procedures prescribed by the manufacturer of the particular instrument used
    - Make a videofluoroscopic examination of the velopharyngeal mechanism; see Videofluoroscopy; follow the procedures prescribed by the manufacturer of the particular instrument used; observe and record the movements of the soft palate, lateral pharyngeal wall, posterior pharyngeal wall, and tongue as the client produces consonant-vowel combinations, two-voiced and voiceless fricatives, and selected phrases
  - Make a complete **Orofacial Examination** (see Standard/Common Assessment Procedures); pay special attention to:
    - Clefts in the lip, hard palate, and soft palate
    - Repaired clefts and a judgment about the adequacy of the repair
    - Racial abnormalities that suggest a genetic syndrome (e.g., micrognathia, macrognathia, hypoplasia)
    - Abnormalities of the external ear
    - Abnormalities of the eyes
    - Observations of the velopharyngeal mechanism

- Note that movements of the soft palate during the sustained production of /a/ may not always indicate soft palate movement in connected speech
- Distinguish between the varieties of velopharyngeal dysfunction
  - Velopharyngeal incompetence: Inadequate movement of the velopharyngeal mechanism; refers to the action, not the structure or tissue mass
  - Velopharyngeal insufficiency: Tissue deficiency in the velopharyngeal mechanism that causes inadequate movement; a term specific to structural deviations
  - Velopharyngeal inadequacy: A general term that suggests a problem in achieving adequate closure regardless of etiology
  - Velopharyngeal mislearning: Inadequate closure of the velopharyngeal closure due to faulty learning, not structural problems

- Assessment of articulation and phonological disorders
  - Record a speech and language sample (see Standard/Common Assessment Procedures) to make an analysis of both the speech and language disorders
  - Have the child count to 20 and recite the alphabet; these tasks can give limited but useful information on connected speech, especially when a young child does not produce much conversational speech in the initial assessment session
  - Sample the production of sounds that are of special relevance to evaluate the effects of clefts on speech; create words and phrases that contain:
    - Stops, fricatives, and affricates (pressure consonants)
  - Have the child produce the sounds in syllables, words, phrases, and sentences
  - Modify or expand A. W. Kummer's (2001) list of sample sentences to assess articulation (as well as resonance characteristics); ask the child to repeat the sentences you model
    - [p] Popeye plays in the pool
    - [b] Buy baby a bib
    - [m] My mommy makes lemonade
    - [w] Wade in the water
    - [y] You have a yellow yo yo
    - [h] He has a big horse
    - [t] Take teddy to town
    - [d] Do it for daddy
    - [n] Nancy is not here
    - [k] I like cookies and cream
    - [g] Go get the wagon
    - [ŋ] Put the ring on her finger
    - [f] I have five fingers
    - [v] Drive a van
    - [l] I like yellow lollipops
    - [s] Sissy sees the sun in the sky
    - [z] Zip up your zipper
    - [ʃ] She went shopping
    - [ʧ] I eat cherries and cheese

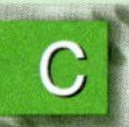

- [j] John told a joke to him
- [r] Randy has a red fire truck
- [ɚ] The teacher and the doctor are here
- [θ] Thank you for the toothbrush

From A. W. Kummer (2001). *Cleft palate and craniofacial anomalies*. Clifton Park, NY: Thomson Delmar Learning. Reproduced with permission.

- Assess the production of pressure consonants because these are significantly affected in children with clefts of the palate
  - Administer the *Iowa Pressure Articulation Test* (a subtest of the *Templin Darley Test of Articulation*; see Articulation and Phonological Disorders) to assess the production of pressure consonants and the nasal emission associated with their production
  - Alternatively, administer the *Bzoch Error Pattern Diagnostic Articulation Test* that samples the production of plosives, fricatives, and affricates that are often the most affected sounds
- Administer one of the articulation and phonological tests to evaluate general errors of articulation; see Articulation and Phonological Disorders
- See Articulation and Phonological Disorders for a description of assessment procedures
- Assess nasal air emission because this is another significant problem associated with speech production by children with palatal clefts
  - During articulation testing and while taking a speech sample, take note of the presence of nasal emission that may be consistent (heard on all pressure consonants), inconsistent (sometimes heard but other times not), or phoneme-specific (consistently occurs only on certain phones)
  - Administer the *Cul-de-Sack Test* by K. R. Bzoch, which helps evaluate nasal air emission (as well as hypernasality and hyponasality)
  - Hold a dental mirror under the nares as the child speaks; take note of any condensation due to nasal air emission
  - Hold a piece of thin paper under the nares as the child produces "**pʌ pʌ pʌ**," "**tʌ tʌ tʌ**," and "**kʌ kʌ kʌ**"; observe the movement of the paper due to nasal emission
  - Use the *See Scape* by Pro-Ed, Austin, which gives a visual representation of nasal emission; it contains a nasal olive, which is placed in the child's nostril and connected to a tube in which a styrofoam stopper moves as the air is emitted through the nose
  - Use a listening tube (one end in the child's nostril and the other end in the clinician's ear) or a stethoscope to assess nasal emission
  - Place one end of an ordinary straw in the child's nostril to hear nasal emission as the child produces syllables or words that contain pressure consonants
- Analyze individual sounds that are in error and a phonological pattern analysis if warranted; see Articulation and Phonological Disorders for a description of procedures; make a separate analysis of errors on pressure consonants (plosives, fricatives, and affricates)
- Take special note of weak production of consonants

- Make a list of compensatory articulation that often involves substitutions and production of sounds at unusual articulatory loci, often more posteriorly in the oral cavity
- Assessment of language disorders
  - Use the recorded speech and language sample to analyze comprehension and production of various semantic, morphological, syntactic, and pragmatic language structures
  - Use procedures of language assessment described under Language Disorders in Children or procedures described under Language Disorders in Infants and Toddlers, depending on the age of the client
  - Administer selected language tests described under Language Disorders in Children or those described under Language Disorders in Infants and Toddlers, depending on the age of the client; assess infants and toddlers at risk for developing speech and language delay
  - Note that assessment of language functions in children with clefts does not significantly differ from such an assessment in children without clefts
  - Summarize the semantic, syntactic, and pragmatic language skills of the child while taking note of deficiencies in each skill area
- Assessment of phonatory disorders
  - Listen to the speech and determine whether a detailed voice assessment is needed; children with clefts have a higher prevalence of voice disorders than those without clefts
    - Use procedures described under Voice Disorders to assess vocal quality deviations (e.g., hoarseness, harshness, breathiness); assess vocally abusive behaviors
    - Evaluate pitch and loudness of voice; see Voice Disorders for procedures; use clinical judgment and rating; if necessary, use instruments to measure pitch and loudness
    - In the case of voice quality deviations, obtain a report from the child's laryngologist; vocal nodules may be the cause of such deviations; if the child has not been seen by a laryngologist, make a referral
- Assessment of resonance disorders
  - Assess hypernasality; make clinical judgments as you listen to the client's speech about the presence of excessive nasality
  - Have two or more clinicians judge and rate hypernasality of connected speech
  - Use procedures described under Voice Disorders including instrumental assessment
  - Assess hyponasality; use procedures described under Voice Disorders including instrumental assessment
  - Administer the *Cul-de-Sack Test* by K. R. Bzoch, which helps evaluate hypernasality, hyponasality, and nasal air emission
  - Modify or expand A. W. Kummer's (2001) list of sample sentences to assess hyponasality, denasality, and cul-de-sac resonance; ask the child to repeat the sentences you model
    - My mama made lemonade for me.
    - My name is Amy Minor.

- My mama takes money to the market.
- Many men are at the mine.
- Ned made nine points in the game.
- My nanny is not mean.
- Nan needs a dime to call home.
- My mom's home is many miles away.
- Many men are needed to move the piano.

From A. W. Kummer (2001). *Cleft palate and craniofacial anomalies.* Clifton Park, NY: Thomson Delmar Learning. Reproduced with permission.

- Note that reliability and validity of resonance ratings are questionable; train observers and constantly monitor reliability and validity; use more than one judge (clinician) whenever possible

### Related/Medical Assessment Data

- Obtain medical and surgical reports to understand the effects of previous medical treatments and to know what additional procedures are planned for the child
- Integrate communication assessment data with those of medical assessment data
- Make assessment or diagnostic decisions as a member of the cleft palate team
- Integrate information about the child's academic performance with communication assessment data
- Obtain psychological assessment data if available and integrate them with your assessment data

### Standard/Common Assessment Procedures

- Complete the Standard/Common Assessment Procedures
- Pay special attention to **Orofacial Examination** to assess all aspects of oral-facial structures and functions
- Pay special attention to any signs of a genetic syndrome because cleft palate is a part of many syndromes; see Syndromes Associated With Communication Disorders

### Analysis of Assessment Data

- Analyze and summarize the child's articulation disorders and phonological patterns if any
- Analyze and summarize the language structures the child uses and those that the child does not
- Analyze and summarize the phonatory and resonatory problems and supplement clinical observations and ratings with the results of instrumental measures
- Analyze and summarize the results of instrumental observations of the velopharyngeal mechanism

### Diagnostic Criteria

- An obvious history of cleft palate and surgical repairs of the cleft is a basis to diagnose and classify the particular kinds of speech disorders
- Communication disorders due to cleft palate should be evident on pressure consonants

- Presence of nasal air emission and hypernasality offer supportive evidence
- Compensatory articulation due to velopharyngeal dysfunction is further evidence
- Characteristic phonatory disorders offer additional evidence

### Differential Diagnosis

- Distinguish articulation disorders due to the cleft and associated physiological problems, including the velopharyngeal dysfunction, from articulation and phonological disorders found in children without clefts
- Take note that a child may have an independent articulation and phonological disorder; in which case the child's misarticulations may not be limited to pressure consonants and phonological patterning may be evident
- Distinguish hypernasality and nasal emission associated with velopharyngeal dysfunction from those that are due to an oronasal fistula (an opening from the oral cavity straight into the nasal cavity); note that unless the fistula is very large, it is unlikely to produce hypernasality; if the degree of nasal air emission is the same on anterior and posterior sounds, then the problem is due to velopharyngeal dysfunction, not the fistula
- Close the fistula with chewing gum and compare the amount of nasal emission with that observed without closing it
- If nasal air emission is limited to a few pressure consonants, but others are produced well, then rule out velopharyngeal dysfunction
- If the child is highly stimulable for misarticulations, or when the child is taught to change the place of articulation and as a consequence nasal emission or hypernasality is reduced or eliminated, then rule out velopharyngeal insufficiency (tissue limitation); such misarticulations may be due to faulty learning

### Prognosis

- Varies across children; presence of multiple handicaps and severe expression of genetic syndromes affect prognosis negatively
- Generally good for improved communication skills in cases of children who only have the clefts that are repaired early in life
- Most children benefit from systematic treatment

### Recommendations

- Early language stimulation if there is evidence of language delay; if the delay or disorder is significant, recommend formal treatment
- Treatment of articulation and phonological disorders; the most likely recommendation for children with clefts of the palate
- Treatment of behaviorally persistent hypernasality after the velopharyngeal function is surgically restored or improved
- Prosthetic aid in cases of persistent hypernasality due to permanent velopharyngeal insufficiency (tissue limitation)
- Repeated assessments before and after various surgical procedures
- See the cited sources and the two companion volumes, *Hegde's PocketGuide to Communication Disorders* and *Hegde's PocketGuide to Treatment in Speech-Language Pathology* (3rd ed.)

Bzoch, K. R. (2004). *Communicative disorders related to cleft palate* (5th ed.). Austin, TX: Pro-Ed

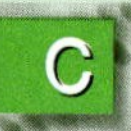

Kummer, A. W. (2001). *Cleft palate and craniofacial anomalies.* Clifton Park, NY: Thomson Delmar Learning.

McWilliams, B. J., Morris, H. L., & Shelton, R. L. (1990). *Cleft palate speech* (2nd ed.). Philadelphia, PA: B. C. Decker.

Moller, K. T., & Starr, C. D. (1993). *Cleft palate: Interdisciplinary issues and treatment.* Austin, TX: Pro-Ed.

Peterson-Falzone, S. J., Hardin-Jones, M. A., & Karnell, M. P. (2001). *Cleft palate speech* (3rd ed.). St. Louis, MO: Mosby Year Book.

Shprintzen, R. J., & Bardach, J. (1995). *Cleft palate speech management: A multidisciplinary approach.* St. Louis, MO: Mosby Year Book.

**Cluttering.** Assessment of cluttering—a disorder predominantly affecting the rate of speech, fluency, and speech intelligibility—may be done with the help of procedures that are appropriate to assess stuttering; see *Hegde's PocketGuide to Communication Disorders* for details on the characteristics and etiological research; see Cluttering under the main entry, Fluency Disorders in this book for specific assessment procedures.

**Computed Tomography.** A radiographic imaging procedure; previously known as *CAT scan* and currently known as CT (computed tomography) scan; the features of the CT scan include:

- An X-ray scanning machine with a camera that rotates around a structure (scans) and takes pictures of sections of that structure; the machine scans tissue density
- A computer analyzes the images generated by the scanning machine and produces pictures of the scanned structure
- It can show internal structures, hemorrhages, lesions, tumors, and other pathologies
- It is an early method of visualizing the brain in living persons; often used in the diagnosis of neuropathology associated with strokes because the method is especially good at detecting recent hemorrhage and both focal and progressive damage
- The method may fail to reveal small lesions
- Although noninvasive, the method carries the risks associated with radiation
- Contrast (picture resolution) may be improved by injecting radiopaque material into the bloodstream with its associated additional risk factors (pain, nausea, kidney problems)

**Concurrent Validity.** Demonstration that a standardized test actually measures what it purports to measure because it is positively correlated with one or more similar tests whose validity is established; an important element in selecting standardized tests for assessing speech, language, and other aspects of communication; see Validity.

**Confrontation Naming.** Naming stimulus items when presented and asked the (typical) question, "What is this?"; a skill that needs to be assessed in most clients with aphasia because this type of naming skill is often impaired in them; see Aphasia for details and assessment procedures.

**Congenital.** Any condition noticed at the time of birth or soon thereafter; may be genetic or acquired; a determination that a condition is *congenital* is mostly made by the knowledge available about it and by the case history information; during assessment:

- All genetic syndromes, familial intellectual impairments (intellectual disabilities), various isolated physical abnormalities, clefts of the palate and lips, and CP, to name a few, are known to be congenital
- Most congenital conditions are observed at the time of or soon after birth; therefore, seek information on prenatal, natal, and postnatal conditions that are associated with the particular clinical condition suspected of being congenital
- Ask whether the parents have noticed the clinical conditions (e.g., cleft of the lip or palate, signs of various genetic syndromes, physical deviations or abnormalities) at birth or soon after the child was born
- Note that the effects of some congenital conditions may be evident only after some time and there may be no observations related to them at or soon after birth (e.g., familial intellectual disabilities, autism, language delay due to intellectual limitations, behavioral deficits due to subtle brain injury during birth, certain genetic conditions whose effects are delayed until early childhood years)

**Congenital Palatopharyngeal Incompetence.** Assessment of velopharyngeal function is an important aspect of diagnosing cleft palate speech and resonance disorders associated with Dysarthria; congenital velopharyngeal incompetence refers to an inadequate velopharyngeal mechanism that cannot close the velopharyngeal port for the production of nonnasal speech sounds; not due to clefts; hard palate may be too short or the nasopharynx may be too deep; speech is hypernasal; depending on the degree of incompetence, resonance (voice) therapy may be ineffective without surgical or prosthetic help; see also Velopharyngeal Dysfunction for differential diagnoses of velopharyngeal incompetence, velopharyngeal insufficiency, and velopharyngeal mislearning for assessment guidelines.

**Consistency Effect.** Stuttering on the same words or same loci when a printed passage is orally read repeatedly; contrasts with the Adaptation Effect; may be assessed in a 5-reading sequence; the diagnostic significance is that the greater the consistency effect, the stronger (more severe) the stuttering on specified loci; see Stuttering; to assess consistency of stuttering on the same loci:

- Select a standard printed prose passage (e.g., *My Grandfather* or *The Rainbow*); have two copies of the passage
- Place a copy in front of the client and instruct the client to read it aloud five times in succession; ask the person to read it in his or her usual manner (discourage too slow a rate)
- As the client reads the passage aloud, mark the occurrence of stutterings on the second copy of the passage; mark them by writing 1 under a word to suggest that the word was stuttered on the first reading; write 2, 3, 4, or 5 to suggest repeated stuttering on the same word during subsequent readings
- Mark dysfluencies between words (e.g., interjections)

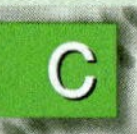

- Calculate the loci on which stuttering occurred only once, twice, three times, four times, and all five times
- Note that the consistency effect shows a gradient of severity: the loci with a single occurrence are least severe and the loci with five occurrences are the most severe; other loci falling between the two extremes
- Possibly, the words on which stuttering occurred most consistently may need special attention during treatment; they may persist the longest in the course of the treatment

**Construct Validity.** Demonstration of the validity of standardized tests by showing that the test results are consistent with certain theoretical constructs or assumptions; see Validity for procedural details.

**Constructional Apraxia.** The same as Constructional Impairment.

**Constructional Impairment.** Difficulty in visuospatial tasks; need to be assessed in clients with brain injury, including those with Traumatic Brain Injury, Right Hemisphere Syndrome, and Apraxia of Speech; to assess:

- Have the client construct a block design that you display (some tests of intelligence have block design subtests)
- Ask the client to construct stick designs that you display
- Ask the client to draw human or geometric figures
- Analyze the errors

**Conversational Repair Strategies.** In evaluating and diagnosing language disorders, it is necessary to assess what two or more conversational partners do when there is breakdown in communication; repair strategies are designed to restore broken communication links; a feature of language disorders in children and adults; assess two main strategies: request for clarification and response to requests for clarification

- Requests for clarification: To assess whether the client would make appropriate requests for clarification
  - Engage the client in conversational speech; with young children, use stimulating stimulus materials (toys, pictures, enacted events while playing with toys)
  - Periodically, make ambiguous statements:
    - Show the picture of three cups and ask the child to "Point to the cup" without specifying which one to see whether the child asks "which one?" or requests clarification nonverbally (e.g., hand or facial gestures)
    - Display three toy cars, each a different color, and ask the child, "Give me the car" to see whether the child asks "Which car?" or requests clarification nonverbally
    - Make unclear statements (e.g., talk too softly, produce incomplete sentences) to see whether the child asks for clarification (e.g., *What did you say? What was that?* or *I didn't hear you*)
    - Count the number of times the child actually requested clarification; may include such statements as "What do you mean?" "I am not sure what you mean," "Can you say it differently?" "I don't understand," "I didn't hear you," or "Can you say it louder?"; analyze the results in relation to the number of

times you made ambiguous statements that should have led to requests for clarification

- Appropriate response to a listener's request for clarification: To assess whether a client would modify his or her statements in response to your request for clarification
  - Engage the child in conversational speech
  - Periodically, pretend that you did not understand what the client said and request for clarification
    - Ask such questions as "What did you say?" "What was that?" or "What do you mean?"
    - Make such statements as "I am not sure what you mean," "I didn't get it," "I didn't hear you," and so forth
    - Count the number of times the client modified his or her statements by saying it differently, by offering explanations or greater descriptions, by giving examples, by saying it more loudly, and so forth; analyze the results in relation to the number of times you requested clarifications

**Craniocerebral Trauma.** Trauma to the head and the brain; often associated with communication disorders, along with behavioral deficits; to assess the effects on communication, see Traumatic Brain Injury.

**Creutzfeldt-Jakob Disease (CJD).** A degenerative, rare, fatal encephalopathy; involves partial degeneration of pyramidal and extrapyramidal systems; associated with Apraxia, Dementia, and Dysarthria; see Dementia for details on assessment.

**Cultural Diversity and Assessment Procedures.** See Ethnocultural Considerations in Assessment.

D

**de Lange Syndrome.** To assess communication disorders associated with this syndrome, which is also known as the *Cornelia de Lange syndrome*, see Syndromes Associated With Communication Disorders.



**Dementia, Progressive.** Assessment of dementia is a multifaceted, team-based task; speech-language pathologists make an important contribution to the assessment of dementia because in many cases impaired speech and language skills are among the early signs and are often necessary to diagnose dementia; it is an acquired neurological syndrome associated with progressive deterioration in intellectual skills, communicative functions, and general behavior; contrasted with forms of impaired intellect and behavior that are temporary (reversible dementia); etiological factors are varied, but often associated with such neurological diseases as Alzheimer's Disease (AD), Huntington's Disease (HD), Parkinson's Disease (PD), Pick's Disease, Progressive Supranuclear Palsy (PS), and Wilson's Disease; also may be due to vascular diseases that result in Vascular Dementia; see the separate entries for these diseases; see also the sources cited at the end of this main entry and the companion volume, *Hegde's PocketGuide to Communication Disorders* for details on epidemiology and ethnocultural variables; neurological, behavioral, and cognitive symptoms; etiologies; neuropathology; and theories of dementia.

### *Assessment of Dementia: General Guidelines*

- Diagnosis and treatment of dementia are a team effort; information is gathered from varied sources, including medical, neurological, and neurodiagnostic evidence; changes in behavior and personality; deterioration in intellectual skills (especially memory skills); and in late stages, varied physical symptoms
- Speech-language pathologists contribute to the diagnostic process by assessing impaired and possibly regressed and progressively deteriorating communication skills
- Diagnosing dementia in its middle and late stages is not as challenging as diagnosing it in its early stages; middle and late stage symptoms are obvious; symptoms of early stage are subtle
- Diagnosis of early-stage dementia is greatly facilitated by a careful assessment of changes in language, cognition, and memory skills because there may be no serious physical symptoms
- Such language and intellectually based tasks as verbal description of everyday objects, storytelling, recall of events, and verbal fluency are especially diagnostic of dementia in its early stages
- Such automatic tasks as pointing to named pictures and reciting alphabets and days of the week are not especially diagnostic of mild dementia
- Syntactic disturbances are not evident in mild dementia; hence they need not be assessed in great detail (except in the case of multi-infarct dementia and dementia associated with Pick's disease)
- Articulation and phonological skills are not diagnostic of early dementia because they are retained until the advanced stage when dementia is obvious
- Sentence repetition skills are not diagnostic of early dementia because they are preserved even when the client cannot comprehend the meaning of repeated sentences

- Language assessment alone will not determine the diagnosis of dementia; deterioration in memory, visuospatial skills, and general intellect also should be demonstrated



### Assessment Objectives

- To assess language, cognitive, memory, and visuospatial skills with a view to diagnose or rule out dementia
- To assess changes in behavior and personality that may support the diagnosis of dementia
- To establish baseline skill levels against which future changes (including deterioration, stabilization even if temporarily, or any improvement associated with treatment and clinical management) can be evaluated
- To identify the strengths and weaknesses of the client with a view to develop an intervention or management plan for the client and family
- To assess the strengths and weaknesses of the family; to identify the support system they need; and to develop a counseling, family education, and treatment plan for the family members
- To have an ongoing assessment plan to track changes in the client's skill levels that may have implications for continuously modifying the treatment or clinical management plan

### Case History/Interview Focus

- See **Case History** and **Interview** under Standard/Common Assessment Procedures
- Concentrate on the detailed history of the client's health, major illnesses, and behavioral changes over time
- Obtain information on the family's resources and support needed because dementia management is often a long-term and expensive process
- Seek family history relative to dementia and progressive neurological diseases
- Get information about the client's education and occupation, interests, hobbies, leisure activities, typical daily activities, intellectual and literary pursuits, and any changes they may have noticed in all these skill areas
- Question the informants about the onset of the symptoms as they see it; the onset of dementia typically refers to a change in the behavior and intellectual skills (especially memory loss) that the family members will have noticed
- Concentrate on the onset of such symptoms as irritability, forgetting to do what the person has been doing routinely (e.g., paying bills), changes in eating or sleeping habits, uncharacteristically eccentric or irrational behavior, deterioration in self-care, and loss or deterioration in skill levels (e.g., cooking, shopping, reading, writing)
- Ask the family members to supply a few premorbid writing samples of the client
- Question the family about any evidence of long-standing psychiatric problems (e.g., schizophrenia, delusions and hallucinations, inappropriate speech and language, anxiety, depression)

D

## *Ethnocultural Considerations*

- See Ethnocultural Considerations in Assessment
- Assess the bilingual status of the client and family; if the client and the family members are bilingual, establish the dominant language and assess the client in that language
- As with clients belonging to any ethnocultural background, assess the family's access to health care and resources needed to sustain care on a long-term basis
- Assess the family's views on such a long-term disability as dementia and take their views and values into consideration in designing the assessment plan and in eventually recommending a treatment or habilitation plan
- Following the assessment, design a family education plan that takes into consideration the strengths and weaknesses of the family as well as the family communication patterns, cultural views, and values related to disability and communication

## *Assessment*

- Assessment parameters include mental status, cognitive or intellectual skills, and communication skills
- Procedurally, both skill-specific tests (e.g., memory or writing) and global dementia assessment tools may help make an evaluation of clients suspected to have dementia
- Many skills may be simply assessed by skill-specific tasks (e.g., asking the person to name as many vegetables as possible, writing a paragraph, copying drawings, adding numbers, or recalling personal experiences)
- Some of the skills may have been evaluated by other professionals (e.g., intellectual functioning by psychologists, self-care and daily living skills by occupational therapists); in such cases, the speech-language pathologist may concentrate on communication skill assessment; nonetheless, the speech-language pathologist must be familiar with all aspects of the assessment

### Assess Mental Status and Cognitive Skills

- Make an initial bedside screening of mental status by asking several questions; appropriateness or inappropriateness of the responses the client gives to questions such as the following will give a preliminary idea about the client's mental status:
  - "What is your name?"
  - "Please name some of the members of your family."
  - "What is the name of your nurse?"
  - "What is the name of your doctor?"
  - "What is today's date?"
  - "What time is it?"
  - "Where are you now?"
  - "When did you get here?"
  - "Who brought you here?"
  - "When did you eat something?"

- "What is going to be your next meal? Breakfast, lunch, or dinner?"
- "What time do you eat lunch?"

- Administer a formal mental status assessment tool
  - Administer the *Mini-Mental Status Examination* by M. F. Folstein, S. E. Folstein, and P. R. McHugh; the screening tools help assess not only basic memory skills, but also some language skills (naming three objects, pointing to named objects, repeating phrases, following commands, writing a sentence) and figure copying
  - Administer the modified and expanded *Mini-Mental Status Examination* by E. L. Teng and K. Chui



### Assess Communication Skills

- Assess articulation and phonological skills
  - Note that articulation and phonological skills are intact in the early phases of dementia
  - Use the conversational speech sample to analyze speech sound productions; take note of any problems
- Assess vocabulary
  - Take a conversational speech sample
  - Use verbal description data to assess correct word usage
  - Assess the variety and specificity of words used in a conversational speech sample and verbal description task
  - Use a standardized measure such as the *Peabody Picture Vocabulary Test (PPVT)* by L. M. Dunn and L. M. Dunn
  - Note that PPVT scores are sensitive to early phases of dementia
- Assess verbal description skills
  - Present a few common objects to the client
  - Ask the client to describe each of them
  - If necessary, model a complete description of an object (such as a pencil)
  - Tape-record the descriptions and transcribe them later
  - Present a picture and ask the client to describe it; consider using the "cookie thief" picture of the Boston Diagnostic Aphasia Examination or similar pictures
  - Take note of the client's memory for words, temporal sequence, logical connections, antecedents and consequences, grammatically of expressions, and topic maintenance as the client describes the presented picture or pictures
  - Note that impaired verbal description tasks can help identify early phases of dementia
- Assess storytelling skills
  - Ask the client to listen carefully to the story you are about to tell
  - Tell the client that he or she will have to retell the story soon after and at the end of the testing session
  - Tell a short story
  - Ask the nonexpressive client to rearrange picture cards to retell the story

- Take note of significant reduction in the number of story elements remembered, wrong temporal order of story elements, missing details, wrong characterization, and so forth
- Assess verbal fluency or generative naming task
  - Ask the client to say as many words as possible that begin with a specific letter; sample responses for at least three letters
  - Allow one minute of response time for each letter
  - Note that generative naming measures help identify early phases of dementia
- Assess appropriate or expected responses in structured conversations
  - Ask an ambiguous question or make an ambiguous request to see whether the client requests more information or clarification
  - Ask for clarifications when the client's statements are not clear
  - Compliment the client to see whether he or she makes a relevant response
  - Judge the presence or appropriateness of responses when you say, "I enjoyed meeting you."
  - Judge the meaningfulness and relevance of sentences produced; consider contexts of utterances
  - Analyze stories or descriptions of clients for contextual and setting information; most clients with dementia omit information on context and setting
- Assess pantomime expression
  - Show common objects or pictures of objects and ask the client to demonstrate their use by gestures
  - Note that a pantomime expression task can help identify mild dementia
- Judge syntactic skills in conversational speech
  - Note that syntactic skills are intact in early phases of dementia
  - Make an informal analysis of sentence types, lengths, and variety; take note of any deviations or deficiencies
  - Assess syntactic skills in detail if clinical judgment warrants it
- Assess pragmatic language skills
  - Take a discourse sample
  - Observe conversational turn taking
  - Observe topic maintenance
  - Observe conversational repair
  - Observe topic initiation
- Assess language comprehension skills
  - Judge language comprehension throughout the interview and assessment duration
  - Administer one or more language comprehension tests (e.g., the *Test for Auditory Comprehension of Language* by E. Carrow-Woodfolk and *Discourse Comprehension Test* by R. Brookshire & L. E. Nicholas)

### Assess Cognitive Functions

- Assess reasoning and event planning skills by asking the client to describe how he or she would:

- Plan a birthday party
- Plan a summer vacation, camping trip, or picnic
- Get an airline ticket
- Obtain a doctor's appointment

- Assess memory skills
  - Use the delayed storytelling procedure in which you tell a short story and have the client recall it after 1 hour
  - Ask the client about his or her past life events and verify the client's description with a family member
  - Ask questions about the known recent events in the hospital setting (e.g., a birthday party the client may have attended, special events organized by the staff, a recent shopping trip or outing)
  - Administer a memory test; many scales of dementia include items to assess memory; in addition, the clinician may administer a dedicated memory test (e.g., the *Benton Visual Retention Test* by A. L. Benton, *Memory Assessment Scales* by J. M. Williams, and the *Wechsler Memory Scale—Revised* by D. Wechsler)
- Assess drawing skills
  - Ask the client to draw some common pictures (e.g., a clock, circle, triangle)
  - Note that clients with even mild dementia perform poorly on this visuospatial task
- Obtain a measure of general intellectual functioning
- Obtain reports from a psychologist about intelligence testing

### Assess Abstract Reasoning

- Ask the client to specify the meaning of a few selected proverbs (e.g., *What is meant by the saying "a stitch in time saves nine"?*)
- Assess whether the client gives a literal or abstract interpretation of such statements

### Assess Reading Performance

- Assess reading comprehension
  - Have the client match printed words with pictures
  - Have the client silently read a story and answer your questions
  - Note that dementia clients are likely to have much more difficulty in comprehending sentences and paragraphs than single words
- Assess oral reading skills
  - Have the client orally read a story and summarize it
  - Have the client read a brief report in a newspaper and summarize it Standardized Tests or Scales of Dementia
- Administer the latest versions of one or more of the following tests or scales to measure behaviors and skills associated with dementia and their changes over time.
- Re-administer the test or the scale to assess deterioration in symptoms

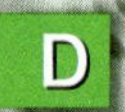


| Test | Purpose |
|---|---|
| *Activities of Daily Living Questionnaire (ADLQ)* (M. Johnson & associates) | To assess the daily living skills with the help of a knowledgeable informant |
| *Alzheimer Disease Assessment Scale (ADAS)* (W. G. Rosen, R. C. Mohs, & K. L. Davis) | To assess cognitive and noncognitive behaviors and their deterioration; widely used in medical settings |
| *Arizona Battery for Communication Disorders of Dementia* (K. A. Bayles & C. Tomoeda) | To assess dementia through 14 subtests and screen it with 4 subtests |
| *Benton Revised Visual Retention Test* (A. L. Benton) | To assess visual memory with figural recall |
| *Blessed Dementia Scale* (G. Blessed & associates) | To rate changes in performance in everyday activities and habits |
| *Brief Cognitive Rating Scale* (B. Reisberg) | To assess cognitive decline due to any reason |
| *Clinical Dementia Rating Scale* (C. P. Hughes & associates) | To rate dementia on a 5-point rating scale; does not assess communication skills |
| *Dementia Deficits Scale (DDS)* (A. Snow & associates) | To assess self-awareness deficits that may lead to dangerous behaviors |
| *Discourse Abilities Profile* (B. Terrel & D. Ripich) | To assess various forms of discourse during conversation with the client and conversation between the client and family members' caregivers |
| *Global Deterioration Scale* (B. Reisberg & associates) | To rate dementia on a 7-point rating scale |
| *Memory Assessment Scales* (J. M. Williams) | To assess memory skills in greater detail than possible with dementia scales |
| *Progressive Deterioration Scale (PDS)* (R. Dejong & associates) | To assess deterioration over time in daily living skills |
| *Wechsler Adult Intelligence Scale—III (WAIS—III)* (D. Wechsler) | To assess general intellectual level and intellectual deterioration |
| *Wechsler Memory Scale—Revised* (E. W. Russell) | To assess various memory functions in greater detail than possible with dementia scales |

- Administer a test of aphasia as found appropriate (see Aphasia), especially the following that have some normative information on clients with dementia as well:
  - *Communicative Abilities of Daily Living* by D. Fromm & A. Holland
  - *The Western Aphasia Battery* by J. Appell, A. Kertesz, & M. Fishman

## Related/Medical Assessment Data

- Obtain copies of medical reports
- Ascertain diagnoses of neurological and other diseases of the client

- Obtain or review available brain imaging and other special diagnostic data
- Obtain copies of social service reports
- Obtain psychological assessment data
- Obtain any other family service information available on the client



### Standard/Common Assessment Procedures

- Complete the Standard/Common Assessment Procedures

### Analysis of Assessment Data

- Analyze the results of the communication assessment
- Analyze the results of the cognition and memory assessment
- Integrate the results of the communication, cognition-memory, medical, social service, and psychological assessment procedures
- Make a summary statement of the significant findings
- Obtain a total picture of the client and his or her strengths and weaknesses
- Integrate the clinical assessment data with those of the case history information

### Diagnostic Criteria

- Generally, impairment should be documented in (1) language; (2) memory; (3) visuospatial skills; (4) emotion, personality, or behavior; and (5) cognition
- The American Psychiatric Association (APA) requires that to diagnose dementia, memory impairments are essential; in addition, at least one of the following also should be documented: language disturbances (aphasia), apraxia, agnosia, or impaired executive functions; the APA definition also requires that impairments should affect occupational and social life to justify a diagnosis of dementia
- Other experts (e.g., Cummings & Benson, 1983) think that memory impairments are not required to diagnose dementia because they may not be evident in early stages and especially in clients with Pick's disease; they also believe that according to the APA criteria, dementia in people who face little or no occupational demands (e.g., the underemployed or unemployed) as well as dementia in people with limited social involvement would be hard to diagnose

### Differential Diagnosis

- Definite diagnosis is possible only with autopsic or biopsic evidence of histopathology
- Differentiate dementia from aphasia
- Differentiate dementia from the language of confusion
- Differentiate dementia from depression (pseudodementia) and other psychiatric conditions
- Differentiate dementia from right hemisphere syndrome
- Distinguish among cortical dementias caused by Alzheimer's Disease or Pick's Disease
- Distinguish among mixed dementias caused by Korsakoff's disease (or syndrome, which is currently considered a form of amnestic disorder); Creutzfeldt-Jakob Disease, or Multi-infarct Dementia.
- Distinguish among subcortical dementias (and possibly dysarthria as well) caused by Huntington's Disease, Parkinson's Disease, Wilson's Disease, or Supranuclear Palsy.

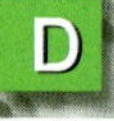

- Note that generative naming problem is a more sensitive early sign of dementia than is confrontation naming
- Note that early stage dementia is characterized by relatively intact phonological and syntactic skills
- Use the following four charts to distinguish dementia from the other potentially confusing disorders

## Dementia or Aphasia?

| Dementia | Aphasia |
|---|---|
| Onset mostly is slow | Onset mostly is sudden |
| Bilateral brain damage | Damage in the left hemisphere |
| Diffuse brain damage in most cases | Focal brain lesions in most cases |
| May be moody, withdrawn, and agitated | Mood usually is appropriate, though depressed or frustrated at times |
| Cognition is mildly or severely impaired, but better language skills until later stages | Impaired language, but generally intact cognition |
| Memory is impaired to various degrees, often severely | Memory typically is intact |
| Behavior often is irrelevant, socially inappropriate, and disorganized | Behavior generally is relevant, socially appropriate, and organized |
| Mentally confused and disoriented to time and space | Mentally alert and oriented to time and space |
| Disorientation to self in later stages | No disorientation to self |
| Progression of deterioration from semantic to syntactic to phonological performance | Semantic, syntactic, and phonological performance simultaneously impaired |
| Fluent until dementia becomes worse | Fluent or nonfluent |
| Relatively poor performance on spatial and verbal recognition tasks | Relatively better performance on spatial and verbal recognition tasks |
| Relatively poor story retelling skills | Relatively better story retelling skills |
| Relatively poor description of common objects | Relatively better description of common objects |
| Relatively poor silent reading comprehension | Relatively better silent reading comprehension |
| Relatively poor pantomimic expression | Relatively better pantomimic expression |
| Relatively poor drawing skills | Relatively better drawing skills |

*Caution: (1) Clients with fluent aphasia are more likely to be confused with dementia than are those with fluent aphasia, (2) aphasia and dementia may coexist, (3) an aphasic client may develop a neurological disease resulting in dementia (Alzheimer's disease), (4) a client with dementia may suffer a stroke, resulting in aphasia.*

## Dementia or the Language of Confusion?

| Dementia | Confusion |
| --- | --- |
| Degenerative diseases are the most common causes | Traumatic brain injury and toxic and metabolic disturbances are the most common causes |
| Reduced range and variety of word usage | No significant problems in word usage |
| Slow onset | Generally more abrupt onset |
| Disorientation to time, place, and person only in more advanced stages | Disoriented to time, place, and persons |
| Progressive worsening of symptoms | More rapid, positive changes in symptoms |

## Dementia or Depression (Pseudodementia)?

| Dementia | Pseudodementia |
| --- | --- |
| Imprecise onset date | More precise onset date |
| Family members often do not know about the symptoms | Family members know about the symptoms |
| Slow progression of symptoms | Rapid progression of symptoms |
| No or rare history of psychiatric problems | History of psychiatric problems |
| Clients do not complain of cognitive problems in detail | Clients complain of cognitive problems |
| Clients try to conceal their problems | Clients highlight their disability, failure, sense of distress |
| Clients struggle to perform | Clients make no or little effort to perform even simple tasks |
| Social skills often preserved until the later stages | Loss of social skills |
| Attentional deficits and poor concentration | No attentional deficits, good concentration |
| Client's response to orientation tests is confusion | Client's response to orientation tests is "don't know" |
| Memory loss for recent events more severe than that for remote events | The same degree of memory loss for both recent and remote events |
| Generalized memory problems | Selective memory problems |
| Consistent difficulty in performing the same task | Variability in performing the same task |

*Note: Pseudodementia is dementia-like symptoms associated with depression; the differentiating characteristics summarized here are based on Wells (1980).*

## Dementia or Right Hemisphere Problems?

| Dementia | Right Hemisphere Problems |
|---|---|
| Significant problems in naming, especially generative naming | Only mild problems in naming, reading, and writing |
| Significant problems in auditory comprehension | Mild problems in auditory comprehension |
| Left-sided neglect not a diagnostic feature | Left-sided neglect a diagnostic feature |
| Prosodic defects less severe | Significant prosodic defect |
| Inappropriate or absent social conventions | Inappropriate humor |
| May retell stories without context or location | May retell only nonessential, isolated details of stories (no integration) |
| Pragmatic impairments less striking until the latter stages | Pragmatic impairments more striking (eye contact, topic maintenance, etc.) |
| Significant linguistic deficits except for syntactic and phonological skills, which also decline in later stages | Pure linguistic deficits are not dominant |

## Cortical Dementias: Dementia of Alzheimer's Disease or of Pick's Disease?

| Alzheimer's Disease | Pick's Disease |
|---|---|
| Gradual onset of the disease | Gradual onset of the disease |
| Diffuse damage associated with senile plaques, neurofibrillary tangles, granulovascular degeneration, neuronal loss, astrocytic gliosis, and amyloid angiopathy | Atrophy in the frontal and temporal regions; Pick bodies (filamentous intracytoplasmic inclusions in neurons) |
| Impairment of semantic and pragmatic language functions in early stages; syntactic and phonological skills preserved until later stages; speech impairment in very later stages | Impaired rate and prosody characterized by slow and deliberate speech; naming problems; syntactic difficulties; auditory comprehension problems |
| Impaired memory, but worse for remote events | Impaired memory, but worse for recent events |
| Willing to perform, tries to perform | Apathetic, shows emotional lability |
| Generally normal motor functions | Impaired motor functions in later stages |

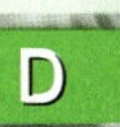


## Mixed Dementias: Dementia of Korsakoff's Disease, Creutzfeldt-Jakob Disease, or Multi-infarct Dementia?

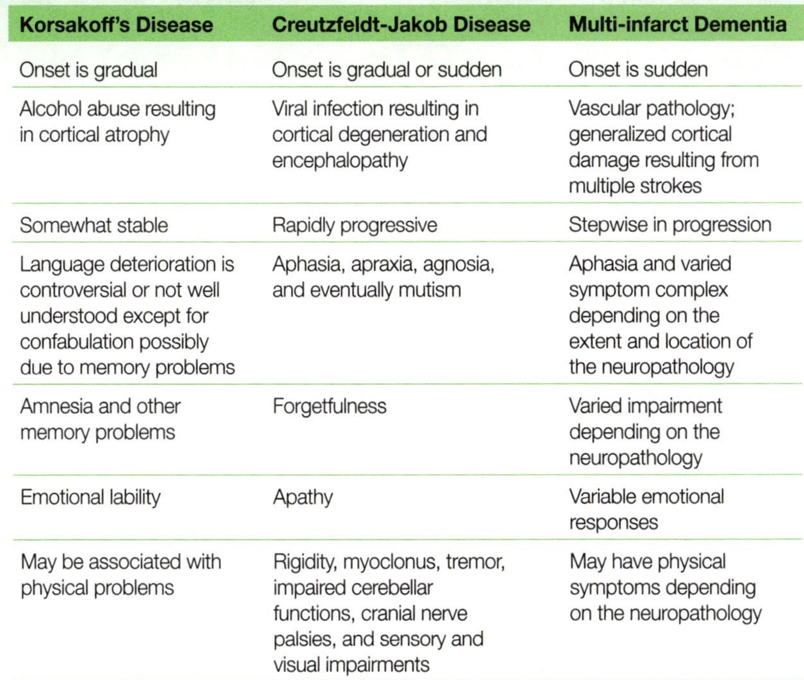

| Korsakoff's Disease | Creutzfeldt-Jakob Disease | Multi-infarct Dementia |
|---|---|---|
| Onset is gradual | Onset is gradual or sudden | Onset is sudden |
| Alcohol abuse resulting in cortical atrophy | Viral infection resulting in cortical degeneration and encephalopathy | Vascular pathology; generalized cortical damage resulting from multiple strokes |
| Somewhat stable | Rapidly progressive | Stepwise in progression |
| Language deterioration is controversial or not well understood except for confabulation possibly due to memory problems | Aphasia, apraxia, agnosia, and eventually mutism | Aphasia and varied symptom complex depending on the extent and location of the neuropathology |
| Amnesia and other memory problems | Forgetfulness | Varied impairment depending on the neuropathology |
| Emotional lability | Apathy | Variable emotional responses |
| May be associated with physical problems | Rigidity, myoclonus, tremor, impaired cerebellar functions, cranial nerve palsies, and sensory and visual impairments | May have physical symptoms depending on the neuropathology |

## Subcortical Dementias: Dementia of Huntington's Disease, Parkinson's Disease, Wilson's Disease, or Supranuclear Palsy?

| Huntington's Disease | Parkinson's Disease | Wilson's Disease | Supranuclear Palsy |
|---|---|---|---|
| Sporadic onset | Insidious onset | Gradual onset | Gradual onset |
| Genetic and nongenetic causes; involvement of substantia negra | Degenerative disease of the CNS; loss of Golgi cells in corpus striatum | Involvement of the basal ganglia; excessive amount of copper in the brain and liver | Involvement of reticular formation, thalamus, or hypothalamus |
| Neuromotor symptoms of shuffling and jerky gait, chorea | Neuromotor symptoms of tremor, rigidity, slowness, bradykinesia, postural instability | Neuromotor symptoms of tremor, rigidity, slowness, bradykinesia, ataxia, dysphagia, mask-like face | Neuromotor symptoms of pseudobulbar palsy, dystonia, rigidity of head and neck and retracted head position |

*(continues)*

(continued)

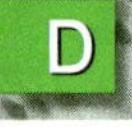

| Huntington's Disease | Parkinson's Disease | Wilson's Disease | Supranuclear Palsy |
|---|---|---|---|
| Depression and significant language impairment even in the early stages; dysarthria; intervals of inappropriate silence | Speech impairment greater than language impairment; weak, breathy voice; dysarthria; abnormal pitch and loudness | Dysarthria; irregular articulatory breakdown; hypernasality; intervals of inappropriate silence | Inaudible speech; harsh sounds; dysarthria |

## Prognosis

- Generally, more favorable for reversible than irreversible dementia
- Prognosis for stopping the course of irreversible dementia is not good; but prognosis for better clinical management, and in most cases, slowing down the course of deterioration in behavior and skills until the last stage is good

## Recommendations

- Communication treatment for clients in the early stages of all dementia
- Treatment directed toward management of problems (including compensatory strategies) in clients with more advanced stages of irreversible dementia
- Counseling for the family members and family-oriented treatment or clinical management for all clients, especially for those in the advanced stages of irreversible dementia
- See the cited sources and the two companion volumes, *Hegde's PocketGuide to Communication Disorders* and *Hegde's PocketGuide to Treatment in Speech-Language Pathology* (3rd ed.)

American Psychiatric Association (1994). *Diagnostic and statistical manual of mental disorders* (4th ed.). Washington, DC: Author.

Bayles, K. A., & Kaszniak, A. W. (1987). *Communication and cognition in normal aging and dementia*. Austin, TX: Pro-Ed.

Brookshire, R. H. (2003). *An introduction to neurogenic communication disorders* (6th ed.). St. Louis, MO: Mosby Year Book.

Clark, C. M., & Trojanowski, J. Q. (2001). *Neurodegenerative dementias*. New York: McGraw-Hill.

Cummings, J. L., & Benson, D. F. (1983). *Dementia: A clinical approach*. Boston, MA: Butterworth.

Hegde, M. N. (2006). *A coursebook on aphasia and other neurogenic language disorders* (3rd ed.). Clifton Park, NY: Thomson Delmar Learning.

Jacques, A., & Jackson, G. A. (2000). *Understanding dementia* (3rd ed.). New York: Churchill-Livingstone.

Lubinski, R. (1991). *Dementia and communication*. Philadelphia, PA: B. C. Decker.

Ripich, D. N. (1991). *Geriatric communication disorders*. Austin, TX: Pro-Ed.

Weiner, M. F. (1996). *The dementias: Diagnosis, management, and research* (2nd ed.). Washington, DC: American Psychiatric Association.

Wells, C. E. (1980). The differential diagnosis of psychiatric disorders in the elderly. In J. Cole & J. Barrett (Eds.), *Psychopathology in the aged* (pp. 19–29). New York: Raven Press.



**Dementia, Reversible.** Assessment of temporary decline in intellectual functions and deterioration in behavior that may be checked or reversed by prompt treatment is essential to distinguish it from reversible decline; this type of dementia is associated with various medical conditions that are not degenerative and may be treated; see the cited sources and *Hegde's PocketGuide to Communication Disorders* for details on epidemiology, etiology, and symptomatology.

### *Assessment of Reversible Dementia*

- Use the general guidelines and procedures described under the previous entry on progressive dementia to assess reversible dementia; because the symptoms bear gross similarities, it is appropriate to use similar assessment procedures to document intellectual and behavioral decline
- Note that although the major dementia symptoms may be common to the two varieties, the differential diagnosis is made on the basis of associated clinical conditions; assess the following to differentially diagnose reversible dementia from the progressive varieties:
  - Review the client record to see whether there is evidence of a neurodegenerative disease (e.g., Alzheimer's disease, Huntington's disease, Pick's disease, Parkinson's disease, Wilson's disease); if so, the dementia is most likely progressive; in such cases, neuromotor disorders associated with those diseases also help establish a progressive form of dementia
  - Review the history to evaluate whether the onset was sudden or slow; if the symptoms had a slow (insidious) onset, then the client's dementia is most likely progressive; if the onset is relatively sudden, then in most clients the dementia may be reversible; among the few exceptions are the dementias due to Creutzfeldt-Jakob disease and traumatic brain injury; both may have a relatively rapid onset and progression; however, in these two instances, a history of possible infection (Creutzfeldt-Jakob disease) or a history of recent brain injury helps distinguish them from progressive neurological disorders
  - Review the case history and medical test results to identify potential drug toxicities; evidence of toxicity due to drugs prescribed, especially for mental illnesses and convulsion disorders, helps establish a diagnosis of reversible versus progressive dementia
  - Review the medical records for evidence of such psychiatric disorders as depression, mania, and schizophrenia that may give the impression of dementia (often described as pseudodementia)
  - Check the medical records to evaluate any evidence for serious vitamin deficiencies (especially B1 and B12) or evidence for metabolic disorders that may help diagnose reversible dementia

**Denasality (Hyponasality).** Assessment of reduced or absent nasal resonance on nasal sounds is important in diagnosing resonance disorders found in clients with Cleft Palate, Dysarthria, and Voice Disorders; see these main entries for assessment procedures.

**Developmental Dysarthria.** This type of motor speech disorder is diagnosed in children with neuromuscular problems; most often diagnosed in children with CP; for assessment procedures, see CP.

D

**Developmental Norms for Phonemes.** Ages at which different phonemes are acquired or mastered by children speaking normally; often used to evaluate whether a child has an articulation disorder; the child who omits or substitutes a sound at an age when others of the same age produce the same sound correctly is said to have an articulation disorder.

- There are wide discrepancies across studies in reported ages at which specific sounds are mastered
- Some or most of the differences may be due to methodological variations across studies; definitions of mastery across investigators vary; it may be defined as:
  - Correct production of a sound in all positions by 75% of the children tested
  - Correct production of a sound by 51% of tested children to derive a *customary age of acquisition*
  - Correct articulation of a sound only in initial and medial word positions
  - Correct production of a sound in all positions
- Limitations of developmental norms, to be taken into consideration during assessment, include the following:
  - Norms belong to the tradition of standardized testing
  - Norms are based on data that are averaged across children; they may or may not apply to an individual child
  - Normative ages of mastery of speech sounds provide only broad guidelines but fail to predict performance of any individual child
  - There are significant individual differences in the age of acquisition of speech sounds
  - Most norms are based on white, monolingual, English speaking, middle class children, although test developers are making efforts to sample children belonging to minority groups
  - Norms developed for ethnocultural minority groups are limited or nonexistent; therefore, exercise caution in using group means in evaluating an individual child's performance, especially if the child belongs to an ethnocultural minority group
- Use the norms in the context of accepted practice within your clinical setting to diagnose an articulation disorder or to determine the need for treatment; the most commonly reported normative data for the English consonants follow:

| Phonemes | Wellman (1934) | Poole (1934) | Templin (1957) | Sander (1972) | Prather (1975) | Arlt & Goodban (1976) |
|---|---|---|---|---|---|---|
| /m/ | 3 | 3–6 | 3 | before 2 | 2 | 3 |
| /n/ | 3 | 4–6 | 3 | before 2 | 2 | 3 |
| /h/ | 3 | 3–6 | 3 | before 2 | 2 | 3 |

*(continues)*

*(continued)*

| Phonemes | Wellman (1934) | Poole (1934) | Templin (1957) | Sander (1972) | Prather (1975) | Arlt & Goodban (1976) |
|---|---|---|---|---|---|---|
| /p/ | 4 | 3–6 | 3 | before 2 | 2 | 3 |
| /f/ | 3 | 5–6 | 3 | 3 | 2–4 | 3 |
| /w/ | 3 | 3–6 | 3 | before 2 | 2–8 | 3 |
| /b/ | 3 | 3–6 | 4 | before 2 | 2–8 | 3 |
| /ŋ/ | – | 4–6 | 3 | 2 | 2 | 3 |
| /j/ | 4 | 4–6 | 3–6 | 3 | 2–4 | - |
| /k/ | 4 | 4–6 | 4 | 2 | 2–4 | 3 |
| /g/ | 4 | 4–6 | 4 | 2 | 2–4 | 3 |
| /l/ | 4 | 6–6 | 6 | 3 | 2–4 | 4 |
| /d/ | 5 | 4–6 | 4 | 2 | 2–4 | 3 |
| /t/ | 5 | 4–6 | 6 | 2 | 2–8 | 3 |
| /s/ | 5 | 7–6 | 4–6 | 3 | 3 | 4 |
| /r/ | 5 | 7–6 | 4 | 3 | 3–4 | 5 |
| /ʧ/ | 5 | – | 4–6 | 4 | 3–8 | 4 |
| /v/ | 5 | 6–6 | 6 | 4 | 4+ | 3–6 |
| /z/ | 5 | 7–6 | 7 | 4 | 4+ | 4 |
| /ʒ/ | 6 | 6–6 | 7 | 6 | 4 | 4 |
| /θ/ | - | 7–6 | 6 | 5 | 4+ | 5 |
| /ʤ/ | - | - | 7 | 4 | 4+ | 4 |
| /ʃ/ | - | 6–6 | 4–6 | 4 | 3–8 | 4–6 |
| /ð/ | - | 6–6 | 7 | 5 | 4 | 5 |

*Note: + sound not mastered by 75% of tested children, - sound not tested or reported.*

- In assessing children with articulation disorders, consider the general trends noted across studies in children's development of consonants
  - By age 3, most children consistently produce /h/, /w/, /m/, /n/, /b/, /p/, and /f/
  - By age 4, most children consistently produce the previously mastered sounds plus /d/, /t/, /j/, /k/, /g/, and /ŋ/
  - By age 6, most children consistently produce the previously mastered sounds plus /l/, /ʤ/, /ʧ/, /ʃ/, and /v/; however, errors on /r/, /s/, /z/, /θ/, /ð/, and /ʒ/ may persist
  - By age 8 to 9, most children's speech sound productions match the adult standard for the production of all consonant sounds
- In assessing children with articulation disorders, consider the consonants that are mastered the earliest and those that are mastered latest

  - Sounds mastered relatively early: /j/, /w/, /m/, /n/, /ŋ/, /p/, /b/, /k/, /g/, /d/, /t/, /f/, /h/
  - Sounds mastered relatively late: /l/, /r/, /ð/, /θ/, /ʧ/, /ʤ/, /ʃ/, /ʒ/, /s/, /z/, /v/
- In assessing children with articulation disorders, consider the following developmental information for English consonantal clusters (blends)
- Note that the mastery criterion is 75% of children producing a cluster correctly

| Age | Initial clusters | Final clusters |
|---|---|---|
| 4–0 | pl, bl, kl, gl<br>pr, br, tr, dr, kr<br>tw, kw<br>sm, sn, sp, st, sk | mp, mpt, mps, ngk<br>lp, lt, rm, rt, rk<br>pt, ks, ft |
| 5–0 | gr, fl, fr, str | lb, lf, rd, rf, rn |
| 6–0 | skw | lk<br>rb, rg, rθ, rʤ, rst, rʧ<br>nt, nd, nθ |
| 7–0 | spl, spr, skr<br>sl, sw<br>ʃr, θr | sk, st, kst<br>lθ, lz<br>ʤd |
| 8–0 | | kt, sp |

- In assessing children with articulation disorders, consider the following developmental information for English vowels and diphthongs:
  - Children within the age range of 1.6 to 1.11 achieve 90% mastery of the following vowels and diphthongs: /ə/, /ʌ/, /ɛ/, /a/, /æ/, /ɔ/, /ɪ/, /i/, /ʊ/, /u/, /ou/, /ai/, /ei/, and /au/
  - The mid-central vowels /ɝ/ and /ɚ/ may not reach the mastery criterion of 90% until the age range of 5–6 to 5–11

Arlt, P. B., & Goodban, M. T. (1976). A comparative study of articulation acquisition as based on a study of 240 normals, aged three to six. *Language, Speech, and Hearing Services in Schools, 7*, 173–180. (Criterion: 75% of children tested in all three word positions).

Poole, I. (1934). Genetic development of consonant sounds in English. *Elementary English Review, 11,* 159–161. (Criterion: 100% of children tested in all three word positions).

Prather, E. M., Hedrick, E. L., & Kerin, C. A. (1975). Articulation development in children aged two to four years. *Journal of Speech and Hearing Disorders, 40*, 179–191. (Criterion: 75% of children tested; average for initial and final word positions).

Sander, E. K. (1972). When are speech sounds learned? *Journal of Speech and Hearing Disorders, 37*, 55–63. (Reanalysis of Templin and Wellman et al.'s data with a criterion of 51%).

Stoel-Gammon, C., & Dunn, C. (1985). *Normal and disordered phonology in children.* Austin, TX: Pro-Ed.

Templin, M. C. (1957). Certain language skills in children. *Institute of Child Welfare Monograph Series No. 26*. Minneapolis, MN: University of

Minnesota Press. (Criterion: 75% of children tested in all three word positions).

Wellman, B., Case, I., Mengert, I., & Bradbury, D. (1931). Speech sounds of young children. *State University of Iowa Studies in Child Welfare, 5* (2). (Criterion: 75% of children tested in all three word positions).

D

**Diadachokinetic Rates.** Also known as the Alternating Motion Rates (AMRs), the diadachokinetic rates refer to the rapidity of coordinated movements of the articulators; assessed in cases of most speech disorders including articulation and phonological disorders, apraxia of speech, and dysarthria; included in assessment of almost all clients as a standard procedure; see Alternating Motion Rates (AMRs); use the following form from Peña-Brooks and Hegde (2007) to make an assessment of diadachokinetic rate and record the results

**Diadochokinetic Syllable Rates Form**

Name: ______________________________

DOB: ________

Age: _____

Grade: ______

Teacher: __________________

Referred by: ______________

Reason for Referral: ____________________

Date of Exam: _____________

____*Pretreatment Assessment*

____*Posttreatment Assessment*

Instruct to the child: "Please take a deep breath and say ______________ as long and as evenly as you can." Model the response for the child to imitate to avoid misunderstanding of the task. Say, "Try doing it like me . . ."

| | | |
|---|---|---|
| [pʌ-pə-pə] | # or repetitions_________ | # of seconds__________ |
| [tʌ-tə-tə] | # of repetitions_________ | # of seconds__________ |
| [kʌ-kə-kə] | # of repetitions_________ | # of seconds__________ |
| [fʌ-fə-fə] | # or repetitions_________ | # of seconds__________ |
| [lʌ-lə-lə] | # or repetitions_________ | # of seconds__________ |
| [pʌ-tə-kə] | # or repetitions_________ | # of seconds__________ |

*(continues)*

*(continued)*

Compare child's performance to the following developmental data:

| Average number of seconds to make | | | | | | | | | |
|---|---|---|---|---|---|---|---|---|---|
| | 20 reps of | | | | | 15 reps of | | | 10 reps of |
| Age | pʌ | tʌ | kʌ | fʌ | lʌ | pʌtə | pʌkə | tʌtə | pʌtəkə |
| 6 | 4.8 | 4.9 | 5.5 | 5.5 | 5.2 | 7.3 | 7.9 | 7.8 | 10.3 |
| 7 | 4.8 | 4.9 | 5.3 | 5.4 | 5.3 | 7.6 | 8.0 | 8.0 | 10.0 |
| 8 | 4.2 | 4.4 | 4.8 | 4.9 | 4.6 | 6.2 | 7.1 | 7.2 | 8.3 |
| 9 | 4.0 | 4.1 | 4.6 | 4.6 | 4.5 | 5.9 | 6.6 | 6.6 | 7.7 |
| 10 | 3.7 | 3.8 | 4.3 | 4.2 | 4.2 | 5.5 | 6.4 | 6.4 | 7.1 |
| 11 | 3.6 | 3.6 | 4.0 | 4.0 | 3.8 | 4.8 | 5.8 | 5.8 | 6.5 |
| 12 | 3.4 | 3.5 | 3.9 | 3.7 | 3.7 | 4.7 | 5.7 | 5.5 | 6.4 |
| 13 | 3.3 | 3.3 | 3.7 | 3.6 | 3.5 | 4.2 | 5.1 | 5.1 | 5.7 |

(*Source:* Fletcher 1972, 1978)

Clinical Impressions and Recommendations: ______________________________

______________________________________________________________

____________________

Speech-Language Pathologist ________________________________________

Peña-Brooks, A., & Hegde, M. N. (2007). *Articulation and phonological disorders: Assessment and treatment resource manual.* Austin, TX: Pro-Ed.

**Diagnosis.** Narrowly defined, a clinical activity designed to find causes of diseases or disorders, especially in medicine and medical speech-language pathology; in a broader sense and especially for communicative disorders with no known physical or neurological cause, diagnosis often is aimed at determining that a disorder exists and then describing and assessing the nature and the degree of severity of the disorder; related clinical activities include making a prognostic statement about the course of the disorder and recommending treatment; requires precise and reliable measurement of communicative behaviors; sometimes means the same as Assessment, although many consider *assessment* a means to make a specific diagnosis; whether considered narrowly or broadly, to diagnose a disorder, the clinician should:

- Take a case history
- Interview the client

- Screen hearing
- Conduct an orofacial examination
- Administer standardized tests that are culturally and linguistically appropriate for the client
- Design and use client-specific procedures
- Take a comprehensive speech-language sample
- Analyze the results to diagnose a disorder and make clinical judgments
- Write a diagnostic report that includes the diagnosis, prognosis, and recommendations

**Differential Diagnosis.** Distinguishing disorders that present some common or similar symptoms and sometimes similar etiological factors with subtle variations; usually done with the help of a symptom complex, and whenever possible, by identifying different underlying factors or causes; an important task of assessment needed to make effective and specific treatment recommendations.

**Diplophonia.** Double voice resulting from differential vibration of the two folds or vibration of both the true and false vocal folds; a disorder of voice; see Voice Disorder for assessment.

**Distinctive Features.** Assessment of distinctive features was once considered a part of assessing speech disorders and finding patterns in articulation errors; distinctive feature analysis has largely given way to phonological process analysis; nonetheless, an understanding of distinctive features is essential to view articulation disorders from varied perspectives; features are unique characteristics of phonemes that distinguish one phoneme from the other; each feature is scored as + (for its presence) or - (for its absence); may be used in economically describing errors of articulation and their changes in treatment; Chomsky-Halle's major distinctive features as applied to consonants are shown in the matrix; the definition of the features follow:

| | Con | Son | Hi | Bck | Rnd | Ant | Cor | Voi | Cnt | Nas | Str |
|---|---|---|---|---|---|---|---|---|---|---|---|
| /p/ | + | - | - | - | - | + | - | - | - | - | - |
| /b/ | + | - | - | - | - | + | - | + | - | - | - |
| /t/ | + | - | - | - | - | + | + | - | - | - | - |
| /d/ | + | - | - | - | - | + | + | + | - | - | - |
| /k/ | + | - | + | + | - | - | - | - | - | - | - |
| /g/ | + | - | + | + | - | - | - | + | - | - | - |
| /f/ | + | - | - | - | - | + | - | - | + | - | + |
| /v/ | + | - | - | - | - | + | - | + | + | - | + |
| /θ/ | + | - | - | - | - | + | + | - | + | - | - |
| /ð/ | + | - | - | - | - | + | + | + | + | - | - |
| /S/ | + | - | - | - | - | + | + | - | + | - | + |

*(continues)*

(continued)

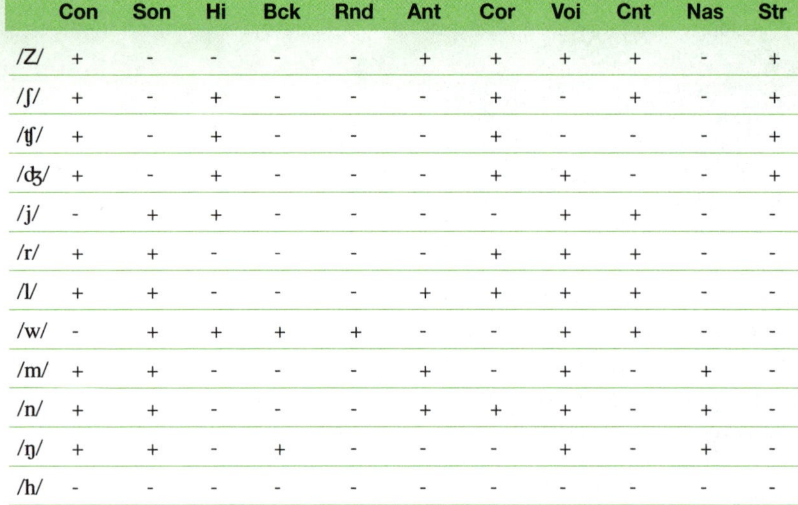

| | Con | Son | Hi | Bck | Rnd | Ant | Cor | Voi | Cnt | Nas | Str |
|---|---|---|---|---|---|---|---|---|---|---|---|
| /Z/ | + | - | - | - | - | + | + | + | + | - | + |
| /ʃ/ | + | - | + | - | - | - | + | - | + | - | + |
| /ʧ/ | + | - | + | - | - | - | + | - | - | - | + |
| /ʤ/ | + | - | + | - | - | - | + | + | - | - | + |
| /j/ | - | + | + | - | - | - | - | + | + | - | - |
| /r/ | + | + | - | - | - | - | + | + | + | - | - |
| /l/ | + | + | - | - | - | + | + | + | + | - | - |
| /w/ | - | + | + | + | + | - | - | + | + | - | - |
| /m/ | + | + | - | - | - | + | - | + | - | + | - |
| /n/ | + | + | - | - | - | + | + | + | - | + | - |
| /ŋ/ | + | + | - | + | - | - | - | + | - | + | - |
| /h/ | - | - | - | - | - | - | - | - | - | - | - |

*Con: Consonant (sounds characterized by vocal tract constriction)*

*Son: Sonorant (sounds with spontaneous voicing because of unobstructed flow of air)*

*Hi: High (sounds produced with elevated tongue position)*

*Bck: Back (sounds produced with the tongue retracted)*

*Rnd: Rounded: sounds made with lip rounding*

*Ant: Anterior (sounds produced with point of constriction being relatively anterior; sounds made in the front of the mouth)*

*Cor: Coronal (sounds produced with raised tongue blade)*

*Voi: Voiced sounds (sounds produced with vocal fold vibration)*

*Cnt: Continuant (sounds produced with partial obstruction of airflow; sounds that can be produced in a continuous manner)*

*Nas: Nasal (sounds produced with nasal resonance)*

*Str: Strident (sounds produced by forcing airstream through a small opening)*

## Development of Distinctive Features

- In assessing distinctive features of speech sound in children with articulation disorders, consider the earliest to latest developing distinctive feature groups as listed:
  - + *nasal*—sounds resonated in the nasal cavity
  - + *grave*—sounds produced at the very front
  - + *voice*—sounds produced with vibration of the vocal folds
  - + *diffuse*—sounds made at the very back
  - + *strident*—sounds made by forcing the airstream through a small opening resulting in the production of intense noise
  - + *continuant*—sounds that are made with an incomplete point of constriction, and thus the flow of air is not stopped entirely at any point
- In assessing distinctive features of speech sound in children with articulation disorders, consider the general sequence of mastery
  - 2-year-olds will have mastered nasal-nonnasal distinctions as well as labial-lingual features

- 3-year-olds will have mastered the vocalic system (vowels)
- 4-year-olds will have mastered the stop-nasal distinction
- 5-year-olds or even those approaching their 5th year will have mastered semivowel features
- 6-year-olds or even those approaching their 6th year will have mastered the continuant features
- 7-year-olds or even those completing their 7th year will have mastered the sibilant features



### *Analysis of Distinctive Features of Articulatory Errors*

- Record a representative, continuous speech sample; follow the procedures described under Articulation and Phonological Disorders
- Transcribe the speech; list all the errors
- For each error, score the distinctive features using the features listed in the matrix; score features that are correctly used for each sound and those that are misused (voicing a voiceless sound is a misuse of the voicing feature)
- Score all features that characterize omitted sounds as incorrect
- Summarize the missing and misused features
- Target the sounds that contain missing or misused features for treatment

### *Limitations of the Distinctive Feature Approach*

- Scoring all features of omitted sounds as incorrect may not be appropriate because the sounds are not even attempted
- Distinctive features based on acoustic analysis may or may not be directly related to articulatory productions that are physiological events
- Errors of sound productions often are not binary events (presence or absence); but are quantitatively varied
- Distinctive features do not account for sound distortions
- Scoring according to the Chomsky-Halle system is extremely time consuming and complex
- Currently, phonological analysis seems to be preferred over distinctive feature analysis
- Note that as you make a phonological analysis, distinctive features that are missing or help group errors may be accomplished to obtain a different view of the error patterns

Bernthal, J. E., & Bankson, N. W. (2004). *Articulation and phonological disorders* (5th ed.). Englewood Cliffs, NJ: Prentice Hall.

Lowe, R. J. (1994). *Phonology: Assessment and intervention applications in speech pathology.* Baltimore, MD: Williams & Wilkins.

Peña-Brooks, A., & Hegde, M. N. (2007). *Assessment and treatment of articulation and phonological disorders in children* (2nd ed.). Austin, TX: Pro-Ed.

Smit, A. B. (2004). *Articulation and phonology: Resource guide for school-age children and adults.* Clifton Park, NY: Thomson Delmar Learning.

Stoel-Gammon, C., & Dunn, C. (1985). *Normal and disordered phonology in children.* Austin, TX: Pro-Ed.

Williams, A. L. (2003). *Speech disorders: Resource guide for preschool children.* Clifton Park, NY: Thomson Delmar Learning.

**Dynamic Aphasia.** To assess this type of aphasia, also known as Transcortical Motor Aphasia, see Aphasia: Specific Types.

D

**Dysarthrias.** Assessment of a group of motor speech disorders resulting from disturbed muscular control of the speech mechanism due to damage of the peripheral or central nervous system is essential to distinguish them from other kinds of speech disorders without a neurophysiological basis; most of the symptoms are due to weakness, incoordination, or paralysis of speech musculature; assessment efforts will be extensive because almost all aspects of speech production, including pitch, loudness, voice quality, resonance, respiratory support for speech, prosody, and articulation may be impaired to varying degrees; assessment of motor speech disorders is a complex process not only because all processes of speech need to be attended to, but also because the impairments are due to varied neuropathologies; dysarthrias are classified into ataxic dysarthria, flaccid dysarthria, hyperkinetic dysarthria, hypokinetic dysarthria, mixed dysarthria, spastic dysarthria, and unilateral motor neuron dysarthria; see the cited sources at the end of this main entry and *Hegde's PocketGuide to Communication Disorders* for information on epidemiology, ethnocultural variables, etiologic factors, general symptoms of dysarthria, and dysarthria of specific types; use this section to make a general assessment of dysarthria and see Dysarthria: Specific Types to distinguish among them.

### *Assessment Objectives/General Guidelines*

- To determine whether dysarthria is the diagnosis of the speech disorder constellation seen in a client
- To describe the specific respiratory, phonatory, articulatory, and prosodic characteristics of speech associated with dysarthria
- To help make an assessment of a potential neuroanatomical basis of dysarthria, although this may not be possible in all cases
- To help make a differential diagnosis; to help distinguish dysarthria from other speech disorders that may be due to structural anomalies unrelated to neuropathology that causes dysarthria, a severe form of articulation disorder, neurogenic stuttering; apraxia of speech, aphasia with dysarthric symptoms, traumatic brain injury, and similar conditions that share a few or more features
- To judge the severity of the disorder that will have implications for management, treatment, future assessments of the same client
- To judge whether further assessment to specify the type of dysarthria is necessary
- To determine potential treatment targets to improve dysarthric speech
- To suggest potential augmentative or alternative forms of communication if the assessment results warrant them
- To suggest a prognosis based on the interpretation of results and a diagnosis (if that were to be feasible) under the given conditions of intervention or no intervention

### *Case History/Interview Focus*

- See **Case History** and **Interview** under Standard/Common Assessment Procedures

- Note that a detailed case history, with an emphasis on the client's speech and changes in speech, is essential to most neurological diagnoses, especially for dysarthria
- Concentrate on a detailed health history; because dysarthria is a symptom associated with neurological disorders, it is essential to either examine the recorded medical history of the client or gather as much information as possible on the various neurological diseases that are associated with this type of motor speech disorder
- Concentrate on the behavioral changes and signs of neurologic disorder
- Seek information from the client's family members on the neurobehavioral consequences of the disorder for which the client is being evaluated



### *Ethnocultural Considerations*

- See Ethnocultural Considerations in Assessment
- Note that the influence of ethnocultural factors in dementia are poorly understood; use the general guidelines specified under Ethnocultural Considerations in Assessment; and pay special attention to the family's:
  - Resources and needed support systems
  - Access to health care and speech-language services
  - Views on long-term disabilities and their rehabilitation efforts
  - Capabilities in working with the client who may have a long-term disability
  - Need for education and information on the client's medical condition and speech-language pathology services

### *Assessment*

- Take a conversational speech sample; note the manner and content of speech as you interview the client
- Record a reading sample; have the client read the *Grandfather* passage
- Assess impairments in speech production with a variety of speech tasks
  - Model syllable productions and ask the client to imitate them
  - Model word, phrase, and sentence productions and ask the client to imitate them
  - Ask the client to take a deep breath and say "ah" as long as possible and note the duration for which the client sustains any steady phonation
  - Note the following minimum and maximum phonation durations (with standard deviations in parentheses) for different groups of individuals; note especially the gender differences in maximum phonation duration
    - Young males: 22.6 (5.5) to 34.6 (11.4)
    - Young females: 15.2 (4.1) to 26.5 (11.3)
    - Elderly males: 13.0 (5.9) to 18.1 (6.6)
    - Elderly females: 10.0 (5.6) to 15.4 (5.8)
- Assess the Diadochokinetic Rate or Alternating Motion Rates (ARMs) and Sequential Motion Rates (SMRs)
- Assess the speech production mechanism during nonspeech activities
  - Observe the face at rest; take note of symmetry, tone, signs of tension, droopiness, expressive or mask-like, and the presence of involuntary movements and tremors

- Observe the movements of the facial structures by asking the client to puff the cheeks; retract and round the lips; bite the lower lip; blow; smack the lips; open and close the mouth; maintain an opened posture of the mouth; and so forth
- Observe the client's emotional expressions
- Take note of the client's jaw at rest; its range of movement and tone; its deviation to one or the other side during movement; resistance offered as you try to close it or open it
- Observe the tongue as you ask the client to protrude, move it from side to side as fast as possible; lick the lips; push the cheeks out with it; resist your attempts to push the protruded tongue back; and so forth
- Observe the velopharyngeal mechanism as the client says "ah"; take note of movement, its symmetry, range, and adequacy; assess nasal airflow by holding a mirror at the nares as the client prolongs the vowel /i/
- Assess laryngeal functions by asking the client to cough; take note of weak cough associated with weak adduction of the cords, inadequate breath support, or both

- Assess respiratory problems
  - Observe the client's posture that might affect breathing; take note of erect or slouched posture
  - Observe the client's breathing habits during quiet and speech; take note of rapid, shallow, or effortful breathing, signs of shortness of breath, and irregularity of inhalation and exhalation
  - Take note of the presence of inhalatory stridor, forced inspiration or expiration, or grunt at end of expiration
- Assess phonatory disorders
  - Have the client to say "ah" after taking a deep breath; ask the client to sustain it as steadily and for as long as the air supply lasts; if the client's pitch or loudness changes, request a more normal repetition of the task; specify whether the client should try to lower or raise the pitch or loudness; see Maximum Phonation Duration for normative values
  - During the interview and conversational speech, take note of the client's pitch level; judge or rate its appropriateness to the client
  - Take note of pitch breaks and abrupt variations in pitch
  - Judge whether pitch variations are normal or absent, resulting in monopitch
  - Take note of voice tremors as the client speaks
  - Assess the presence of diplophonia
  - Judge the appropriateness of vocal loudness; take note of too soft or too loud voice; take note of loudness that is highly variable
  - Take note of loudness decay and alternating changes in loudness
  - Judge the quality of voice; take note of hoarseness, harshness, and breathiness; take note of their severity and consistency
  - Judge whether the voice production is strained or effortful
  - Take note of sudden cessations of voice
- Assess articulation disorders
  - Use the speech sample and standardized test results

- Rate or evaluate consonant productions; judge the precision with which they are produced
- Evaluate the duration of speech sounds; take note of prolongation of phonemes
- Record the frequency of phoneme repetitions
- Take note of irregular breakdowns in articulation
- Assess the precision with which vowels are produced; take note of distortions
- Judge the adequacy of pressure consonantal productions

- Assess prosodic disorders
  - Measure the rate of speech; judge whether the rate is normal, slower than normal, or excessively fast
  - Judge whether the speech rate is highly variable; take note of progressive increase in rate in segments of speech
  - Measure phrase lengths in selected portions of speech; judge their adequacy
  - Evaluate stress patterns in speech; take note of inappropriate stress patterns including even stress, lack of stress, and undue stress on normally unstressed syllables
  - Take note of pauses or silent periods in speech; judge whether they are at appropriate or inappropriate junctures and whether they are too long
  - Take note of any short rushes of speech
- Assess resonance disorders
  - Make clinical judgments as you listen to the client's speech or make an instrumental analysis; see Voice Disorders
  - Take note of hypernasality, hyponasality, and nasal emission
- Assess other characteristics
  - Assess the client's proneness to general fatigue or deterioration in speech with prolonged conversation; ask the client to read an extended passage to note deterioration in all aspects of speech production
  - Take note of palilalia; evaluate the rate at which repetitions occur; observe whether loudness of such repetitions decreases as the rate increases
  - Assess a concomitant apraxia of speech; generally, such tasks as repeating speech sounds, words, sentences, counting to 10, reciting the days of the week, singing a familiar song, and a test of alternating motion rates will help assess verbal apraxia; see Apraxia of Speech for assessment procedures
- Assess the global characteristics of communication
  - Assess speech intelligibility; note that intelligibility may not always be negatively affected in dysarthria
  - Make a clinical judgment of intelligibility, which may be adequate in many cases; estimate the percentage of words or phrases that you understand
  - Administer a rating scale to assess intelligibility; use a scale such as the one Duffy (2005) describes
  - Use a rating scale, such as the one Duffy (2005) describes, to more formally evaluate speech disorders associated with dysarthria
  - Assess the client's overall communicative effectiveness; use a questionnaire of the kind given in Yorkston, Beukelman, Strand, and Bell (1999)

D

### *Standardized Tests*

- Note that there are very few comprehensive tests of dysarthric speech; therefore, it is essential to design client-specific procedures to assess clients with dysarthria
- Administer the latest edition of one or more of the following tests:

| Test | Purpose |
|---|---|
| *Assessment of the Intelligibility in Dysarthric Speakers* (K. M. Yorkston & D. Beukelman) | To assess single-word and sentence intelligibility and rate of speech |
| *Computerized Assessment of the Intelligibility of Dysarthric Speakers* (K. M. Yorkston, D. Beukelman, & C. D. Traynor) | To assess dysarthric speech intelligibility through computerized analysis and judgment |
| *Dysarthria Examination Battery* (S. S. Drummond) | To assess severity of dysarthria and functional communication |
| *Frenchay Dysarthria Assessment* (P. M. Enderby) | To assess speech-related structures and function in dysarthric speakers and to distinguish different types of dysarthria |
| *Phonetic Intelligibility Test* (R. D. Kent, G. Weismer, J. F. Kent, & J. C. Rosenbek) | To assess the intelligibility of dysarthric speech by examining the relationship between phonetic and perceptual properties of speech |

### *Related/Medical Assessment Data*

- Ascertain the client's medical-neurological diagnosis
- Find out the client's current medication(s) and its side effects
- Understand the current and future medical treatment plans for the client
- Know the client's medical prognosis (e.g., Parkinson's disease, Pick's disease, amyotrophic lateral sclerosis, vascular diseases) that may be associated with different types of dysarthria
- Review the client's radiological and brain imaging data that might be integrated or correlated with speech diagnosis
- Understand the physical rehabilitation plans that might affect communication treatment
- Obtain the results of audiologic assessment that might be integrated with communication assessment

### *Standard/Common Assessment Procedures*

- Complete the Standard/Common Assessment Procedures
- Pay special attention to the orofacial examination to fully understand weakness or paralysis in the orofacial muscles that contribute to dysarthric speech

### *Analysis of Assessment Data*

- Analyze and summarize the assessment data to determine the nature of physiological (speech movement related), respiratory, articulatory, prosodic, phonatory, and resonance disorders
- Integrate the findings with medical-neurological assessment data to obtain a comprehensive profile of the client's physiological, neurological, and behavioral (including communication) performance

### *Diagnostic Criteria*

- Clear evidence of peripheral or central nervous system damage
- An associated medical-neurological diagnosis with clear evidence of disturbed strength, speed, range, steadiness, tone, and accuracy of movement patterns, although in some cases dysarthria may be diagnosed in the absence of a clear neurological or physical diagnosis
- Speech characteristics that support a diagnosis of dysarthria, including disturbed phonation, articulation, prosody, and resonance, and supplemented by disturbed respiratory support for speech

### *Differential Diagnosis*

- Initially, determine whether the diagnosis is dysarthria
- If dysarthria, then proceed to make further assessment to determine the type of dysarthria (see Dysarthria: Specific Types)
- Find out whether the medical, neurological, radiological, and brain imaging data suggest a specific etiology that might support a particular type of dysarthria; however, take note that:
    - Many etiological conditions are the same for different types of dysarthria; therefore, just the knowledge of a neuropathology (e.g., vascular pathology, which can cause different types of dysarthria) is not sufficient to diagnose a particular type
    - Dysarthria may exist even when a reliable neuropathological diagnosis is not possible and neuropathology remains doubtful
- To make a differential diagnosis of a particular type of dysarthria, consider the overall picture of the client with an emphasis on the dominant neuropathological problems and communication deficits
    - Diagnose flaccid dysarthria if:
        - Neuromotor weakness, hypotonia, and diminished reflexes are the dominant neuromotor symptoms
        - Hypernasality, continuous breathiness, nasal emission, audible inspiration, and short phrases are the dominant communication problems
        - The presence of amyotrophic lateral sclerosis (ALS) and surgical trauma involving ear, nose, throat, and chest offer strong supportive evidence
    - Diagnose spastic dysarthria if:
        - Spasticity is the dominant neuromotor sign
        - Imprecise consonants, harshness of voice, low pitch, slow rate, short phrases, and pitch breaks are the dominant communication problems
        - The presence of ALS, vascular diseases (especially nonhemorrhagic strokes) offer strong supportive evidence
    - Diagnose ataxic dysarthria if:
        - Uncoordination is the dominant neuromotor sign
        - Excess and equal stress, irregular articulatory breakdowns, distorted vowels, prolonged phonemes, and excess loudness variations are the dominant communication problems
        - The presence of hypothyroidism, toxic drug effects, multiple sclerosis, and cerebellar diseases offer additional supportive evidence, although ataxic dysarthria has many possible causes and none that is especially strong or frequent causes

D

- Diagnose hypokinetic dysarthria if:
  - Rigidity and reduced range of movement are the dominant neuromotor signs
  - Monopitch, monoloudness, reduced stress, inappropriate silences, short rushes of speech, variable or increased rate, and repetitions of phonemes are the dominant communication problems
  - The presence of Parkinson's disease and Pick's disease offers strong supportive evidence
- Diagnose hyperkinetic dysarthria if:
  - Involuntary movements are the dominant neuromotor sign
  - Prolonged intervals, variable rate, inappropriate silences, excess loudness variations, prolonged phonemes, sudden forced inspiration or expiration, voice stoppages, and transient breathiness are the dominant communication problems
  - The presence of toxic drug effects offers supportive evidence, although hyperkinetic dysarthria has many causes but few that are exclusive to it
- Diagnose unilateral upper motor neuron dysarthria if:
  - A combination of weakness and spasticity seems to be the dominant neuromotor symptom
  - Imprecise articulation, slow diadochokinetic rate, and harshness are the dominant communication problems
  - The brain imaging data suggest unilateral lesions involving the upper motor neurons
  - The presence of vascular diseases (especially aneurysm rupture and nonhemorrhagic strokes) offers strong supportive evidence
- Diagnose mixed dysarthria if:
  - Multiple neuromotor characteristics are evident
  - Heterogeneous cluster of communication disorders is present
  - The presence of diseases or clinical conditions that are frequently associated with each type that is mixed in a case offers supportive evidence
- See the separate alphabetical entries for different types of dysarthria for assessment procedures

- Using the following differential diagnostic grids, distinguish:
  - Dysarthria from apraxia of speech and other neurogenic speech disorders
  - Dysarthria from aphasia
  - Dysarthria from dementia
  - Dysarthria from language of confusion
  - Dysarthria from other relevant disorders based on the following characteristics:

### Dysarthria or Apraxia of Speech?

| Dysarthria | Apraxia of Speech (AOS) |
|---|---|
| The cause is muscle weakness, paralysis, or incoordination | The cause is motor programming deficit, not muscle weakness |

*(continues)*

*(continued)*

| Dysarthria | Apraxia of Speech (AOS) |
|---|---|
| Lesions in supratentorial and other areas (including posterior fossa, spinal structures, or peripheral nerves) | Lesions often in the supratentorial level of the brain |
| Huntington's chorea, parkinsonism, Pick's disease, and ALS *are* associated with dysarthrias | Huntington's chorea, parkinsonism, Pick's disease, and ALS are *not* associated with apraxia |
| Often associated with abnormalities of orofacial mechanism and function | Can be associated with normal orofacial mechanism and function (except for nonverbal oral apraxia [NVOA]) |
| NVOA not typically associated with dysarthrias | NVOA may be associated with AOS |
| Presence of dysphagia | Absence of dysphagia |
| Consistent misarticulations (except for ataxic dysarthria in which articulatory breakdowns are irregular) | Variable misarticulations |
| The same problems with automatic and propositional productions | Better production of automatic utterances than propositional productions |
| Word length (except for in ataxic dysarthria), meaningfulness, frequency of occurrence are *not* significant variables | Word length, meaningfulness, frequency of occurrence are significant variables |
| Distortions and simplification of speech gestures are dominant | Besides distortions, complications of speech gestures may be noticeable |
| Less frequent and less variable dysfluencies | More frequent and more variable dysfluencies |
| Articulatory groping not characteristic | Frequent articulatory groping |
| Few, if any, attempts at self-correction | Many attempts at self-correction |
| Respiratory, phonatory, and resonance problems as significant as articulatory and prosodic problems | Respiratory, phonatory, and resonance problems *not* as significant as articulatory and prosodic problems |
| Most forms (except for unilateral upper motor neuron [UUMN] dysarthria) infrequently associated with aphasia | Frequently associated with aphasia |

## Dysarthria or Aphasia?

| Dysarthria | Aphasia |
|---|---|
| Neurogenic speech disorder | Neurogenic language disorder |
| Lesions in the central nervous system, peripheral nervous system, or both | Lesions in the dominant or left hemisphere language areas and related subcortical structures |
| Weakness, paralysis, incoordination of orofacial muscles are a distinguishing characteristic | Except in cases of facial paralysis, normal oral mechanism |

*(continues)*

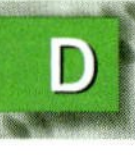

*(continued)*

| Dysarthria | Aphasia |
|---|---|
| Does not affect auditory comprehension and reading | Affects auditory comprehension and reading |
| No significant word finding problems | Word retrieval and related language problem |
| No problems in language formulation or interpretation | Significant problems in language formulation and interpretation |
| Prosodic problems are characteristic | Prosodic problems not dominant, especially in fluent aphasias |

## Dysarthria or the Language of Dementia?

| Dysarthria | Dementia |
|---|---|
| A neurogenic speech disorder | A neurogenic language/cognitive disorder |
| Motor system affected from the beginning | Motor system is spared until the final stages of the disease |
| Many clients with dysarthria do not exhibit dementia | Many clients with dementia may exhibit dysarthria, especially in the later stages |
| Impaired speech functions | Impaired language |
| Intact cognition | Impaired cognition |
| Intact reading comprehension | Disturbed reading comprehension |
| Intact semantic and syntactic functions | Semantic and syntactic errors in the initial stages |
| Errors of articulation prominent from the beginning | Errors of articulation not predominant; such errors appear only in later stages |
| Behavior is relevant, socially appropriate, and not disorganized | Behavior often is irrelevant, socially inappropriate, and disorganized |
| Mentally not confused and not disoriented to time and space | Mentally confused and disoriented to time and space |
| No disorientation to self | Disorientation to self in later stages |

*Note: There is less information on the relationship between dysarthria and dementia. In later stages, clients with dementia exhibit motor speech disorders; dysarthria in such cases may be of the mixed variety. Early stages of subcortical dementias may be associated with dysarthria.*

## Dysarthria or the Language of Confusion?

| Dysarthria | Language of Confusion |
|---|---|
| A neurogenic speech disorder | A neurogenic language disorder |
| More varied etiology including traumatic brain injury and toxic and metabolic disturbances | Traumatic brain injury and toxic and metabolic disturbances in most cases |

*(continues)*

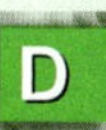


*(continued)*

| Dysarthria | Language of Confusion |
|---|---|
| Typically relevant | Typically irrelevant |
| Attentional deficits not the most striking | Attentional deficits are the most striking |
| Symptoms are more stable | Symptoms are more transient |
| Greater number of articulation problems | Fewer articulation problems |
| Speaking problems dominant; no significant writing problems | Writing problems often greater than speaking problems |
| No confabulation | Confabulation |
| No disorientation | Disoriented to time, place, and persons |
| Normal behavior | Significant behavioral change |

*Note: In cases of dementing dysarthrias, disorientation and behavioral changes may be present; in cases of traumatic head injury, dysarthria and language of confusion may coexist. However, dysarthria due to head injury may have a better chance of improvement.*

## Dysarthria or Neurogenic Stuttering?

| Dysarthria | Neurogenic Stuttering |
|---|---|
| Dysfluencies occur mostly on initial sounds and syllables | Dysfluencies can occur on final and medial sounds as well as on syllables |
| Dysfluencies consistent with other symptoms of dysarthria (e.g., reduced range of movement, rapid rate) | Dysfluencies may not be consistent with other symptoms of dysarthria. |
| Dysfluent productions are characterized by imprecise articulation | Imprecise articulation may not be a characteristic of neurogenic stuttering in the absence of dysarthria |

*Note: Both dysarthria and neurogenic stuttering are speech disorders. Dysfluencies are often present in hypokinetic dysarthria; they are not characteristic of flaccid dysarthria. Information on different varieties of neurogenic stuttering and characteristics of dysfluencies in dysarthria is limited.*

## Dysarthria or Palilalia?

| Dysarthria | Palilalia |
|---|---|
| Varied sites of lesions in the central and peripheral nervous systems | Bilateral lesions typically in the basal ganglia |
| Typically, sound and syllable dysfluencies without necessarily increasing rate and decreasing loudness | Typically, word and phrase repetitions with increasing rate and decreasing loudness |
| Dysfluencies at the beginning of utterances | Dysfluencies at the end of utterances |

*Note: Palilalia is more commonly associated with hypokinetic dysarthria than any other type. In such cases, make a dual diagnosis of dysarthria and palilalia. Dysarthric speakers may have dysfluencies that do not suggest palilalia; just describe those dysfluencies.*

### Prognosis

- Highly variable, depending on the underlying neuropathology, its severity, course, general health, and medical and rehabilitative treatment potential of individual clients
- Potential to maintain, improve, augment, or supplement communication skills is good enough in most cases to recommend treatment

### Recommendations

- Communication treatment based on the individual patent's needs and strengths
- See the cited sources and the two companion volumes, *Hegde's PocketGuide to Communication Disorders* and *Hegde's PocketGuide to Treatment in Speech-Language Pathology* (3rd ed.), for details


Darley, F. L., Aronson, A. E., & Brown, J. R. (1975). *Motor speech disorders*. Philadelphia, PA: W. B. Saunders.

Duffy, J. R. (2005). *Motor speech disorders: Substrates, differential diagnosis, and management* (2nd ed.). St. Louis, MO: Elsevier Mosby.

Freed, D. (2000). *Motor speech disorders*. Clifton Park, NY: Thomson Delmar Learning.

Kent, R. D., Duffy, J. R., Slama, A., Kent, J. F., & Clift, A. (2001). Clinicoanatomic studies in dysarthria: Review, critique, and directions for research. *Journal of Speech, Language, and Hearing Research*, *44*, 535–551.

Kent, R. D., Kent, J. F., Weismer, G., & Duffy, J. R. (2000). What dysarthria can tell us about the neural control of speech. *Journal of Phonetics*, *28*, 273–302.

Kent, R. D., Vorperian, K. K., Kent, J. F., & Duffy, J. R. (2003). Voice dysfunction in dysarthria: Application of the Multi-Dimensional Voice Program. *Journal of Communication Disorders*, *36*, 281–306.

Paslawski, T., Duffy, J. R., & Vermino, S. (2005). Speech and language findings associated with paraneoplastic cerebellar degeneration. *American Journal of Speech-Language Pathology*, *14*, 200–207.

Soliveri, P., Piacentini, S., Carella, F., Testa, D., Ciano, C., & Girotti, F. (2003). Progressive dysarthria: Definition and clinical follow-up. *Neurological Science, 24*, 211–212.

Spencer, K. A., & Rogers, M. A. (2005). Speech motor programming in hypokinetic and ataxic dysarthria. *Brain and Language*, *94,* 347–366.

Stolberger, C., Finsterer, J., Bran, E., & Taschabitscher, D. (2001). Dysarthria as the leading symptom of hypothyroidism. *American Journal of Otolaryngology*, *22*(1), 70–72.

Teasell, R., Foley, N., Doherty, T., & Finstone, H. (2002). Clinical characteristics of clients with brainstem strokes admitted to a rehabilitation unit. *Archives of Physical Medicine and Rehabilitation, 83*(7), 1013–1016.

Vogel, D., & Cannito, M. P. (2001). *Treating disordered speech motor control* (2nd ed.). Austin, TX: Pro-Ed.

Yorkston, K. M., Beukelman, D. R., Strand, E. A., & Bell, K. R. (1999). *Management of motor speech disorders in children and adults* (2nd ed.). Austin, TX: Pro-Ed.

**Dysarthria: Specific Types.** Assessment of variations in etiological factors and symptoms of dysarthria that allow for a typological classification is essential for differential diagnoses among the different types and to recommend appropriate treatment strategies; consider the general assessment procedures described under Dysarthria along with features unique to specific types described under this entry

***Ataxic Dysarthria.*** A type of motor speech disorder caused by damage to the cerebellar system; characterized by slow, inaccurate movement and Hypotonia; distinguished from other types by its dominant articulatory and prosodic problems; use the assessment procedures described under Dysarthrias and focus on the following that apply especially to ataxic dysarthria:

### Special Assessment Considerations

- Examine the medical records for evidence of bilateral or generalized cerebellar lesions, degenerative ataxia including Friedreich's ataxia and olivopontocerebellar atrophy, cerebellar vascular lesions, tumors, traumatic brain injury, toxic conditions including alcohol abuse, drug toxicity, and such inflammatory conditions as meningitis and encephalitis
- Observe and review the neurological examination results to document the presence of abnormal stance and gait; instability of the trunk and head, involving tremors and rocking motions; rotated or tilted head posture; hypotonia
- Observe such movement disorders as over- or undershooting of targets; discoordinated movements; jerky, inaccurate, slow, imprecise, and halting movements
- Assess the following speech characteristics from the conversational speech samples and tests of dysarthria:
  - Articulation disorders: Imprecise production of consonants, irregular breakdowns in articulation, and distortion of vowels
  - Prosodic disorders: Excessive and even stress; prolonged phonemes and intervals between words or syllables; slow rate of speech; a drunker speech quality
  - Phonatory disorders: Monopitch, monoloudness, and harshness

### Diagnostic Criteria

- Clear evidence of cerebellar damage and a supportive neurological diagnosis
- Listed speech characteristics

### Differential Diagnosis

- Possible confusion between ataxic dysarthria and hyperkinetic dysarthria
  - The two are distinguished by involuntary movements of the jaw, face, and tongue (present in hyperkinetic dysarthria, absent in ataxic dysarthria)
  - Strained-strangled voice quality, audible inspiration, voice tremor, and voice stoppages of hyperkinetic dysarthria are not prominent in ataxic dysarthria
- Possible confusion between ataxic dysarthria and unilateral upper motor neuron (UMN) dysarthria
  - The two are distinguished by unilateral lower facial and lingual weakness (present in UMN dysarthria and absent in ataxic dysarthria)

- Distorted vowels, prolonged phonemes, and prosodic problems of ataxic dysarthria are not prominent in UMN dysarthria

### Recommendations

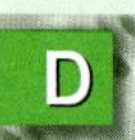

- Communication treatment with an emphasis on modifying rate and prosody

***Flaccid Dysarthria.*** A type of motor speech disorder due to damage to the motor units of cranial or spinal nerves that supply speech muscles (lower motor neuron involvement); use the assessment procedures described under Dysarthrias and focus on the following that apply especially to flaccid dysarthria:

### Special Assessment Considerations

- Review medical records and neurological symptoms for evidence of damage to such cranial nerves as the trigeminal (cranial V), facial (cranial VII), glossopharyngeal (cranial IX), vagus (cranial X), accessory (cranial X), and the hypoglossal (cranial XII)
- Check for evidence of spinal nerve lesions, which may affect respiration
- Review medical records and neurological symptoms for evidence of such degenerative diseases as motor neuron diseases, progressive bulbar palsy, and ALS; vascular diseases and brainstem strokes; infections including polio, secondary infections in AIDS clients, and herpes zoster (a viral infection that tends to affect the nerve ganglia of the cranial nerves V and VII); demyelinating diseases including Guillain-Barré syndrome; surgical trauma during neurosurgery, laryngeal and facial surgery, and chest/cardiac surgery; and injury to the laryngeal branches of the vagus nerve
- Assess such neurological symptoms as muscle weakness, hypotonia, muscle atrophy, and diminished reflexes, fasciculations (isolated twitches of resting muscles) and fibrillations (contractions of individual muscles), rapid and progressive weakness with use and recovery with rest (especially with neuromuscular junction diseases)
- Assess the following speech characteristics from the conversational speech samples and tests of dysarthria
  - Respiratory disorders: Respiratory weakness in combination with cranial nerve weakness
  - Phonatory disorders: Breathy voice; audible inspiration; short phrases
  - Resonance disorders: Hypernasality; imprecise consonants (mostly due to resonance problems); nasal emission; and short phrases
  - Phonatory-prosodic disorders: Harsh voice; monopitch, and monoloudness
  - Articulation disorders: May be significant, especially with lesions of cranial nerves V, VII, and XII

### Diagnostic Criteria

- Evidence of lesion in one or more of the cranial nerves; an associated medical-neurological diagnosis when appropriate; and the listed dominant phonatory and resonatory speech problems

### Differential Diagnosis

- Breathiness, audible inspiration, and short phrases that characterize flaccid dysarthria are less pronounced in other types of dysarthria

- Hypernasality that occurs in spastic and hypokinetic dysarthrias is much more prominent in flaccid dysarthria
- Short phrases that occur in spastic and hyperkinetic dysarthria are not associated with other kinds of evidence of vocal cord weakness that are present in flaccid dysarthria
- Audible nasal emission that characterizes flaccid dysarthria is rare in other types
- Rapid speech deterioration and recovery after rest found in flaccid dysarthria are rare in other types of dysarthria

### Recommendations

- Treatment to improve communication

***Hyperkinetic Dysarthria.*** A type of motor speech disorder dominated by prosodic disturbances caused by damage to basal ganglia (extrapyramidal system); use the assessment procedures described under Dysarthrias and focus on the following that apply especially to hyperkinetic dysarthria:

### Special Assessment Considerations

- Review medical records and neurological symptoms for evidence of degenerative, vascular, traumatic, infectious, neoplastic, and metabolic factors; also caused by neuroleptic and antipsychotic drugs that cause dyskinesia and dystonia and such degenerative diseases as Huntington's disease
- Review medical records and neurological symptoms for evidence of damage to the basal ganglia control circuit
- Note that the causes may be unknown in a majority of cases
- Assess such movement disorders as orofacial dyskinesia; myoclonus; tics of the face and shoulders; tremors; chorea; ballism (abrupt and severe contractions of the extremities); athetosis (writhing, involuntary movements, often in hands); dystonia; spasmodic torticollis (intermittent dystonia and spasm of the neck muscles); blepharospasm (forceful and involuntary closure of the eyes due to spasm of the orbicularis oculi muscle); and tonic or clonic muscle spasms
- Assess the following speech characteristics from the conversational speech samples and tests of dysarthria; note that the constellation of communication disorders depends on whether the dominant neurological condition is chorea, dystonia, athetosis, spasmodic torticollis, and so forth
  - Phonatory disorders: Voice tremor; intermittently strained voice; voice stoppage; vocal noise; harsh voice
  - Resonance disorders: Intermittent hypernasality
  - Prosodic disorders: Slower rate; excessive loudness variations; prolonged inter-word intervals; inappropriate silent intervals; equal stress
  - Respiratory problems: Audible inspiration; forced and sudden inspiration/expiration
  - Articulation disorders: Imprecise consonants; distortion of vowels; inconsistent articulatory errors

### Diagnostic Criteria

- Evidence of lesion or disease resulting in chorea, dystonia, athetosis, spasmodic torticollis, and so forth; associated medical-neurological diagnosis when appropriate
- Listed communication disorders

### Differential Diagnosis

- Involuntary movements of the face and mouth distinguish hyperkinetic dysarthria from other types
- Regularity of vocal tremor and stoppages in conjunction with movement disorders also help distinguish hyperkinetic dysarthria from other types

### Recommendations

- Treatment to improve communication

***Hypokinetic Dysarthria.*** A type of motor speech disorder caused by damage to basal ganglia (extrapyramidal system); caused by varied factors including the most typical form produced by Parkinson's disease; use the assessment procedures described under Dysarthrias and focus on the following that apply especially to hypokinetic dysarthria:

### Special Assessment Considerations

- Review the client's history, medical records, and neurological symptoms for evidence of such degenerative diseases as progressive supranuclear palsy, Parkinson's disease (much more commonly), Alzheimer's disease, and Pick's disease; vascular disorders causing multiple or bilateral strokes; repeated head trauma; inflammation; tumor; antipsychotic or neuroleptic drug toxicity; and normal pressure hydrocephalus
- Review medical records and neurological symptoms for evidence of tremor at rest (tremor in relaxed facial, mouth, and limb structures that diminish when moved voluntarily; pill-rolling movement between the thumb and the forefinger); rigidity; bradykinesia; hypokinesia; lack of facial expression (mask-like face); infrequent blinking; lack of smiling; reduced hand and facial movements during speech; slow walking, changing into rapid, short, shuffling steps; postural disturbances; and swallowing problems and possible drooling
- Assess the following speech characteristics from the conversational speech samples and tests of dysarthria
    - Phonatory disorders: Monopitch; monoloudness; harsh voice; continuously breathy voice; low pitch
    - Prosodic disorders: Reduced stress; inappropriate silent intervals; short rushes of speech; variable and increased rate in segments; short phrases
    - Articulation disorders: Imprecise consonants; repeated phonemes; resonance disorders; mild hypernasality (in about 25% of the cases)
    - Respiratory problems: Reduced vital capacity, irregular breathing, and faster rate of respiration
    - Writing problems: Micrographic writing (small print)

### Diagnostic Criteria

- Evidence of lesion in the basal ganglia and the listed neurological symptoms
- An associated medical-neurological diagnosis when appropriate
- Listed dominant speech disorders and writing problems

### Differential Diagnosis

- Hypokinesia, bradykinesia, and other neuromotor symptoms of hypokinetic dysarthria are not prominent in other types of dysarthria
- Dominant phonatory and prosodic problems, including monopitch, monoloudness, reduced loudness, reduced stress, inappropriate silent intervals, variable rate, short rushes of speech, and in some cases, increased rate distinguish hypokinetic dysarthria

### Prognosis

- Varies with the associated neurological disease and other factors listed under Dysarthrias

### Recommendations

- Treatment to improve communication

***Mixed Dysarthria.*** A type of motor speech disorder that is a combination of two or more pure dysarthrias; the neuropathology is varied and often multiple; any and all combinations of pure dysarthrias are possible; use the assessment procedures described under Dysarthrias and focus on the following that apply especially to mixed dysarthria:

### Special Assessment Considerations

- Note that the flaccid-spastic dysarthria is the most common (42% of the mixed cases), followed by ataxic-spastic (23%); note also that mixed types are more common than any single pure type
- Review medical records and neurological symptoms for evidence of various diseases that are associated with dysarthrias; in many cases, look for diseases and conditions associated with flaccid, spastic, and ataxic types of dysarthria
- Assess the constellation of symptoms that characterize the client and identify those that are a part of different varieties of dysarthria to diagnose the mixed type

### Diagnostic Criteria

- Evidence of lesion, often in multiple sites and an associated medical-neurological diagnosis when appropriate
- Constellation of communication disorders as listed

### Differential Diagnosis

- Differentiate the types of dysarthrias that are mixed; use the guidelines given under specific types of dysarthria

### Recommendations

- Treatment to improve communication

***Spastic Dysarthria.*** A type of motor speech disorder caused by bilateral damage to the upper motor neuron (direct and indirect motor pathways), resulting predominantly in spasticity and slow rate of speech combined with a strained voice quality; use the assessment procedures described under Dysarthrias and focus on the following that apply especially to spastic dysarthria:

### Special Assessment Considerations

- Review medical records and neurological symptoms for evidence of multiple lesions in cortical areas, basal ganglia, internal capsule, pons, and medulla
- Review medical records and neurological symptoms for evidence of degenerative, vascular, traumatic, metabolic, toxic, and other factors that are associated with spastic dysarthria
- Observe the clinical symptoms of spasticity; increased muscle tone, weakness, especially bilateral facial weakness; however, normal jaw strength and less pronounced lower face weakness; reduced range of movements; slowness of movement; slow nonspeech alternating motion rates; hyperadduction of vocal folds and inadequate closure of the velopharyngeal port
- Assess the following speech characteristics from the conversational speech samples and tests of dysarthria
  - Prosodic disorders: Excess and equal stress; slow rate; monopitch; monoloudness; reduced stress; short phrases
  - Articulation disorders: Imprecise production of consonants; distorted vowels
  - Phonatory disorders: Continuous breathy voice; harshness; low pitch; pitch breaks; strained-strangled voice quality; short phrases; slow rate
  - Resonance disorders: Hypernasality

### Diagnostic Criteria

- Evidence of damage to the direct and indirect activation pathways of the upper motor neuron and the resulting physical symptoms listed previously
- An associated medical-neurological diagnosis when appropriate
- Dominance of slow rate, strained-strangled voice quality, and slow alternating speech-related movements that support a diagnosis of spastic dysarthria

### Differential Diagnosis

- Abnormal reflexes, dysphagia, drooling, and uncontrolled crying or laughter support the diagnosis of spastic dysarthria
- The strained-strangled voice quality of hyperkinetic dysarthria is distinguished by its less frequent association with slow alternating motion rates and decreased speech rate, which characterize spastic dysarthria
- Slow rate found in other dysarthrias is less frequently associated with strained-strangled voice quality except in spastic dysarthria
- Slow rate and excess and equal stress are found in both spastic dysarthria and ataxic dysarthria; however, ataxic dysarthria is not associated with strained-strangled voice

### Recommendations

- Treatment to improve communication

***Unilateral Upper Motor Neuron (UUMN) Dysarthria.*** A type of motor speech disorder caused by damage to the upper motor neurons that supply cranial and spinal nerves involved in speech production; use the assessment procedures described under Dysarthrias and focus on the following that apply especially to UUMN dysarthria as described by Duffy (2005):

### Special Assessment Considerations

- Review medical records and neurological symptoms for evidence of various diseases that are associated with dysarthrias, especially vascular disorders that are the most common causes
- Review medical records and assess such neurological symptoms as unilateral lower face weakness; unilateral tongue weakness; unilateral palatal weakness; hemiplegia/hemiparesis
- Assess the following speech characteristics from the conversational speech samples and tests of dysarthria
  - Articulation disorders: Imprecise production of consonants; irregular articulatory breakdowns
  - Phonatory disorders: Harsh voice; reduced loudness; strained-harshness
  - Prosodic disorders: Slow rate; increased rate in segments; excess and equal stress; monopitch, monoloudness, low pitch, and short phrases may be present in some cases
  - Resonance disorders: Hypernasality
  - Assess dysphagia, aphasia, apraxia, and right hemisphere syndrome that are often associated with UUMN

### Diagnostic Criteria

- Evidence of upper motor neuron lesion
- An associated medical-neurological diagnosis when appropriate
- Dominant communication disorders as listed

### Differential Diagnosis

- The presence of central facial weakness on either the right or left side helps distinguish UUMN dysarthria from other types, except for flaccid dysarthria
- Overall, mild and temporary communication problems of UUMN dysarthria help distinguish it from other types
- Most difficult to distinguish UUMN dysarthria from flaccid and ataxic varieties because all three share imprecise articulation; however, infrequent occurrence of voice and resonance problems in UUMN dysarthria help distinguish it from these two varieties
- More regular alternating movement rates of UUMN dysarthria may help distinguish it from ataxic dysarthria

### Recommendations

- Treatment to improve communication
- See the cited sources and *Hegde's PocketGuide to Treatment in Speech-Language Pathology* (3rd ed.) for details

Darley, F. L., Aronson, A. E., & Brown, J. R. (1975). *Motor speech disorders*. Philadelphia: W.B. Saunders.

D

Duffy, J. R. (2005). *Motor speech disorders: Substrates, differential diagnosis, and management* (2nd ed.). St. Louis, MO: Elsevier Mosby.

Freed, D. (2000). *Motor speech disorders*. Clifton Park, NY: Thomson Delmar Learning.

Kent, R. D., Duffy, J. R., Slama, A., Kent, J. F., & Clift, A. (2001). Clinicoanatomic studies in dysarthria: Review, critique, and directions for research. *Journal of Speech, Language, and Hearing Research, 44*, 535–551.

Kent, R. D., Kent, J. F., Weismer, G., & Duffy, J. R. (2000). What dysarthria can tell us about the neural control of speech. *Journal of Phonetics, 28*, 273–302.

Kent, R. D., Vorperian, K. K., Kent, J. F., & Duffy, J. R. (2003). Voice dysfunction in dysarthria: Application of the Multi-Dimensional Voice Program. *Journal of Communication Disorders, 36,* 281–306.

Paslawski, T., Duffy, J. R., & Vermino, S. (2005). Speech and language findings associated with paraneoplastic cerebellar degeneration. *American Journal of Speech-Language Pathology, 14*, 200–207.

Soliveri, P., Piacentini, S., Carella, F., Testa, D., Ciano, C., & Girotti, F. (2003). Progressive dysarthria: Definition and clinical follow-up. *Neurological Science, 24*, 211–212.

Spencer, K. A., & Rogers, M. A. (2005). Speech motor programming in hypokinetic and ataxic dysarthria. *Brain and Language, 94*, 347–366.

Stolberger, C., Finsterer, J., Bran, E., & Taschabitscher, D. (2001). Dysarthria as the leading symptom of hypothyroidism. *American Journal of Otolaryngology, 22*(1), 70–72.

Teasell, R., Foley, N., Doherty, T., & Finstone, H. (2002). Clinical characteristics of clients with brainstem strokes admitted to a rehabilitation unit. *Archives of Physical Medicine and Rehabilitation, 83*(7), 1013–1016.

Vogel, D., & Cannito, M. P. (2001). *Treating disordered speech motor control* (2nd ed.). Austin, TX: Pro-Ed.

Yorkston, K. M., Beukelman, D. R., Strand, E. A., & Bell, K. R. (1999). *Management of motor speech disorders in children and adults* (2nd ed.). Austin, TX: Pro-Ed.

**Dysfluencies.** Assessment of behaviors that interrupt fluency is essential to diagnose stuttering and other forms of fluency disorders; see Stuttering under Fluency Disorders for a description of different forms of dysfluencies and their assessment.

**Dysgraphia.** Assessment of writing problems associated with recent neuropathology is important in understanding the total symptom complex associated with various clinical conditions, including aphasia and other neurologically based communication disorders; also known as *agraphia* and need to be distinguished from childhood writing problems that may be due to variables other than a clearly established neuropathology; see Agraphia for assessment.

D

**Dysphagia.** Assessment of disorders of swallowing due to a variety of physical diseases, disorders, and surgical consequences is a responsibility of speech-language pathologists because of their expertise; dysphagia includes problems in the execution of the oral, pharyngeal, and esophageal stages of swallow; includes problems in chewing the food, preparing it for swallow, initiating the swallow, propelling the bolus through the pharynx, and in passing the food through the esophagus; speech-language pathologists assess and treat oropharyngeal disorders of swallowing; esophageal swallowing disorders are handled medically, although speech-language pathologists play a role in their overall clinical management; see the cited sources at the end of this main entry and the companion volume, *Hegde's PocketGuide to Communication Disorders* for epidemiology, normal swallow, and etiology and description of swallowing disorders.

### *Assessment Objectives/General Guidelines*

- To assess the functioning of the different stages of swallow and their dynamic interactions
- To assess various swallowing disorders
- To assess potential causes of the disorders to the extent possible
- To make both clinical and instrumental assessment of the symptom complex
- To assess the types and consistencies of food that are safe to swallow
- To make dietary recommendations to the health care staff and the client's family
- To help develop clinical staff and client education materials specific to the client
- To assess various treatment options and potential
- To suggest specific treatment or clinical management strategies

### *Case History/Interview Focus*

- See **Case History** and **Interview** under Standard/Common Assessment Procedures
- Concentrate on the client's medical history and medical records to obtain information that suggests the presence of dysphagia, including any evidence of dysarthria; drooling; frequent coughing; choking on food and sputum; difficulty in chewing; excessively slow eating; weight loss; and painful swallow
- Review the client's medical history and examination reports to find evidence of diseases associated with dysphagia, including brainstem and anterior cortical strokes; any type of aphasia; such neurological diseases as Parkinson's disease, amyotrophic lateral sclerosis, multiple sclerosis, myasthenia gravis, muscular dystrophy, and dystonia; tumors in the oral cavity or the pharynx; surgical treatment of oral, pharyngeal, and laryngeal cancer; any form of head, neck, and gastrointestinal surgery; radiation therapy for oral, pharyngeal, and laryngeal cancer; neurosurgery; traumatic brain injury; cervical spine disease; and chronic, obstructive, pulmonary disease

### *Ethnocultural Considerations*

- See Ethnocultural Considerations in Assessment
- Assess dietary habits of the family and especially the client; check for vegetarianism, religious beliefs about food and eating, religious holidays

and their restrictions on eating (e.g., restrictions on eating during day time) and client's food preferences

### Assessment of Dysphagia



- Assess client's mental status
  - Because dysphagia is associated with various neurological diseases, it is necessary to assess the mental status of the client; ask questions about:
    - Time, date, year, and place
    - His or her name; names of family members
    - What he or she ate for breakfast or lunch
    - What he or she did (in the morning, afternoon, evening, yesterday)
    - Why he or she is in the hospital
  - Administer, if preferred or necessary, a test of mental status (e.g., the *Mini-Mental Status Examination* by M. F. Folstein, S. E. Folstein, and P. R. McHugh); see Dementia for details on mental status examination
- Screen speech, voice, language, and writing skills
  - Note that it is essential to screen communication skills because the client with swallowing disorders also may have accompanying communication disorders that may complicate dysphagia or its clinical management
  - Screen articulation as you interview the client
    - Take note of any errors
    - Measure the diadochokinetic rate
    - Make a more detailed assessment if necessary; see Articulation and Phonological Disorders
  - Screen voice
    - Judge the quality of voice as the client talks to you (take note of hoarseness, harshness, and breathiness)
    - Ask the client to sustain a vowel; measure the duration and take note of the vocal quality
    - Take note of the pitch and loudness of voice
    - Take note of hyponasality and hypernasality
  - Screen the client's language comprehension; give a series of:
    - Simple verbal commands to assess their comprehension
    - Written commands to assess their comprehension
  - Screen naming responses; have the client:
    - Name a few common objects and geometric forms
    - Name pictures of family members
  - Screen spelling and writing skills; ask the client to:
    - Copy a few printed words
    - Write words and phrases as you dictate them
    - Write a paragraph about anything
  - Screen comprehension of abstract meaning; ask the client to:
    - Tell the meaning of a few proverbs
    - Tell the meaning of a few common phrases (e.g., *go overboard, come out of the closet, elbow room, lame duck, top brass*)
    - Define a few abstract terms (e.g., *honesty, truthfulness, good, bad*)
  - Screen visual-perceptual skills; ask the client to
    - Copy geometric forms (e.g., *a square, triangle, circle, rectangle*)

- Make a laryngeal examination
  - With indirect laryngoscopy and/or endoscopic examination:
    - Inspect the base of the tongue, vallecula, epiglottis, piriform sinuses, vocal folds, and ventricular folds
    - Evaluate the vocal cord functioning during such tasks as quiet breathing, forced inhalation, and phonation
  - Refer the client to an otolaryngologist for a medical examination
- Administer test swallows
  - Take note of the client's posture, alertness, intubation, ability to follow direction, language comprehension, and readiness for examination
  - Use case history, medical charts, initial indications of the type of swallowing problems, and results of your observation to plan test swallows
  - Collect the necessary materials: laryngeal mirror, tongue blade, cup, spoon, straw, syringe; and various foods of different consistency (described later)
  - Use an appropriate posture during the test swallows
    - In the case of tongue weakness and bolus manipulation problems, ask the client to tilt the head downward as food is placed in the mouth and tilt the head backward when the swallow is initiated
    - In the case of hemilaryngectomy, delayed triggering of swallowing reflex, and inadequate laryngeal closure, ask the client to tilt the head downward to hold the food in the valleculae until the reflex is triggered
    - Ask the client with pharyngeal paralysis to turn the head toward the affected side during swallowing
    - Ask the client to tilt the head toward more normal side in case of unilateral oral or lingual weakness or paralysis; have the client tilt the head before placing food in the mouth
  - Make appropriate placement of foods in the mouth
    - Place food in the more normal side of the mouth
    - Use a straw or a syringe to place liquids posteriorly
    - Use a tongue blade to place thicker foods on various places on the tongue
  - Use different kinds of foods in evaluating test swallows
    - Use liquid foods or foods of thin consistency when the client has limited oral control
    - Use liquid foods when the client has reduced pharyngeal peristalsis or impaired functioning of the cricopharyngeus muscle
    - Use foods of thicker consistency when the client's swallowing reflex is delayed or laryngeal closure is inadequate
    - Modify food consistency to suit a client who has a combination of problems
  - Give appropriate instructions
    - Give the client any special instructions (e.g., head tilting)
    - Place food appropriately
    - Ask the client to swallow the material
  - Manually examine the swallowing movements
    - Place your index finger just below the chin, middle finger on the hyoid, and the third and fourth fingers at top and bottom of the thyroid; do not press the structures

    - Take note of the submandibular, hyoid, and laryngeal movements during swallowing
    - Take note of lack of laryngeal movement causing aspiration
    - Take note of abnormally low position of the larynx in some elderly clients
    - Ask the client to phonate a vowel soon after swallowing; take note of gargling sounds indicative of food material on the vocal cords
    - Ask the client to pant for several seconds to shake loose foods in the pharyngeal recesses; ask the client to vocalize
    - Take note of coughing and expectoration that suggest aspiration
    - Be aware that lack of signs of aspiration does not mean no aspiration; videofluorography is more definitive
- Instrumental assessment: general guidelines
  - Note that a clinical swallow examination may not reveal aspiration and, therefore, it is essential to conduct one or more instrumental assessments
  - Note that instrumental assessment may require medical collaboration and equipment
  - Medical professionals including radiologists, otorhinolaryngologists, gastroenterologists, and other specialists may have to collaborate with the speech-language pathologist to conduct various instrumental assessments
  - Select the instrumental assessment procedures described here and in the cited sources, but always seek the medical collaboration needed in your professional setting
- Arrange for still radiographic assessment
  - Use the still radiographic procedure if videofluorography is not available
    - Take lateral still radiographs 2 seconds after you instruct the client to swallow
    - Take note of food residue in the valleculae, pyriform sinuses, or food coating on the pharyngeal wall that indicate swallowing problems
    - Note that still radiographic assessment provides only limited information on the nature of the disorder
- Make videofluorographic assessment
  - Note that a videofluorographic assessment (modified barium swallow: MBS) of oropharyngeal swallow function is essential for a more complete assessment and diagnosis of dysphagia
  - Complete both lateral and anterior-posterior (A-P) plane examinations; note that the lateral examination provides the most information and the A-P examination provides information on the symmetry of the swallow
  - Note that the procedure uses radiation and may be contraindicated in some cases; do not use the procedure if:
    - No new information is likely to emerge
    - The client is not alert and mouth feeding is not practical
    - The client has no swallowing response at all
  - If the client is severely ill and the procedure is still judged necessary, request the presence of a physician, nurse, or respiratory therapist during the test
  - Note that a regular barium procedure is necessary to diagnose esophageal disorders; it should follow MBS and not be done simultaneously

- Begin with the lateral plane examination and then switch over to (A-P) plane examination; give calibrated boluses:
  - Begin with liquid barium: 1 ml, 3 ml, 5 ml, 10 ml, and drinking from a cup
  - Pudding: 1 ml
  - Cookie: 1/4 of a butter cookie
  - Thicker liquids or foods of thicker consistencies
  - Place the food in the mouth with a spoon or a syringe
  - Ask the client to hold the food in the mouth until asked to swallow; use gestures; check the client's understanding of your instructions
- Let the client try two swallows of each kind/quantity
  - Examine the anatomy and physiology of swallowing structures
  - Identify swallowing disorders; take note of food residues in various structures; coughing; and aspiration
- In completing the assessment and interpreting the results, use a standard and detailed set of instructions and follow the prescribed procedures carefully; see Logemann (1993)

- Make a Fiberoptic Endoscopic Examination of Swallowing (FEES)
  - Note that this technique helps assess the pharyngeal and laryngeal motor and sensory integrity through a flexible endoscope inserted transnasally through the pharynx; the end of the scope is suspended above the epiglottis
  - Ask the client to ingest liquid and food items that have been colored blue or green
  - Lower the scope to view laryngeal structures, including the vocal folds, and into the subglottic area to assess aspiration
  - Take note of any premature spillage of the bolus over the base of the tongue, delay in the initiation of the swallow, and laryngeal penetration, aspiration, and pooling; timing of airway closure also can be assessed
- Make a Fiberoptic Endoscopic Examination of Swallowing with Sensory Testing (FEESST)
  - Note that FEESST is both a sensory and motor test of swallowing
  - In this test, the sensory testing component is added to the basic endoscopic evaluation of swallowing
  - Note that FEESST helps assess supraglottic and pharyngeal sensation using air pulses and examines both airway protection reflex triggered by the brainstem (the sensory part) and the bolus transport (the motor component)
  - Insert the transnasal flexible laryngoscope with a sensory stimulator into the most patent side of the nasal cavity
  - Pass the scope into the posterior portion of the nasal cavity, where velopharyngeal opening and closure can be assessed by having the client say "cookie"
  - Directed the scope inferiorly to observe the base of the tongue, valeculla, and supraglottic structures, and the anatomy and physiology of the larynx
  - Test the laryngeal sensory function involved in airway protection, deliver calibrated puffs of air to the supraglottic larynx and pharynx with the help of a specially designed flexible nasopharyngoscope
  - Observe the air pulse-elicited laryngeal adductor reflex that protects the airway

  - Note that the absence of the airway protection reflex suggests a high risk for airway penetration and aspiration
  - Assess swallowing as the final portion of the FEESST; present various consistencies of food and liquid dyed green or blue; observe any pharyngeal pooling; laryngeal residue, penetration, or aspiration; and reflux
- Make a flexible fiberoptic esophagoscopy
  - Assess the functioning of the esophagus with the flexible fiberoptic esophagoscopy
  - Assess potential esophageal neoplasms that are potential causes of the swallowing disorder
  - Ascertain from the client if there is any pain while swallowing (odynophagia)
  - Note that gastroesophageal reflux and esophageal ulcers also may be assessed with this procedure
- Arrange for an assessment with scintigraphy
  - Use this nuclear medicine procedure to assess the bolus movement through the oropharynx, pharynx, larynx, and trachea
  - Note that the method requires the presentation of food or liquid that is tagged with radioactive material and hence contains the risks of radiation
  - Assess residual bolus and trace aspiration and use the method for repeated measurement of aspiration
  - Note that the client should be cognitively competent, free from any movement disorders, and be able to sit or stand in front of the scanning camera.
- Make a manometric assessment
  - Note that an esophageal manometer measures pressure in the upper and lower esophagus
  - Have the client swallow three small pressure-sensitive tubes that are positioned at the upper esophageal sphincter, within the esophagus, and at the lower esophageal sphincter
  - Measure pressure changes associated with various swallows
  - Take note of pressure deviations (disruptions in peristaltic waves) and esophageal disorders associated with them
  - Note that manometry may be conducted simultaneously with videofluoroscopy
- Make an electromyographic assessment
  - Note that an electromyographic examination is done by attaching electrodes on structures of interest (e.g., oral, laryngeal, or pharyngeal muscles)
  - Note that the electrical activity of the muscles involved in swallow can be measured with this technique
  - Note that muscle weakness or paralysis can be identified with this technique
  - Use the procedure described in the manual of the electromyographic instrument used in the assessment
- Make an ultrasound examination
  - Note that ultrasound equipment helps measure oral tongue movement and hyoid movement
  - Place the ultrasound sensor under the chin
  - Give measured foods of different amount and thickness

- Record the reflected and converted sound waves on tape
- Take note of the movements of the tongue and hyoid bone

## Related/Medical Assessment Data



- Consider the medical conditions associated with swallowing disorders
- Integrate the results of all medical, surgical, and radiological examinations with the results of dysphagia assessment, including clinical examination and instrumental assessment results
- Consider the client's current physical condition and urgent nutritional needs

## Standard/Common Assessment Procedures

- Complete the Standard/Common Assessment Procedures; pay special attention to the:
  - Muscles of facial expression
  - Muscles of mastication
  - Tongue mobility and strength
  - Lip closure
  - Movement of the soft palate
  - Oral sensation (stimulate with hot and cold stimuli and with pressure; note that reduced oral sensation is rarely a cause of dysphagia)
  - Dryness or the amount of moisture in the mouth
  - Presence of drooling

## Analysis of Results

- Analyze the results of the clinical and bedside examination to make a preliminary assessment of dysphagia and its potential loci and causes
- Integrate the results of the clinical examination with those of the instrumental assessment (e.g., videofluoroscopy, EMG, manometry, endoscopy)
- Describe the specific symptoms and causes of dysphagia
- Analyze the types and consistencies of food that seem to help promote better swallowing and nutritional intake

## Diagnostic Criteria/Guidelines

- Relate symptoms to the different phases of swallow and their anatomical and physiologic loci and physiologic and anatomical (if any) deviations
- Note that the presence of aspiration clinically observed or observed through instrumental assessment (silent aspiration) is a significant diagnostic feature of dysphagia

## Differential Diagnosis

- Greater difficulty with liquids may suggest neurological involvement (general weakening of the muscle movements)
- No or little difficulty with liquids but greater difficulty with solids may suggest physical obstructions including tumor
- Difficulty with both liquids and solids may suggest a greater involvement of esophageal structures
- Differential effects of cold and hot food (e.g., esophageal spasms or reduction of esophageal peristalsis due to cold food) may suggest esophageal stage problems

- Pain associated with swallowing (odynophagia) may help rule out dysphagia of neurological origin
- Hyperactive gag reflex, tongue thrusting, and tonic bite may suggest neurological impairment
- Nasal penetration of food suggests velopharyngeal closure problems
- Chest pain may suggest esophageal motor disorder
- Dysphagia caused by drugs may help rule out esophageal involvement (because esophagus is rarely affected by drugs)
- Normal speech and voice may suggest swallowing problems due to cricopharyngeal (late pharyngeal stage) or esophageal dysfunction
- Normal eating and swallowing when food is presented without verbal instructions but difficulty in swallowing when such instructions are given suggest the presence of swallowing apraxia

### *Prognosis*

- Varies, depending on the underlying anatomical and physiological causes, associated diseases and their natural course, physical and mental condition of the client, and the past, present, and future medical and surgical treatment planned for the client
- Most clients with oropharyngeal dysphagia with good mental condition are candidates for dysphagia treatment
- Clients with esophageal dysphagia may be candidates for clinical management strategies to be combined with medical management

### *Recommendations*

- Treatment for oropharyngeal dysphagia by speech-language pathologist trained in dysphagia management
- Medical management for esophageal dysphagia and suggestions for clinical management strategies
- See the cited sources and the two companion volumes, *Hegde's PocketGuide to Communication Disorders* and *Hegde's PocketGuide to Treatment in Speech-Language Pathology* (3rd ed.)


Aviv, J. E., & Murry, T. (2005). *Flexible endoscopic evaluation of swallowing with sensory testing*. San Diego, CA: Plural Publishing.

Carrau, R. L., & Murry, T. (2006). *Comprehensive management of swallowing disorders*. San Diego, CA: Plural Publishing.

Corbin-Lewis, K., Liss, J. M., & Sciortino, K. L. (2005). *Clinical anatomy and physiology of the swallow mechanism.* Clifton Park, NY: Thomson Delmar Learning.

Groher, M. E. (Ed.) (1997). *Dysphagia: Diagnosis and management.* Boston, MA: Butterworth-Heinemann.

Huckabee, M. L., & Pelletier, C. A. (1999). *Management of adult neurogenic dysphagia*. San Diego, CA: Singular Publishing Group.

Langmore, S. E., & McCulloch, T. M. (1997). In A. L. Perlman & K. S. Schulze-Delrieu (Eds.), *Deglutition and its disorders: Anatomy, physiology, clinical diagnosis, and management* (pp. 201–225). San Diego, CA: Singular Publishing Group.

Logemann, J. A. (1998). *Evaluation and treatment of swallowing disorders*. (2nd ed.). Austin, TX: Pro-Ed.

Logemann, J. A. (1993). *A manual of videofluoroscopic evaluation of swallowing* (2nd ed.). Austin, TX: Pro-Ed.

Miller, R. M. (1992). Clinical examination for dysphagia. In M. E. Groher (Ed.), *Dysphagia: Diagnosis and management* (pp. 143–162). Newton, MA: Butterworth-Heinemann.

Murry, T., & Carrau, R. L. (2006). *Clinical Management of Swallowing Disorders*. (2nd ed.). San Diego, CA: Plural Publishing Inc.

Perlman, A., & Schultze-Delrieu, K. (1997). *Deglutition and its disorders: Anatomy, physiology, clinical diagnosis and management*: San Diego, CA: Singular Publishing Group.

Provencio-Arambula, M., Provencio, D., & Hegde, M. N. (2007a). *Assessment of dysphagia: Resources and protocols in English and Spanish*. San Diego, CA: Plural Publishing.

Provencio-Arambula, M., Provencio, D., & Hegde, M. N. (2007b). *Treatment of dysphagia: Resources and protocols in English and Spanish*. San Diego, CA: Plural Publishing.


**Dysphonia.** To assess any voice disorder with the exception of Aphonia, see Voice Disorders.

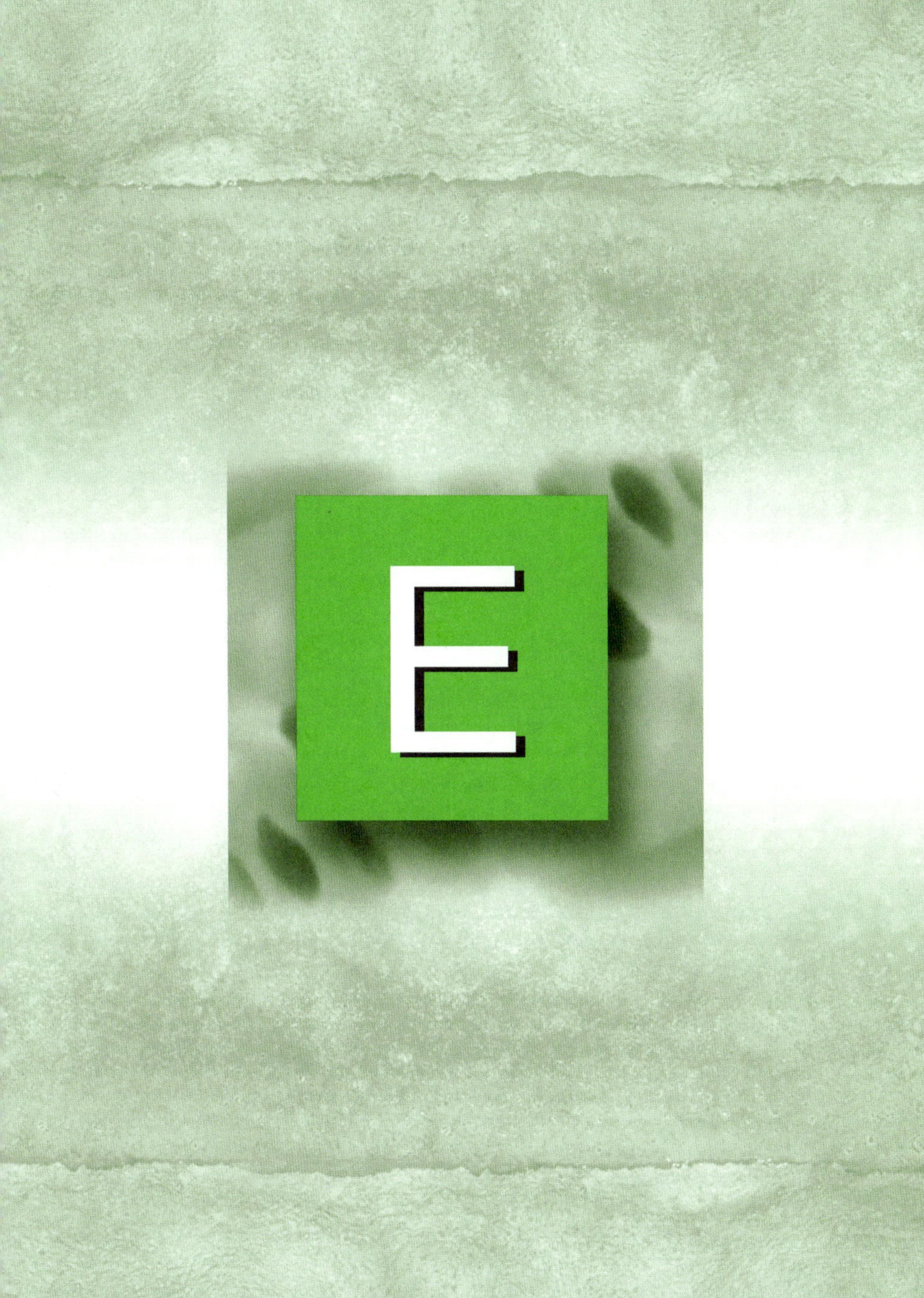
E

**Echolalia.** Assessment of parrot-like repetition of what is heard is important in certain disorders of communication, especially in persons with autism and in clients with aphasia, Pick's disease, various dementias including Alzheimer's disease, and Tourette's syndrome; echolalia's communicative value is doubtful in most cases, except that in cases of autism, it may serve limited communicative function; to assess echolalia and its communicative function:

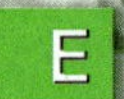

- Question the family members about echolalic behavior at home; find out if the client echoes what is just heard (immediate echolalia), echoes what has been heard in the past (delayed echolalia), or exhibits both kinds of echolalia
- Ask the family members if echolalic behavior has ever meant as a request, comment, or question
- Ask whether the client has ever echoed a question such as, "Do you want something to eat?" and then showed either an expectation of receiving food or proceeded to accept some food that is offered; in such cases, the echolalic response is thought to be *communicative*
- Take note of immediate or delayed echolalic responses throughout the assessment period
- When appropriate, offer something implied in an echolalic response to judge whether it is indeed a request; for example, when the child echoes you when you ask, "Do you want to play with this toy?," offer the toy; if the child accepts and begins to play, perhaps the echoic response was a request
- Withhold something that may have been requested through an echolalic response; if the child shows signs of disappointment or grabs the object withheld, infer that the echolalic response was indeed a request
- Distinguish echolalia from imitative responses; in imitation, the clinician models a response and asks the client to reproduce it; thus, there is a contingent and planned relationship between the clinician's model and the client's imitation; there is no such relationship in echolalic response; also, typically, echolalic responses are not reinforced (unless one is sure of its communicative function), whereas imitative responses are reinforced

**Electroencephalogram (EEG).** An established neurodiagnostic method; a method to record the electrical impulses of the brain by surface electrodes; can show different patterns of cerebral electrical discharge (brain waves) associated with different kinds of activity (e.g., listening, talking, thinking); abnormal electrical activity indicates cerebral pathology, including focal lesions in the brain.

**Electroglottography (EGG).** A noninvasive, electrical method to study the behaviors of the vocal folds; also called the laryngograph; in this procedure:

- Electrodes are attached on either side of the thyroid alae to record the electrical activity of the folds generated by their movement and vibration
- Recorded waveforms (Lx waveform) represent vocal fold opening (increased resistance to electrical conductance) and closing (decreased resistance)
- Different phases of opening and closing and the degree and duration of fold closures may be observed
- The generated waveforms may be affected by several factors including the placement of the electrodes, tissue thickens in the neck area, and gender of the client (more difficult to obtain representative Lx waveforms in women)

- Significant vocal fold lesions, mucous across the glottis, and paralysis of the folds reduce the reliability of assessment

**Endoscopy.** A fiberoptic instrument to view internal bodily structures; naso- or oropharyngolaryngoscopes are of special interest to otorhinolaryngologists and speech-language pathologists because they permit viewing of the laryngeal or pharyngeal structures; the essential features of endoscopic procedures and their diagnostic usefulness are as follows:



- Endoscopes can be inserted either through the nose (nasal endoscopy) or mouth (oral endoscopy) to view structures within the body and their functions
- Endoscopic examination of the laryngeal structures is useful in diagnosing laryngeal pathologies, vocal fold vibrations, and associated voice disorders; see Voice Disorders
- Endoscopic examination of the pharyngeal structures is useful in observing the velopharyngeal structures and functions and thus useful in assessing these mechanisms in clients with clefts and velopharyngeal incompetence
- Endoscopic examination of the laryngeal and pharyngeal structures and functions helps evaluate swallowing functions and aspiration; see Dysphagia
- Endoscopic examinations are invasive procedures, although trained speech-language pathologists working in medical settings may perform them
- Endoscopes may be connected to a stroboscope, which is a thin bundle of fibers that carry light and illuminate the structures to be observed; another set of fibers bring the image back to a monitor; may be connected to a video recorder for recorded images
- Endoscopes should not be used as the sole data source for diagnosis because some distortions may be common

**Ethnocultural Considerations in Assessment.** Assessment of factors related to the individual's cultural, ethnic, social, family, and personal variables that may affect communication and its disorders is important to make nonbiased and valid diagnoses of speech and language impairments; often assumed to be of importance in assessing ethnic or cultural minority group members, but relevant to all individuals, including those belonging to majority ethnic or cultural groups; consider the following in designing appropriate assessment procedures for clients of all ethnocultural groups; note that the suggestions are only illustrative, not exhaustive:

- Understand the differences in prevalence rates of different disorders or related medical conditions in different ethnocultural groups
  - Note that in African Americans:
    - High prevalence of hypertension and strokes
    - High prevalence of multi-infarct dementia, but possibly a low incidence of Alzheimer's disease
    - A high prevalence of head injury, especially due to gunshot wounds in the youth
    - A high prevalence of laryngeal, lung, and esophageal cancers
    - A low incidence of cleft palate, especially cleft lip
    - Generally low smoking rate

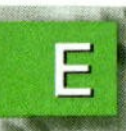

- Note that in American Indians:
  - High prevalence of otitis media
  - High prevalence of cleft palate
  - Generally high smoking rate
  - High prevalence of alcoholism and fetal alcohol syndrome
  - Generally low prevalence of lung cancer
- Note that in Asian Americans:
  - High prevalence rate of strokes
  - Low prevalence of Alzheimer's disease, especially in Chinese Americans
  - High prevalence of cleft palate, especially in Chinese and Japanese
  - High prevalence of nasopharyngeal cancer in Chinese Americans
  - Generally low smoking rate
  - Generally low rate of alcoholism
- Note that in Hispanics:
  - Higher prevalence of strokes and diabetes than in whites
  - High prevalence of cardiovascular diseases, especially correlated with low income
  - Low prevalence of esophageal cancer
  - Generally low smoking rate

- Take note of gender differences in the prevalence of various diseases or disorders
  - High prevalence of high blood pressure in older nonwhite women, especially older African American women
  - High prevalence of laryngeal cancers in African American males
  - Higher prevalence of laryngeal cancer in African American females compared to white females
  - Higher prevalence of high blood pressure and arteriosclerosis in Hispanic women than in Hispanic men
  - Higher prevalence of multiple strokes in Hispanic men than in Hispanic women
  - Generally higher incidence of laryngeal pathologies in males than in females
  - High prevalence of vocal nodules in white *male* children and in African American *female* children
  - Higher prevalence of stuttering in males than in females
  - Higher prevalence of articulation and phonological disorders in males than in females
- Explore during the interview the different views and dispositions regarding diseases and disorders
  - Understand how the client's culture views the etiology, effects, and social significance of diseases and disorders of interest
  - Understand how the client's culture views treatment and rehabilitation for congenital or acquired deficiencies or disabilities
- Explore during the interview the different views and dispositions regarding communication and communication disorders
  - Understand how the client's cultural milieu views communication, its importance, and its need for social survival
  - Understand how language is used in different cultural groups and how the use of language varies depending on the communication partners

- Understand how the parents of children being evaluated view communication problems for which they seek help
- Note that in some minority cultures early cognitive changes associated with dementing diseases may be attributed to the normal aging process or folk illnesses
- Understand any social stigma attached to all or certain disorders of communication

- Explore during the interview the different views and dispositions regarding assessment and treatment of communicative disorders
  - Understand how the family views assessment and treatment and what expectations they have of clinical services
  - Explore the level of support the family members seem to offer for assessment and treatment of the client
- Observe the client carefully and take note of the client's and accompanying persons':
  - General behavioral disposition
  - Level of ease and comfort in interacting with you
  - Use of language with you and among themselves
  - Expressed opinions about communication disorders, etiology, assessment, treatment, and clinical expectations
- Explore during the interview different geographic and socioeconomic barriers to access to, and underuse of clinical services
  - Note that lack of access to health care and clinical services (including speech-language pathology services) may be a critical barrier that many minority families face
  - Note that probably due to health care access problems, dementia and other neurodegenerative diseases may be underdiagnosed in nonwhite populations
  - Note that undiagnosed depression in some elderly may be mistaken for dementia
  - Note that many diseases and associated disorders may be in a more advanced stage in minority groups because of lack of access to health care that leads to an early diagnosis
  - Seek appropriate services for clients and families; educate the family about resource and support systems that may be available to them
- Study and understand dialectal differences including Black English
  - Understand the semantic, morphological, syntactic, and pragmatic differences of African American English (Black English)
  - Understand variations in English dialects as influenced by the client's primary language
  - Develop your own resources on the phonological and language characteristics of such languages as Spanish, a Native American language, Chinese, or other languages that are spoken in your service area
  - Be aware of differences in the same primary language (e.g., Spanish spoken by Mexican Americans or Cuban Americans; dialectal variations of Chinese)
- Avoid cultural stereotypes; consider individual uniqueness
  - Understand cultural patterns, but always treat a client as a unique individual

- Explore to what extent a member of a cultural group is different from the majority of that group (e.g., an African American who does not speak the Black English dialect or a southern rural white person who does)
- Understand that foreign-born individuals of minority groups who live in the United States will have changed to varying degrees
- Consider the client's home environment and past experiences before formulating interview or assessment questions
- Consider the client's home environment and past experiences before selecting stimulus items to be used during assessment (e.g., exposure to certain kinds of toys, television shows, books)

- Select assessment tools that are ethnoculturally appropriate for the client
  - Consider the bilingual, multilingual, or bidialectal status of the client; select assessment tools that are appropriate for the language or dialectal status of the client
  - Select standardized tests that have, in their standardization process, sampled the ethnocultural group to which the client belongs; do not use a standardized test if it did not include persons from the client's ethnocultural background in its standardization process
  - Avoid testing information about practices or events that are not culturally maintained or reinforced (e.g., not celebrated anniversaries or birthdays)
  - If culturally appropriate standardized tests are not available, design Client-Specific Assessment Procedures; consider alternative methods of assessment, including Authentic Assessment, Criterion-Referenced Assessment; Dynamic Assessment, and Portfolio Assessment
  - Use trained interpreters in assessing bilingual/multilingual clients
- Make appropriate diagnostic decisions
  - Determine whether a communication disorder exists in the primary language, the second language (which may be English), or both
  - Do not diagnose an articulation disorder based solely on a dialect influenced by the client's primary language
  - Do not diagnose a language disorder in English unless the client's primary language characteristics are taken into account
  - Note the possibility of misclassification of minority children as being learning disabled or intellectually impaired; taking such misdiagnoses at their face value might unduly influence your assessment of communication disorders and prognosis for improvement; help correct such misdiagnoses with a detailed communication skill assessment
  - Try to avoid both the kinds of errors in assessment and diagnosis: and failing to make a diagnosis when a problem does exist, or making a diagnosis when there is no problem

Battle, D. E., (2002). *Communication disorders in multicultural populations* (3rd ed.). Boston, MA: Andover Medical Publishers.

Cheng, L. L. (1995). *Integrating language and learning for inclusion.* San Diego, CA: Singular Publishing Group.

Goldstein, B. A. (2004). *Bilingual development and disorders in Spanish-English speakers.* Baltimore, MD: Paul H. Brookes.

Gutierrez-Clellen, V., & Pena, E. (2001). Dynamic assessment of diverse children: A tutorial. *Language, Speech, and Hearing Services in Schools*, *32*, 212–224.

Hegde, M. N., & Maul, C. A. (2006). *Language disorders in children: An evidence-based approach to assessment and treatment.* Boston, MA: Allyn and Bacon.

Kamhi, A. G., Pollock, K. E., & Harris, J. L. (1996). *Communication development and disorders in African American Children.* Baltimore, MD: Paul H. Brookes.

Kayser, H. (1998). *Assessment and intervention resources for Hispanic children.* San Diego, CA: Singular Publishing Group.

Payne, J. C. (1997). *Adult neurogenic language disorders: Assessment and treatment.* San Diego, CA: Singular Publishing Group.

Roseberry-McKibbin, C. (2002). *Multicultural students with special language needs* (2nd ed.). Ocean Side, CA: Academic Communication Associates.

Schraeder, T., Quinn, M., Stockman, I., & Miller, J. (1999). Authentic assessment as an approach to preschool speech-language screening. *American Journal of Speech-Language Pathology, 8,* 195–200.

**Expressive Aphasia.** To assess this type of nonfluent aphasia, also known as Broca's aphasia; see Aphasia: Specific Types.

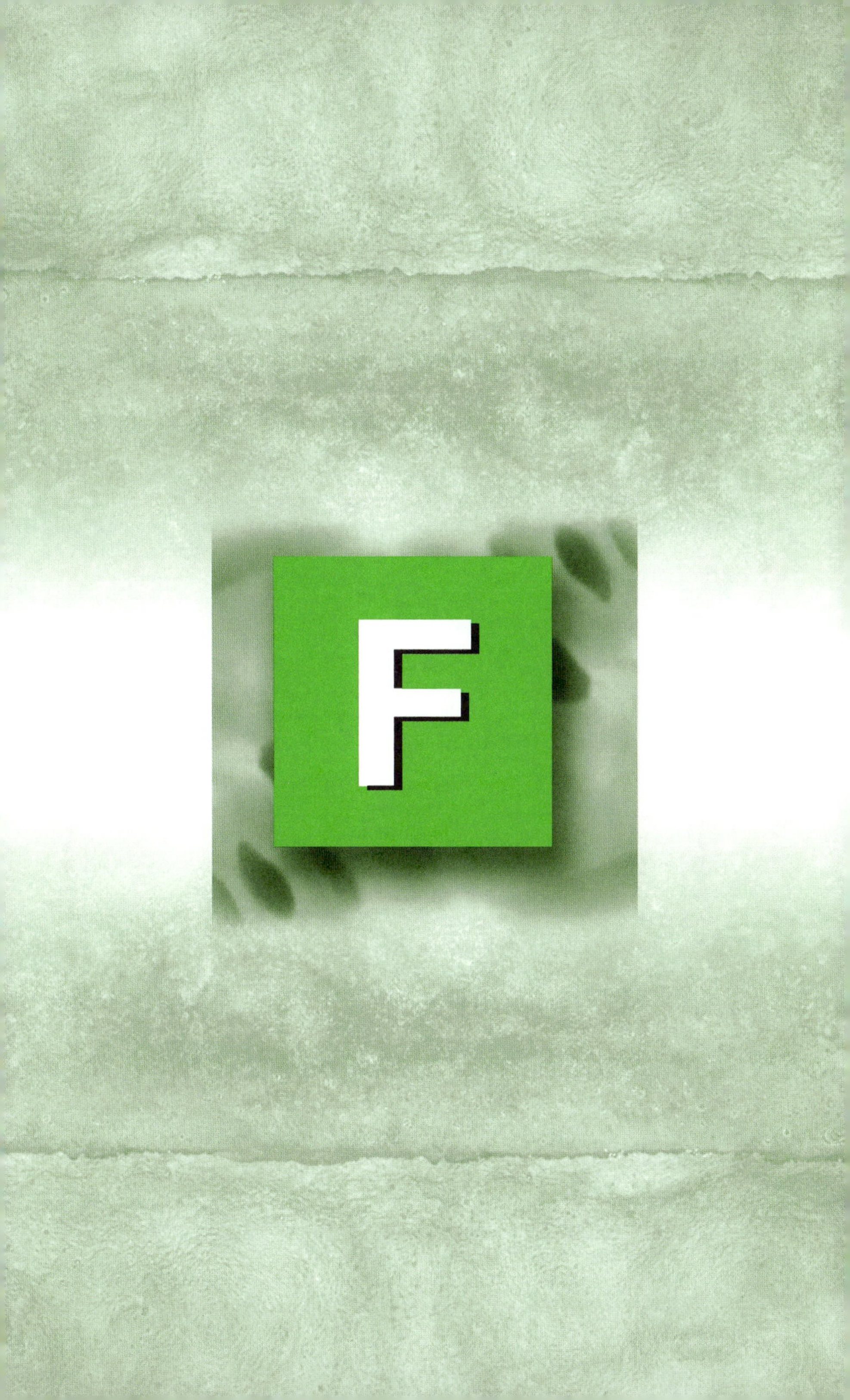
F

**Facio-Auriculo-Vertebral Syndrome.** To assess this syndrome, also known as the *Goldenhar syndrome*, see Syndromes Associated With Communication Disorders.

**First and Second Bronchial Arch Syndrome.** To assess this syndrome, also known as the *Goldenhar syndrome,* see Syndromes Associated With Communication Disorders.

F

**Flaccid Dysarthria.** A variety of motor speech disorder with lesions in the lower motor neurons; see Dysarthria for general assessment procedures and Dysarthria: Specific Types for assessment of flaccid dysarthria.

**Fluency Disorders.** Assessment of several speech disorders whose main characteristic is impaired fluency requires a differential diagnosis of Cluttering, Stuttering, and Neurogenic Stuttering; stuttering is the most researched and commonly assessed and treated fluency disorder; each fluency disorder has certain unique features, but an increase in the amount or duration of dysfluencies is a feature that is common to most fluency disorders; see the sources cited at the end of this main entry and the companion volume, *Hegde's PocketGuide to Communication Disorders* for details on epidemiology, symptomatology, and etiological theories of fluency disorders.

***Cluttering.*** A fluency disorder characterized by an excessively fast rate of speech that causes hurried and indistinct speech with too many dysfluencies; may also involve abnormal language and thought processes; similar to Stuttering but its unique features are significant; see the sources cited at the end of this main entry and the companion volume, *Hegde's PocketGuide to Communication Disorders* for symptomatology and etiology; clinicians assess cluttering as they would stuttering, but pay special attention to assessing the unique features of cluttering.

#### Assessment Objectives/General Guidelines

- To assess behaviors that suggest cluttering
- To assess any coexisting stuttering
- To suggest treatment options

#### Case History/Interview Focus

- See **Case History** and **Interview** under Standard/Common Assessment Procedures
- During the interview, explore the reasons why the client, especially an older student or an adult, is seeking clinical services
- Take note of any expressed or implied lack of motivation to seek services; the client may have come to the clinic because of the urging of family members or work place supervisors; unlike people who stutter, people who clutter show a lack of motivation to seek help
- Explore whether the client is concerned about his or her speech problem; unlike people who stutter, those who clutter may be less concerned about their speech problem
- Explore whether people have complained about not understanding the client's speech and if so, how did the client handle it; people who clutter

tend to dismiss such complaints and tend not to take effective corrective actions (e.g., speaking more slowly)
- Seek information on previous assessment and treatment; an adult who stutters is likely to have been more often assessed and treated than a person of comparable age who clutters

## Ethnocultural Considerations

- See Ethnocultural Considerations in Assessment

## Assessment



- Assess types and frequency of dysfluencies
  - Obtain a conversational speech sample to analyze the types and frequency of stuttering
  - The same kinds of dysfluencies are found in people who stutter and people who clutter; use the procedures under Stuttering
  - Ask the person to read a well-known text and have the person relax and speak; there may be a tendency for increased frequency of dysfluencies under these conditions
  - Take note of the degree of muscular effort associated with dysfluencies; possibly, in some people who clutter, the dysfluencies may be relatively effortless (unless there is a coexisting stuttering, which is often associated with increased effort)
  - Ask questions that require brief or short answers and alternate such questions with those that require longer responses; note the reduced rate of dysfluencies while giving short answers (not necessarily the case with people who stutter)
- Assess articulatory performance
  - Note that an assessment of articulatory performance—rate of speech and breakdowns in intelligibility—is more important in assessing cluttering than it is in assessing stuttering
  - Screen articulation to assess or rule out misarticulations; note that technically, cluttering is not an articulation disorder; articulation problems associated with cluttering may not be revealed in isolated word productions; however, a person who clutters may have an independent articulation disorder as well
  - Evaluate articulation in conversational speech and oral reading when the client used his or her typical rate of speech
  - If a normally slow rate is not spontaneously exhibited (a likely event), model a slower rate of speech and ask the person to imitate that rate to assess production of speech sounds; make sure the rate is actually reduced because persons who clutter have difficulty imitating a slower rate of speech
  - Have the client repeat progressively longer words (*love, loving, lovingly; thick, thicken, thickening*); take note of deterioration in articulation as the word length increases
  - Take note of improved articulation when the rate is slowed down; any errors still remaining may suggest an independent articulation disorder; if such errors are evident, consider administering a test of

articulation; see Articulation and Phonological Disorders for assessment procedures and standardized tests
    - Take note of unique articulatory breakdowns seen in people who clutter; in addition to the more typical omissions of sounds, they may omit syllables and entire words while speaking rapidly; they may transpose sounds, telescope syllables, and invert the order of sounds in words
- Assess rate of speech
    - Assess both the overall rate of speech and the articulatory rate; see Stuttering for procedures
    - Assess intelligibility in relation to the rate of speech; judge speech intelligibility when the client is talking in his or her usual manner; judge again when you manipulate the rate by asking the client to slow down the rate for a period of time; take note of the typical improvement in intelligibility at slower rates
    - Take note of progressively faster speech; even those who manage to reduce the rate soon after a request is made may speed it up very soon
    - Take note of fast and short bursts of speech during conversation
    - Take note of rate variations and irregular rates in different segments of speech
- Assess language skills
    - Use the conversational speech sample to assess the client's production of various morphologic, syntactic, and pragmatic structures
    - In the case of children who clutter, administer a standardized language test if judged appropriate and necessary; see Language Disorders in Children
    - In the case of adults who clutter, make judgments of grammaticality of sentences produced and correct use of grammatical morphemes; assess whether client produces varied types of sentences
    - Judge whether the client produces run-on sentences and misuses pronouns or prepositions
    - Assess pragmatic language skills; during conversation, take note of the frequency with which the client introduced a topic, interrupted conversation or inappropriately took turns, or terminated conversation abruptly
    - Assess whether the client exhibited appropriate conversational repair strategies because this may give a significant clue to the client's awareness of his or her speech problems and willingness to modify speech to help the listener; frequently request for clarification (suggesting a problem in comprehending what the client said) and evaluate whether the client modified his or her productions (such as speaking more slowly)
    - Take note of fluency and rate breakdowns as the complexity of language tasks increases
- Assess oral reading skills
    - Select a fairly easy prose passage for the client to read; in the case of children, select material that is at least one grade below their academic level; select materials that are ethnoculturally appropriate for the client

    - Ask the client to read the passage aloud and take note of word omissions, sound distortions, sound telescoping, sound transpositions, and so forth during oral reading
    - Take note of the rate of reading; it is likely to be too rapid for the listener's comprehension
- Obtain a writing sample
    - Ask the client to write two short paragraphs to dictation
    - Ask the client to spontaneously write a short passage (about one's school, friends, vacations, work, hobby, etc.)
    - Take note of the errors including spelling errors, letter formation, organization of paragraphs, transition within and across paragraphs, margins, punctuation, and so forth
- Assess voice and resonance
    - During the interview, informally assess voice and resonance qualities
    - Take note of any voice quality deviations and any resonance problems
    - If an independent voice disorder is suspected, make a more complete assessment of voice and resonance; use procedures described under Voice Disorders



### Related/Medical Assessment Data

- Obtain any available neurologic and medical assessment reports; take note of any allergies
- Obtain psychological and neuropsychological assessment reports
- Obtain reports from teachers about academic performance

### Standard/Common Assessment Procedures

- Complete the Standard/Common Assessment Procedures
- Make a thorough orofacial examination to rule out any muscle weakness or structural anomalies

### Analysis of Assessment Data

- Analyze the types and frequency of dysfluencies; calculate the percent dysfluency rate; see Stuttering
- Analyze the speech rate data; calculate the speech rate and articulatory rate
- Analyze the articulation assessment data; make a list of errors of articulation
- Analyze any improvement or deterioration in articulation depending on the rate of speech and articulatory rate
- Analyze any errors of articulation that may be independent of the rate problem (errors in slower speech; errors in single word productions)
- Judge the intelligibility of speech for running conversational speech, speech produced at a slower rate, and for individual words and phrases
- Analyze language skills; take note of morphologic, syntactic, and pragmatic problems; take note of any indication of language formulation problems and disorganized thought processes; take note of conversational repair strategies the client uses to gauge the client's awareness of, or concern about, the speech problem

- Analyze the reading and writing problems; relate them to the teacher's reports and data from any educational assessment (e.g., learning disabilities)
- Summarize voice and resonance problems, if any
- Make judgments about the client's awareness of his or her speech problem, or more likely, the level of concern he or she expresses about it or indirectly implies (e.g., by not slowing down the speech or modifying it in other ways when a request for clarification is made)

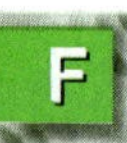


### Diagnostic Criteria

- The most critical diagnostic features that may be more common across clients than other features include an excessively fast rate associated with sound omissions, substitutions, transpositions, and word telescoping resulting in reduced intelligibility of speech
- Excessive amount of dysfluencies
- Other listed symptoms that may be present in some cases; note that disorganized thought and reading and writing problems may not be found in all those who clutter

### Differential Diagnosis

- Differentiate between cluttering and Stuttering; cluttering and Neurogenic Stuttering
- Note that people who stutter are more aware and more concerned with their speech difficulty than are those who clutter
- People who stutter tend to exhibit more negative emotions and avoidance behaviors related to speech and speaking situations than those who clutter
- Dysfluencies of people who stutter may be associated with a greater degree of muscular effort than the dysfluencies of people who clutter
- People who stutter are more likely to stutter on short responses (e.g., saying one's own name, giving their telephone number or address, greeting people, saying *good bye*) than those who clutter
- Neurogenic stuttering is of late (adult) onset whereas both cluttering and stuttering are diagnosed in childhood years, although the diagnosis of cluttering may be a bit more delayed than the diagnosis of stuttering
- People who have neurogenic stuttering have a recent history of neurological impairment including strokes, tumors, and other forms of cerebral insults; they exhibit neurological symptoms that people who clutter do not
- Some people with neurogenic stuttering also may have aphasia, dysarthria, or apraxia that is typically not associated with cluttering (or stuttering of early onset)
- See also Stuttering and Neurogenic Stuttering for additional distinguishing features
- Note that when cluttering and stuttering often coexist, the distinction may be blurred, but the special features of cluttering would still be needed to make a differential diagnosis of both the disorders

### Prognosis

- No hard data to predict prognosis
- Impression of many clinicians is that it is generally more difficult to treat cluttering than stuttering, possibly due to reduced motivation and reduced awareness or concern
- Generally, greater clinical effort is needed to promote self-monitoring skills in people who clutter

### Recommendations

- Treatment designed to induce slower rate of speech, careful formulation of language expression when warranted, and procedures to increase awareness and self-monitoring
- See the cited sources at the end of this main entry and the two companion volumes, *Hegde's PocketGuide to Communication Disorders* and *Hegde's PocketGuide to Treatment in Speech-Language Pathology* (3rd ed.)



***Neurogenic Stuttering.*** A disorder of fluency that has a demonstrated neurological basis; also known as *acquired stuttering*, although this term is confusing because the early onset stuttering with no neurological basis also may be acquired; often associated with aphasia; may be associated with apraxia of speech; may be associated with strokes in the absence of aphasia; re-emergence of stuttering in a person who had stuttered but was fluent for years until the onset of the neurological condition is also included in this category, though somewhat controversially; may be persistent or transient; see the cited sources at the end of this main entry and the two companion volumes, *Hegde's PocketGuide to Communication Disorders* and *Hegde's PocketGuide to Treatment in Speech-Language Pathology* (3rd ed.)

### Assessment Objectives/General Guidelines

- To assess all aspects of the neurogenic communication disorder
- To assess the types and frequency of dysfluencies that help distinguish neurogenic stuttering from other kinds of fluency disorders
- To assess the unique characteristics of neurogenic stuttering that would help make a differential diagnosis and distinguish it from stuttering of early onset and cluttering
- To suggest treatment strategies if a diagnosis is made

### Case History/Interview Focus

- See **Case History** and **Interview** under Standard/Common Assessment Procedures; see also Stuttering
- In taking the case history and in reviewing the client's medical records, concentrate on the onset of the various medical conditions that may be associated with neurogenic stuttering
- Check the case history and medical records and question the family members about strokes and the onset of aphasia, clinical conditions that cause Apraxia of Speech, Dysarthria (especially hypokinetic dysarthria), head trauma, such extrapyramidal diseases as Parkinson's disease, progressive supranuclear palsy, brain tumors, brain surgery, seizure

disorders, dialysis dementia, drug toxicity, cerebral anoxia, and so forth; see *Hegde's PocketGuide to Communication Disorders* for details on etiological or associated disease conditions

- Review medical and neurodiagnostic assessment results to ascertain brain lesions; likely to be in the left cerebral hemispheres in a majority of cases
- If possible, ascertain whether the lesion is bilateral or unilateral because of their differential prognostic significance
- Ascertain that the onset of the fluency problem was subsequent to the onset of the medical problem
- Take a detailed history to document normal fluency during early childhood days or if early stuttering was documented, document regained normal fluency until the late onset of neurogenic stuttering

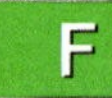


### Assessment

- Assess associated Aphasia, Apraxia of Speech, Dementia, or other neurogenic communication disorders with which neurogenic stuttering may be associated
- Assess types and frequency of dysfluencies; see Stuttering
- Assess associated motor behaviors; see Stuttering
- Assess variability in stuttering; see Stuttering
- Assess the unique and differentially diagnostic features of neurogenic stuttering
- Assess Adaptation in oral reading
- Assess the dysfluency rates under masking noise
- Assess the dysfluency rates during choral reading
- Take note of dysfluency rates on function and content words
- Assess dysfluencies when the person speaks to a metronomic rhythm
- Take note of dysfluencies on medial and final syllables in words

### Related/Medical Assessment Data

- Study the medical history of the client as described
- Obtain all available neurological and neurodiagnostic reports
- Obtain speech-language pathology reports on aphasia, apraxia, dementia, dysarthria, and related neurologically based speech or language disorders if an assessment for those disorders has already been made

### Standard/Common Assessment Procedures

- Complete the Standard/Common Assessment Procedures
- Make a thorough orofacial examination to evaluate orofacial muscle weakness or paralysis that may be associated with a coexisting dysarthria

### Diagnostic Criteria

- Clear evidence of a neurological disease, trauma, or toxicity is essential to make a neurogenic stuttering diagnosis
- Neurological symptoms consistent with the underlying condition or the disease; for instance, various movement disorders in the case of dysarthria
- Evidence of aphasia and stroke if dysarthria and apraxia are ruled out; note, though, that neurogenic stuttering may or may not be accompanied

by aphasia, but the evidence of stroke or other adverse neurological event will have to be documented

- Late onset of fluency problems and convincing information suggesting lack of stuttering of childhood onset
- Dysfluency characteristics that are diagnostic of neurogenic stuttering

### Differential Diagnosis

- See Stuttering for differential diagnostic guidelines
- To distinguish nonfluent aphasia from neurogenic stuttering, rule out word retrieval problems that may also induce dysfluencies; dysfluencies may precede words that are hard to recall; they may be heard on persistent errors on the wrong word being produced; clients with word retrieval problems will find it hard to generate word lists; see Aphasia for these and other characteristics of word retrieval problems that are not characteristic of strict neurogenic stuttering
- Be aware that neurogenic dysfluencies that are due to word-finding problems may coexist in a client; try to separate them to the extent possible
- Take note of stuttering on medial and final syllables; dysfluent production of function words (versus content words); dysfluencies in imitated speech; lack of adaptation effect; few or less remarkable associated motor behaviors or avoidance behaviors; little or no effect of delayed auditory feedback, masking noise, rhythmic speech, and choral reading; little or no anxiety about stuttering that helps distinguish neurogenic stuttering from early-onset stuttering
- Note, however, that neurogenic stuttering in clients with extrapyramidal diseases may show the adaptation effect
- People with neurogenic stuttering are likely to show evidence of brain injury on such tasks as copying and drawing, tapping to rhythm; not evident in people with early-onset stuttering
- The presence of dysphagia and other fluency disorders may also suggest neurogenic stuttering

### Prognosis

- Variable, depending on the underlying neurological disease or trauma
- No specific information on the prognostic variables although it is known that people with bilateral damage may have more persistent stuttering than those with unilateral damage

### Recommendations

- Treatment to improve fluency
- See the cited sources at the end of this main entry and *Hegde's PocketGuide to Treatment in Speech-Language Pathology* (3rd ed.) for details

***Stuttering.*** A speech problem characterized by impaired fluency and rhythm of speech; a speech disorder of early childhood onset; although there is no universally agreed-upon definition, clinicians usually have no difficulty diagnosing well-established stuttering in adults when they see its visual features and hear its audible characteristics; may be difficult to diagnose at the time of onset and in some individuals of any age, mostly because of its variability across time and situations; the problem may not be evident during a particular assessment session; needs to be distinguished from cluttering and neurogenic stuttering; many clinicians measure the types and number of dysfluencies in speech to diagnose stuttering, although additional features are important to consider; the final diagnosis is based on multiple factors including the types, amounts, and the characteristics of dysfluencies, avoidance and negative emotions, and struggle and tension associated with dysfluent speech production; see the sources cited at the end of this main entry and the companion volume, *Hegde's PocketGuide to Communication Disorders* for epidemiology and ethnocultural variables, symptomatology, and theories of stuttering.



### Assessment Objectives/General Guidelines

- To assess the types and frequency of dysfluencies or stutterings in conversational speech and oral reading
- To assess associated motor behaviors
- To assess variability in stuttering across speaking situations
- To assess avoidance and negative emotional reactions
- To diagnose stuttering of early childhood onset
- To distinguish stuttering of early onset from neurogenic stuttering and cluttering
- To suggest treatment options and counsel parents of children who stutter

### Case History/Interview Focus

- See **Case History** and **Interview** under Standard/Common Assessment Procedures
- During the interview, concentrate on the onset and course of stuttering; note that the onset typically occurs between the ages of 2.5 and 6 years; therefore, family members are the main source of information on the onset
- Find out what the parents did when they first noticed stuttering in their child; ask about any suggestions they may have offered the child (e.g., *Speak slowly, Think before you talk*, etc.) and the effects the suggestions had on the child's stuttering
- Obtain information on previous assessment and treatment; get the details about the treatment procedures from the previous clinician
- Ask the parents about the course of the disorder: variable, constant, progressively deteriorating, or gradually improving; any specific conditions that may provoke more stuttering or situations that help improve fluency
- Question the parents about the child's avoidance and negative emotional experiences associated with speech; the child may avoid one or more conversational partners (it may be one of the parents) or speaking situations
- Obtain information on family history of stuttering
- In the case of school-age children, get information on the child's academic performance, peer reactions, and teacher reactions to stuttering

## Ethnocultural Considerations

- See Ethnocultural Considerations in Assessment
- Explore the family members' views on speech fluency, speech and language competence, speech disability, and treatment options
- Ascertain whether the child is bilingual, and if so, determine which language is predominant (primary) and make preparations to assess the child's stuttering in both languages
- Assess the family resources for sustained treatment and find out about the needs of the family and the support system they may need
- Gauge the family members' sophistication in conducting home treatment and the extent of training they may need



## Assessment of Stuttering

- Assessment of stuttering is multidimensional; it typically includes the assessment of dysfluencies, associated motor behaviors, avoidance reactions, negative emotions, rate of speech, breathing abnormalities associated with dysfluent speech, variability across situations, adaptation and consistency (likely an optional procedure), and characteristics of fluent production
- When there is doubt about the existence of stuttering, repeated assessment will be necessary; often, the clients or their parents may submit home speech samples, recorded over a period of time, that capture stuttering behaviors for clinical analysis
- Generally speaking, when an adult or parents of a child report stuttering, there usually is stuttering; some parents may miss stuttering for a while in their child, but once they conclude their child stutters, they are typically right about it
- False negatives (the wrong conclusion that there is no problem when there is one) are more likely than false positives (the wrong conclusion that there is a problem when there is none)
- Assess frequency and types of dysfluencies or stutterings
  - Conversational speech with the clinician
    - Take an extended conversational speech sample

    In the case of young children, have toys, books, objects, and other materials to evoke speech; see Speech and Language Sample under Standard/Common Assessment Procedures
    - In the case of adults, use the interview as a means of conversational speech sampling
    - Tape-record the speech sample and the interview with the client for later analysis of dysfluencies or stutterings
    - Take note of associated motor behaviors during the interview and speech sampling; write down the specific kinds of associated motor behaviors the client exhibited
    - If you are trained or want to train yourself to do it reliably, count the dysfluencies as you interview the client; until the reliability of your measures are established, consider repeated counting of the

dysfluencies on the audiotape or videotape as the more reliable measure (see Analysis of Assessment Data for additional suggestions)

- Conversational speech with a family member
  - Ask the accompanying family member to engage the client in conversation
  - In the case of children, let the parent or other family member use toys, pictures, objects, and storybooks to stimulate and maintain conversation for about 10 minutes
  - Audiotape the conversation for later analysis of dysfluencies
- Oral reading sample
  - Select a printed passage that is appropriate for the client's age, education, cultural background, and general interest
  - Have the client read it aloud in his or her usual manner
  - Tape-record the oral reading for later analysis of dysfluencies or stutterings
  - Count the number and types of dysfluencies as the client reads if you are trained to do that reliably or wish to train yourself to do that reliably
  - If you wish to count dysfluencies during the session, have a copy of the printed passage in front of you and mark dysfluencies on the page itself; until the reliability of your measures are established, consider counting dysfluencies from repeated listening of the audio- or video-tape as the more reliable measure



- Assess speech, language, and voice
  - Use the conversational speech for making clinical judgments about speech, language, and voice
    - Take note of errors of articulation; children who stutter may have a coexisting articulation disorder
    - Take note of the client's language production including grammatical, syntactic, and pragmatic structures; take note of limitations or deviations; children who stutter may have a coexisting language disorder
    - Take note of voice quality, intensity, loudness, and resonance characteristics
    - Make a detailed assessment of articulation and phonological disorders, language disorders, and voice disorders if clinical judgment indicates a need; see Articulation Disorders, Language Disorders, and Voice Disorders for procedural details including information on selected standardized tests (especially for testing articulation and language skills)
- Assess associated motor behaviors
  - Note that for most clinical purposes, it is sufficient to describe associated motor behaviors and make judgments about their general frequency levels (e.g., *frequent nose wrinkling, an occasional foot tapping*); systematic counting may be necessary only for research purposes
    - Take notes during the interview and oral reading on all the associated motor behaviors
    - Give clear and specific descriptions of them

    - Have a checklist of associated motor behaviors on which you record the occurrence of specific behaviors
- Assess avoidance behaviors
  - Note that most avoidance behaviors are self-reported by the client; parents of children may report some of the obvious avoidance reactions (e.g., the child's overstatement, *I don't want to talk*, or an obvious avoidance of one or more conversational partners)
    - Explore avoidance behaviors during the interview; take note of frequent word changes or substitutions, beating around the bush (circumlocution), use of less precise synonyms, changing syntax in the middle of a sentence, and easy and fluent repetitions or long periods of silent pauses that are followed by severe dysfluencies (such repetitions or pauses may be attempts at avoiding or postponing ensuing severe dysfluencies)
    - Ask the client to make a list of sounds or words that are especially difficult
    - Ask the client to make a hierarchy of most difficult (e.g., speaking to the boss) to least difficult (speaking to a close friend) speaking situations
    - Ask the client to expand and refine the difficult sounds/words list and the hierarchy of situations during the next few days and give them back to you on the next visit
    - Ask the family members or friends who accompany the client to describe avoidance reactions they have observed
- Assess frequency and types of dysfluencies in nonclinical situations
  - At home
    - Ask the client or a family member to audiotape three conversational samples over the following few days and submit them for evaluation
    - Ask the family member to watch your method of recording the conversational speech sample
    - In the case of children, ask the parents to use your method of recording a speech sample
  - At school
    - Obtain a verbal report from teachers about the amount and types of dysfluencies the client exhibits in the classroom
    - Audiotape the client's conversation with a peer
    - Have the teacher audiotape a brief conversational speech sample and submit for analysis
    - Have the teacher audiotape a reading sample and submit for analysis
  - At work
    - If practical, have the client audiotape a sample of conversation with a colleague
    - Note that such assignments often are more readily completed when treatment is started, a good working relationship is established, and you have convinced the client about their necessity and importance
- Assess overall rate of speech
  - Use the speech sample to assess the rate of speech

  - Take at least three 2-minute samples from the total speech sample; select one sample from the beginning, one from the middle, and one more from the final portion of the interview
  - With a digital stopwatch, calculate the number of words/syllables spoken per minute
  - Discount pauses in calculating the rate of speech
- Assess articulatory rate
  - Use the three 2-minute samples selected from the larger sample
  - Discount all dysfluencies or stuttering including pauses that exceed 2 seconds
  - Count the number of syllables produced per minute to obtain the articulatory rate
- Assess variability in stuttering and establish reliability of measures
  - Obtain verbal reports from the client about variability in stuttering across different situations and over time
  - Obtain verbal reports from family members regarding variability in stuttering across time and situations
  - Compare the frequency of dysfluencies produced at home with the frequency obtained in the clinic
  - If the clinic and the home samples are widely discrepant, repeat both; question the client, family members, or both to evaluate the representativeness of the amount of dysfluencies exhibited in all speech and reading samples
- Assess fluency characteristics
  - Use the recorded speech sample for this assessment
  - Find out the longest fluent utterance (measured in words or syllables)
  - Find out the most frequently occurring fluent interval (measured in seconds or minutes)
  - Find out the most frequently occurring fluent response (measured in words or syllables)
- Assess negative emotional reactions
  - During the interview, explore the various negative emotional reactions listed earlier; ask the client to describe his or her feelings about speech, speaking situations, listeners, and self
  - Administer a comprehensive assessment battery to evaluate the negative emotions and attitudes associated with stuttering (e.g., the *Behavior Assessment Battery* by G. Brutten & M. Vanryckeghem; the *S-Scale* by R. L. Erickson; and the modified version by G. Andrews & J. Cutler)
  - Ask the spouse, parents, or other family members about negative emotions the client typically expresses
- Assess breathing abnormalities
  - Take note of all breathing abnormalities exhibited during the assessment session (e.g., trying to speak on inhalation, trying to speak when the expiratory air is already exhausted, impounding the inhaled air in the lungs by abrupt and hard glottal closure)
  - Take note of the different kinds of dysfluencies with which specific breathing abnormalities may be associated

- Assess adaptation effect and consistency effect
  - Consider these as optional measures; they help gauge the severity of stuttering on certain sounds and words with some treatment implications
  - Have the client read a printed passage aloud five times in succession (e.g., the *Rainbow Passage* for adults and *Arthur the Young Rat* for children)
  - On a copy of the printed passage, mark the words stuttered during each of the five oral readings; take note of the words or loci on which stuttering was repeated twice, thrice, four times, and five times
  - Count the number of dysfluencies separately for each reading trial
  - Chart the frequency of dysfluencies across oral readings; take note of the degree of adaptation
  - Make a list of words and sounds on which stuttering was most consistent
  - Make a list of words and sounds on which stuttering was least consistent (i.e., stuttered only once; most adapted)
  - Use the data to identify words on which stuttering is most and least likely; expect the most likely (most severe) stuttering to be lingering in the later stages of treatment, which will then have to be handled with special attention
- Assess stimulability (potential treatment probes)
  - Ask the client to reduce the speech rate dramatically; model a slow rate with continuous phonation; take note of the effects on dysfluencies
  - Ask the client to initiate sounds softly and gently; take note of the effects on dysfluencies
  - Ask the client to inhale and exhale a small amount of air before starting to speak; model the behaviors; take note of the effects on dysfluencies
  - Try such other treatment contingencies as pause-and-talk (time-out) or response cost to evaluate their potential usefulness

### Related/Medical Assessment Data

- Integrate any medical information of relevance with your assessment data; if there is evidence of neurological involvement, investigate this further and re-examine the age of onset in an adult client; consider the possibility of neurogenic stuttering (not stuttering of early childhood onset)
- Integrate educational and occupational information with your assessment data
- Integrate case history information and reports from other professionals with your assessment data

### Standard/Common Assessment Procedures

- Complete the Standard/Common Assessment Procedures
- Pay special attention to the onset and development of stuttering and information on previous assessment and treatment information

### Analysis of Assessment Data

- Analyze all speech and oral reading samples for the frequency and types of dysfluencies or stutterings
- List the types of dysfluencies and their frequencies separately for each sample

- Count the number of words in a speech or reading sample
- Calculate either the percent dysfluency rate or the number of dysfluencies per 100 words spoken or read (percent dysfluency rate = number of dysfluencies divided by the total number of words spoken or read and multiplied by 100)
- Measure the durations of at least the 15 longest dysfluencies and 15 shortest dysfluencies to give a range of durations
- Note that the following kinds of dysfluencies are especially difficult to measure and that you need to train yourself to measure them reliably:
  - Silent pauses (tendency is to ignore them)
  - Different types of dysfluencies that are clustered, combined, or produced in rapid succession; in such a cluster, one or more dysfluencies may be missed
  - Interjections, especially the schwa (tendency is to ignore them)
  - Word repetitions (tendency is to ignore them)
  - Any dysfluency that is extremely brief, fleeting, and softly produced (e.g., a brief sound prolongation or a weak schwa)
  - Silent prolongations on audiotapes (tendency is to not to recognize them as silent prolongations and to consider them as insignificant pauses)
- Summarize the associated motor behaviors, avoidance behaviors, negative emotional reactions, and situational variability in stuttering
- If desired, rate the severity of stuttering; consider using the *Stuttering Severity Instrument* by G. Riley

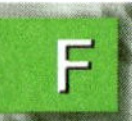


### Diagnostic Criteria

- Use one of several primary diagnostic criteria
  - An operationally defined excessive amount of dysfluencies when all types of dysfluencies are counted (e.g., 5% dysfluency rate based on the number of words spoken)
  - Part-word repetitions, sound prolongations, and broken words at less than 5% of the words spoken because of lower social threshold of tolerance for these dysfluency types (perhaps only 3%)
  - Clinically judged excessive duration of dysfluencies when neither of the first two criteria is met
- Consider other assessment data in conjunction with the primary diagnostic criteria
  - Rapidity of dysfluencies; note though, that some young children close to the time of onset may produce multiple repetitions of syllables, words, and phrases at a normal rate
  - The number of repetition units in an instance of part-word and word repetitions (the greater the number of units, the higher the chance that the repetitions will be judged as stutterings)
  - Tension and effort associated with dysfluencies; note, though, that some young children may produce multiple dysfluencies with little or no tension
  - Associated motor behaviors; not critical for diagnosis, but when they are observed in conjunction with dysfluencies, diagnosis of stuttering is supported

- Negative emotional experiences associated with speech and speaking situations; not critical to diagnose stuttering, partly because many preschool children at the time onset either do not exhibit them or cannot describe them reliably; when present, they are important to support the diagnosis and plan for treatment
- Avoidance of speaking situations, certain conversational partners, and sounds and words; not critical for diagnosis of stuttering because many children at the time of onset may not have clearly established avoidance reactions



### Differential Diagnosis

- Differentiate stuttering from normally fluent speech
  - Note that normally fluent speech also contains dysfluencies (although at a lower level)
  - Note that normally fluent individuals also may avoid certain people or speaking situations for reasons unrelated to stuttering; one might avoid talking to people who are boring, overbearing, or offensive
  - Note that not only those who stutter, but those who have other kinds of communication disorders also may be concerned about their speech and minimize talking (e.g., a child with limited language skills, an adult with aphasia)
  - Use one of the diagnostic criteria specified above to diagnose stuttering; increased frequency of dysfluencies and possibly changes in their topography (added tension and rapidity of production) distinguish normally fluent speech from stuttering
  - Use such associated features of stuttering as emotional reactions, avoidance, and breathing abnormalities that are not typical of normally fluent speech to support a diagnosis of stuttering
- Differentiate stuttering from cluttering on the basis of
  - Consider the overall symptom complex: stuttering as a fluency disorder and cluttering as more than a fluency disorder
  - Rate of speech: excessively fast or somewhat erratic in cluttering, which is not a distinguishing feature of stuttering
  - Indistinct articulation and lack of intelligibility: possibly due to excessively fast or rate burst associated with cluttering, which is not a distinguishing feature of stuttering
  - Disorganized language and thinking in some individuals with cluttering: may not be found in all persons who clutter, but when it is evident, it supports the diagnosis of cluttering (along with other critical features); a language disorder associated with stuttering is not likely to be described as disorganized with an implication of disorganized thinking; it will more likely resemble Language Disorders in Children without stuttering
  - Awareness of the problem: high in people who stutter and low in those who clutter
  - Concern about the speech or speech problem: little or none in people who clutter and much, to the extent of being fearful, in people who stutter

- Concern about listener reactions: low in people who clutter and high in those who stutter
- Speaking under stress: possibly better in people who clutter and worse in those who stutter
- Speaking while relaxed: possibly worse in people who clutter and better in those who stutter
- Giving short answers: possibly better in people who clutter and worse in those who stutter
- Reading a well-known text: possibly worse in people who clutter and better in those who stutter
- Reading an unknown text: possibly better in people who clutter and worse in those who stutter
- Motivation for therapy: generally poor in people who clutter and generally good in people who stutter

- Differentiate Stuttering of Childhood Onset (SCO) from Neurogenic Stuttering (NGS) on the basis of:
  - Age of onset: stuttering during early childhood and NGS in later years, often in older people
  - Neurological symptoms: prominent in NGS and absent or extremely subtle in SCO
  - Repetitions of medial and final syllables in words: rarely if ever in SCO and may be observed in NGS
  - Dysfluent production of function words: less common in older children and adults with SCO and may be more common in NGS; note, though that children under 7 or 8 may produce significant amounts of dysfluencies on function words (e.g., conjunctions, prepositions, pronouns)
  - Etiology: largely unknown and no specific cause detected in most cases with SCO but the presence of such neurological-medical conditions as stroke, tumors, traumatic brain injury, parkinsonism, dialysis dementia in NGS
  - Adaptation effect: may be absent or less pronounced in NGS than in SCO
  - Problems in copying and drawing: may be a distinguishing feature of NGS, but not SCO
  - Problems in copying block designs: may be a distinguishing feature of NGS, but not SCO
  - Problems in sequential hand positions: may be a distinguishing feature of NGS, but not SCO
  - Problems in tapping out rhythms: may be a distinguishing feature of NGS, but not SCO

## Prognosis

- Prognosis for improved fluency is good with systematic treatment in most children and adults who stutter
- Maintenance of fluency in adults is good, but only with systematic follow-up and periodic booster treatment; maintenance of fluency is generally better when children are treated
- Early intervention is especially effective

### Recommendations

- Treatment for all clients and at all age levels when a diagnosis of stuttering is made
- See the cited sources and the two companion volumes: *Hegde's PocketGuide to Communication Disorders* and *Hegde's PocketGuide to Treatment in Speech-Language Pathology* (3rd ed.) for details

Bloodstein, O. (1995). *A handbook on stuttering.* San Diego, CA: Singular Publishing Group.

Conture, E. G. (2001). *Stuttering: Its nature, diagnosis and treatment.* Boston, MA: Allyn and Bacon.

Culatta, R., & Goldberg, S. A. (1995). *Stuttering therapy: An integrated approach to theory and practice.* Boston, MA: Allyn and Bacon.

Curlee, R. F. (1999). *Stuttering and related disorders of fluency* (2nd ed.). New York: Thieme.

Daly, D. A. (1986). The clutterer. In K. O. St. Louis (Ed.), *The atypical stutterer: Principles and practices of rehabilitation.* Orlando, FL: Academic Press.

Daly, D. A., & Burnett, M. L. (1999). Cluttering: Traditional views and new perspectives. In R. F. Curlee (Ed.), *Stuttering and related disorders of fluency* (2nd ed.), pp. 222–254. New York: Thieme.

Duffy, J. R. (2005). *Motor speech disorders: Substrates, differential diagnosis, and management* (2nd ed.). New York: Elsevier Mosby.

Gregory, H. (2003). *Stuttering therapy: Rationale and procedures.* Boston, MA: Allyn and Bacon.

Guitar, B. (2006). *Stuttering: An integrated approach to its nature and treatment* (3rd ed.). Baltimore, MD: Williams & Wilkins.

Helm-Estabrooks, N. (1986). Diagnosis and management of neurogenic stuttering. In K. O. St. Louis, (Ed.). *The atypical stutterer* (pp. 193–217). New York: Academic Press. *Journal of Fluency Disorders,* Volume 21, Issues 3–4, September–December 1996. [A special issue devoted to cluttering.]

Market, K. E., and associates (1990). Acquired stuttering: Descriptive data and treatment outcome. *Journal of Fluency Disorders, 15*, 21–31.

Myers, F. L., & St. Louis, K. O. (1992). *Cluttering: A clinical perspective.* Kibworth, England: Far Communications.

Rosenbek, J. C. (1984). Stuttering secondary to nervous damage. In R. F. Curlee & W. H. Perkins (Eds.), *Nature and treatment of stuttering* (pp. 31–48). Austin, TX: Pro-Ed.

Silverman, F. H. (2004). *Stuttering and other fluency disorders* (3rd ed.). Long Grove, IL: Waveland Press.

Van Riper, C. (1982). *The nature of stuttering* (2nd ed.). Englewood Cliffs, NJ: Prentice Hall.

Yairi, E., & Ambrose, N. G. (2005). *Early childhood stuttering.* Austin, TX: Pro-Ed.

**Fluent Aphasias.** In assessing several syndromes of aphasia, the clinician should measure normal-sounding or even excessive fluency with impaired meaning; generally associated with more posterior cerebral lesions; see Aphasia for general assessment procedures; and see Aphasia: Specific Types for special assessment considerations related to the following types of fluent aphasias: anomic aphasia, conduction aphasia, transcortical sensory aphasia, and Wernicke's aphasia.

**Foreign Accent Syndrome.** Assessment of speech articulatory and prosodic characteristics that are alien to the client's native language is essential in diagnosing some forms of communication impairment associated with neuropathological conditions; characteristics that are not necessarily pathological, but different from the client's native language; a controversial syndrome associated with neuropathological factors; may be a feature of aphasia or apraxia in some individuals; see the cited sources at the end of this entry and the companion volume, *Hegde's PocketGuide to Communication Disorders* for details on symptomatology and etiology; to assess:

- Keep the native language prosodic and articulatory features as the reference point to make clinical judgments about the presence of a foreign accent syndrome
- Judge patterns of intonation in relation to that found in the client's native language; misplaced rising or falling pitch that are not characteristic of the language
- Assess vowel production to identify their distortions or insertion of epenthetic vowels
- Assess the linguistic stress patterns of the client and compare them with those that are typical of the native language
- Note any changes in timing and rhythm of speech
- Diagnose a foreign accent syndrome when a neurological disease or disorder and the presence of other communication disorders (e.g., aphasia, apraxia, or dysarthria) have been confirmed

Blumstein, S. E., & Kurowski, K. (2006). The foreign accent syndrome: A perspective. *Journal of Neurolinguistics, 19*(5), 346–355.

Moen, I. (2000). Foreign accent syndrome: A review of contemporary explanations. *Aphasiology, 14,* 5–15.

Scott, S. K., Clegg, F., Rudge, P., & Burgess, P. (2006). Foreign accent syndrome, speech rhythm and the functional neuronatomy of speech production. *Journal of Neurolinguistics, 19*(5), 370–384.

**Frontotemporal Dementia (FTD).** Assessment and diagnosis of dementia associated with frontal and temporal lobe pathology has been evolving in recent years; the relatively new syndrome of dementia now includes Pick's disease; in fact, Pick's disease is the dominant entity within the FTD; during the assessment, the clinician needs to look for the symptoms of cortical dementia associated with degeneration in both the frontal and temporal regions of the brain; FTD is a major form of non-Alzheimer type of dementia; the clinician needs to note significant changes in behavior and social conduct in the initial stages of the disease to diagnose FTD; the diagnostic category of FTD is still evolving; several variants of the syndrome have been identified; therefore, the clinician needs to keep abreast of research literature on this syndrome.

## Case History/Interview Focus

- Take a detailed case history to document the initial changes in behavior and language because they may be the earliest of the symptoms of FTD
- Find out from the informants if general behavioral changes suggestive of right-sided atrophy or language changes suggestive of left-sided atrophy were the dominant initial symptoms
- Look for evidence of uninhibited and inappropriate social behavior and repetitive and meaningless actions, combined with a lack of insight



## Ethnocultural Considerations

- Assess the family communication patterns, family resources, and needed support systems because the management of clients with dementia almost always taxes the family's financial and emotional resources

## Assessment of Frontotemporal Dementia

- Assess behavioral changes and psychiatric symptoms
  - Through the **Case History** and **Observation**, assess uncharacteristically inappropriate and uninhibited social behavior (including sexual jokes) and excessive jocularity, and exaggerated self-esteem
  - Document excessive eating and weight gain with a craving for carbohydrates
  - Take note of such psychiatric symptoms as apathy, depression and euphoria; delusions without feelings of persecution
- Assess symptoms of dementia
  - Through assessment and case history, establish that behavioral changes preceded intellectual deterioration
  - Assess memory and orientation that may be better preserved than in clients with dementia of the Alzheimer type
  - Assess impaired judgment, thinking, constructional skill, planning, and abstraction; difficulty recognizing familiar faces suggestive of right-sided brain atrophy
  - Take note of repetitive, ritualistic, and meaningless behavior
- Assess communication disorders
  - Establish through case history that reduced speech output was an early sign with a progressive decrease in the size of expressive vocabulary
  - Assess anomia, impaired confrontation naming, nonfluent speech with verbal paraphasia; see Aphasia for procedural details
  - Assess reduced spontaneous conversation, echolalia, and verbal stereotypes
  - Muteness suggests the final stages of the disease

## Standardized Tests

- Consider administering a test of Dementia

## Related/Medical Assessment Data

- Review the case history and medical records for evidence of dementia and frontotemporal pathology

## Standard/Common Assessment Procedures

- Complete the Standard/Common Assessment Procedures

## Diagnostic Criteria

- Evidence of neuropathology in the frontal, temporal, or both regions of the brain

- Evidence of Pick bodies and Pick cells if the diagnosis is Pick's disease
- Evidence of gliosis if it is a non-Pick variation of the syndrome
- Characteristic neurobehavioral and language problems

### *Differential Diagnosis*

- Review medical, neurological, and neurodiagnostic records for evidence of frontotemporal atrophy
- Check for evidence of differential pathology: predominantly frontal pathology in some clients and temporal pathology in others
- Distinguish FTD from dementia of the Alzheimer type (DAT); behavioral changes precede intellectual deterioration in FTD, a trend opposite to what is seen in DAT; unlike in DAT, memory and orientation are better preserved in FTD; clients with FTD may also have better preserved reading and writing skills until more advanced stages

F

### *Prognosis*

- Complete muteness and severe dementia in the final stages
- Fair prognosis for clinical management of symptoms in the initial and intermediate stages

### *Recommendations*

- Clinical management of behavioral symptoms and language skills
- Family counseling and management strategies for the family members

Dickson, D. W. (2001). Neuropathology of Pick's disease. *Neurology, 56* (Suppl 4), S16–S18.

Hodges, J. R. (2001). Frontotemporal dementia (Pick's disease): Clinical features and assessment. *Neurology, 56* (Suppl 4), S6–S9.

Rossor, M. N. (2001). Pick's disease: A clinical overview. *Neurology, 56* (Suppl 4), S3–S5.

**Functional Assessment.** Assessment of functional communication skills in naturalistic, socially meaningful contexts; whether a person achieves certain effects through whatever the means (verbal, nonverbal, instrument-assisted, written) is the main focus of assessment; some assessment devices, and perhaps an increasing number, include functional components; several procedures within the traditional assessment can help target functional communication

- Observe the client's communication with family members during the assessment
- Always arrange a mother-child interaction that approximates their usual play-oriented interaction to observe more naturalistic communication than would be possible under typical testing conditions
- Whenever possible, with children and adolescents, arrange for a peer interaction situation and observe communication patterns; interview a peer on how the client communicates in social contexts
- Obtain one or more home speech and language samples; instruct the family to record natural and everyday communication interactions
- In educational (school) settings, observe the child in the classroom, in the playground, in the cafeteria, and so forth; obtain information from teachers about the child's communication skills; focus on target communication skills (e.g., fluency, language structures, voice quality, articulation)

- In medical settings, observe the client's interaction with family members and health caregivers; interview them and obtain information on how the client communicates with them (e.g., how does the client communicate with the nurse? With the physician? With the physical therapist?)
- With adults, always interview at least one person with whom the client regularly interacts (spouse, friend, colleague)
- Place emphasis on conversational speech; never make judgment based solely on purely imitative tasks or picture-naming tasks; note, however, that such tasks are diagnostic and necessary in many cases (e.g., in assessing clients with dysarthria, apraxia, aphasia)
- Record a conversational speech (or at least observe speech) outside the clinic room and in more naturalistic situations
- To the extent possible, structure assessment tasks that are meaningful (e.g., instead of having the client repeat sentences that have no bearing to his or her life, select sentences that include activities the client enjoys, the names of family members, and so forth)
- Document variations in the disorder in natural settings (e.g., in assessing a person who stutters, document the degree of fluency in such naturalistic contexts as ordering in a restaurant, purchasing at counters, talking on the telephone)
- Place an emphasis on the effects the communicative attempts produce rather than the language structure that the traditional assessment is often concerned with (e.g., whether a brain-injured or stroke client can successfully communicate his or her basic needs may be, at a certain stage in assessment, more important than how it is done); take note, however, that this does not suggest that the assessment of language structures is unimportant
- In essence, take note that functional assessment requires the clinician to make targets, procedures, and settings of assessment to be as naturalistic as possible
- Select standardized methods or tests that are functionally oriented
- See ASHA FACS for adults as an example and develop similar procedures for your clients (American Speech-Language-Hearing Association: *Functional Assessment of Communication Skills for Adults* by C. M. Frattali, C. K. Thompson, A. L. Holland, C. B. Wohl, & M. M. Ferketic)

# G

**Gestural Communication.** Movements of body structures (e.g., smiling and nodding, eye movements, hand gestures, specific postures) that normally accompany oral communication; may be a primary means of communication for people who cannot speak; may augment limited oral communication in some individuals; for assessment procedures, see Augmentative and Alternative Communication (AAC).

**Glossing.** In articulation assessment, interpreting the word the child was presumably trying to produce; adult interpretation of a child's misarticulated word (e.g., the child says *wawa* and the clinician's gloss of it is *water*).



**Grammatical Morphemes of Language.** Assessment of small grammatical features of language is essential to diagnose language disorders in children and agrammatic speech in clients with aphasia; these morphemes have a grammatical value and change or modulate meaning; they include such inflections as the regular plural or possessive and such grammatical elements as articles and conjunctions; an element that is usually omitted or misused by children who exhibit language disorders and those who speak agrammatically and telegraphically (as do some clients with aphasia); an important element of language assessment in all clients, especially in children with language disorders; See Language Disorders in Children for assessment procedures; see also Aphasia.

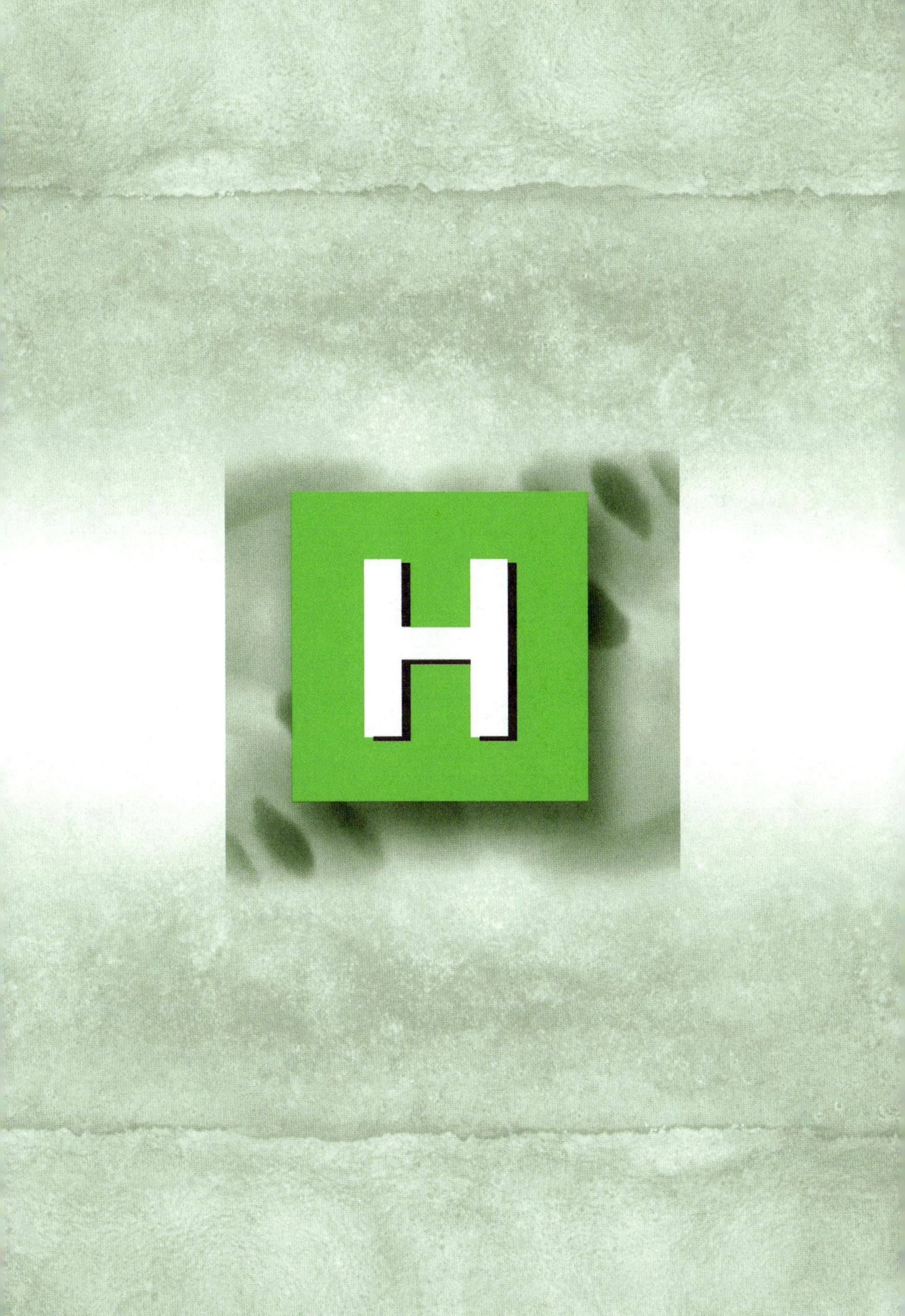
H

**Hearing Impairment.** Assessment of oral communication disorders associated with reduced hearing acuity is the professional responsibility of the speech-language pathologist whereas the assessment of hearing loss is the responsibility of the audiologist; hearing impairment is a hearing loss that is greater than 25 dB HL in the case of adults and 15 dB HL in the case of young children who still are learning language; includes the Hard of Hearing who may need amplification but are able to learn oral language and the Deaf whose hearing level is insufficient to acquire oral language; variety of pathologies cause hearing impairment; clients with significant Hearing Loss may exhibit a variety of oral communication disorders although the deaf individuals may be competent sign language communicators; the role of the speech-language pathologist in the rehabilitation of people with hearing loss is to assist oral language acquisition with or without the help of amplification as requested by the family of a young child or by an adult; requires the assessment of all aspects of oral speech and language production because significant levels of hearing loss will affect speech, language, voice, and fluency; even a mild loss of 15 dB HL during infancy and early childhood may cause a delay in speech and language learning; see the sources cited at the end of this entry and *Hegde's PocketGuide to Communication Disorders* for the epidemiology, symptomatology, and etiology of hearing impairment; in assessing the communication disorders in children and adults with hearing impairment, use the procedures described under Language Disorders in Children, Articulation and Phonological Disorders, and Voice Disorders; take into consideration the following special features of assessing individuals with hearing impairment:



### *Assessment Objectives/General Guidelines*

- To assess all aspects of oral communication, including speech, language, voice, and fluency characteristics
- To take note of the nonverbal communication skills of the individual
- To assist the audiologist and special education personnel in developing an oral communication rehabilitation program for a child with hearing impairment based on the assessment results
- To counsel the family members regarding the communication needs of the individual with the hearing loss and the education and clinical treatment options that are based on the assessment results

### *Case History/Interview Focus*

- See **Case History** and **Interview** under Standard/Common Assessment Procedures
- Concentrate on hearing loss, its onset, and effects on communication
- Seek information on medical conditions that are associated with hearing impairment (e.g., maternal alcoholism, otitis media, noise exposure, anatomical abnormalities of the ear, otosclerosis, tumors of the middle ear, ototoxicity, evidence of auditory nerve damage or tumors, and many other conditions)
- Seek information on early signs of hearing impairment (e.g., lack of infant's response to sound and the mother's voice, failure to babble or sustain babbling, delayed acquisition of speech sounds)
- Explore the family's reaction to hearing impairment in their child and the early measures they took to help the child

## *Ethnocultural Considerations*

- See Ethnocultural Considerations in Assessment
- Assess the family's cultural values related to disabilities in general and hearing impairment in particular
- Gauge the family resources and the need for support systems (e.g., can the family afford a hearing aid?)
- Assess the family's ability to access medical services (e.g., has the child been seen by an otologist? Audiologist?)

## *Assessment*

- An audiologist makes an evaluation of the type and degree of hearing loss
- The client may have been examined by an otologist for a medical diagnosis
- A speech-language pathologist makes an assessment of communication disorders associated with hearing loss
- Hearing impairment affects all aspects of oral communication; it is essential to make a comprehensive assessment of speech, voice, language, and fluency



### Assess Speech

- Take a comprehensive speech and language sample (see Standard/ Common Assessment Procedures)
- Pay special attention to the kinds of speech problems a hearing-impaired person is likely to exhibit
  - Take note of the omission of sounds in initial and final positions, especially the /s/
  - Assess the reduction of clusters
  - Assess the substitution of voiced sounds for the unvoiced, nasal sounds for the oral sounds, and any vowel substitutions or hypernasal vowel productions
  - Take note of distortions of most speech sounds, especially the stops and fricatives
  - Measure the duration of vowels, which tend to be excessively long
  - Take note of any insertion of extraneous sounds
- Use the procedures described under Articulation and Phonological Disorders
- List the kinds of *articulation problems the client exhibits*
- If useful, make a phonological pattern analysis; see Articulation and Phonological Disorders

### Assess Language

- Use the recorded speech and language sample to make an analysis
- Take note of observed deviations during the interview and speech-language sampling
- Pay special attention to the kinds of language problems a hearing-impaired person is likely to exhibit
  - Ask parents about lack of babbling or sustained babbling
  - Judge the size of the oral vocabulary, ask parents or other family members for their opinion on the adequacy of their child's oral vocabulary compared to children of similar age

  - Judge the comprehension of speech during the assessment; ask parents about speech comprehension deficits
  - Assess the understanding of abstract and metaphoric language (e.g., proverbs, similes, and slang); hearing loss tends to negatively affect abstract language comprehension and production
  - Assess the production of all grammatical morphemes because they tend to be negatively affected
  - Evaluate the sentence types and variety of syntactic structures in the conversational speech sample
  - Assess any deviant prosodic features (improper rhythm of speech, inappropriate linguistic stress patterns)
  - Evaluate narrative skills, conversational turn taking, topic initiation and maintenance, and conversational repair strategies



- Use the additional procedures described under Language Disorders in Children
- List the kinds of semantic, morphological, syntactic, and pragmatic problems the client exhibits

### Assess Fluency

- Use the recorded speech and language sample
- Use the assessment procedures described under Stuttering
- Count the number of individual dysfluencies and the number of words in the speech sample
- Calculate the percent dysfluency rate
- Describe the overall rhythm of speech

### Assess Voice

- Use the recorded speech and language sample
- Note that voice deviations are highly characteristic of hearing impairment, especially significant impairment
- Use the procedures described under Voice Disorders to make an assessment of voice and resonance problems
- Observe and take note of voice deviations during the interview and speech and language sample
  - Assess overall voice quality
  - Take note of high-pitched, harsh, and often hoarse voice
  - Assess breathiness that may be present
  - Judge the adequacy of vocal intensity
- Take note of resonance problems
  - Take note of hyponasality on nasal sounds
  - Take note of hypernasality on oral sounds
- List the voice and resonance problems of the client

### Assess Nonverbal Communication

- Observe and take note of the client's nonverbal communication skills
- Take note of whether the client is a competent user of an organized nonverbal communication form (e.g., the American Sign Language)

### Assess Literacy Skills

- Obtain a report from the special education specialist if the literacy skills have been assessed in a school-age child with hearing impairment
- Assess reading skills by:
  - Having the child read aloud a passage of a story or book that is appropriate to his or her grade level
  - Asking the child to retell or summarize what has been read
  - Taking note of reading errors as the child reads aloud the text (e.g., omission of sounds and words, substitution of sound and words, struggling to read, silent pauses during reading)
- Assess writing skills by:
  - Having the child write a passage to dictation
  - Having the child write a brief essay on his or her personal experience
  - Analyzing an extended writing sample you may obtain from the child or the child's teacher
  - Taking note of writing problems that usually parallel the oral language problems (syntactic errors, omission of grammatical morphemes, telegraphic writing, limited information offered, plus frequent misspellings)



## *Standardized Tests*

- Administer selected tests listed under Articulation and Phonological Disorders and Language Disorders in Children

## *Related/Medical Assessment Data*

- Obtain the otological report from the client's otologist
- Obtain the audiological assessment report from the child's audiologist
- Obtain reports from the child's regular teacher or special education specialist including the educator of the deaf
- Obtain psychological assessment reports
- Obtain any general medical reports that shed light on the child's health and hearing

## *Standard/Common Assessment Procedures*

- Complete the Standard/Common Assessment Procedures
- Obtain the audiological and otolaryngological examination reports

## *Analysis of Results*

- Analyze and summarize the results of the communication assessment; highlight the significant problems in speech and language production; emphasize the unique articulation, voice, resonance, reading, and writing problems
- Relate communication assessment results with those of the audiological, otological, general medical, educational, and psychological reports
- Take note of the client's strengths (including the use of a nonverbal system of communication) and limitations

## *Diagnostic Criteria/Guidelines*

- An independent diagnosis of hearing impairment (including its type and severity level) based on the otological and audiological examinations is essential

- The pattern of unique oral communication disorders (especially the articulation, voice, and resonance problems) that support the diagnosis is important

### *Differential Diagnosis*

- Differentiate communication disorders associated with hearing impairment from those associated with intellectual disabilities
  - Characteristic articulation, voice, and resonance problems associated with hearing impairment are less marked in individuals with intellectual disability, although omission of grammatical morphemes and limited syntactic structures will be common features
  - An independent diagnosis of hearing impairment will support the distinction between the communication disorders in the two groups
  - An independent diagnosis of intellectual deficiency also will support the distinction between the two kinds of communication disorders

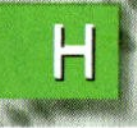


- Differentiate communication disorders associated with hearing impairment from those associated with cerebral palsy
  - Compare the characteristic articulation, voice, and resonance problems of individuals with hearing impairment with those of children with cerebral palsy to make the distinction; children with cerebral palsy present obvious neuromuscular deficits that are not present in children with hearing loss; take note that hypernasality or a degree of hyponasality may be found in both populations
  - Support the distinction between the neuromotor problems found in individuals with cerebral palsy with their absence in individuals with hearing loss
- Differentiate the communication disorders associated with hearing impairment from those associated with autism
  - Compare the characteristic articulation, voice, and resonance problems of individuals with hearing impairment with those of individuals with autism to make the distinction
  - Support the distinction between the observed deviant or eccentric behaviors of individuals with autism with their absence in individuals with hearing impairment
- Differentiate the communication disorders associated with hearing impairment from those associated with specific language impairment
  - Distinguish the two kinds of disorders by the absence of the characteristic voice, articulation, and resonance problems associated with hearing impairment in individuals with specific language impairment
  - Note that specific language impairment is limited to an obvious and dominant language disability without serious intellectual or sensory problems

### *Prognosis*

- Prognosis for oral communication depends on the individual client's or family members' philosophy of communication and emphasis on, and acceptance of, oral modes of communication
- Prognosis for oral communication also depends on the degree of hearing loss; the less severe the loss, the better the prognosis for sustained oral communication skills

- Prognosis for oral communication is generally good for children who are hard of hearing (not deaf)
- Prognosis for sustained nonverbal means of communication (such as the American Sign Language) is generally good for persons who are deaf

### *Recommendations*

- Early speech and language intervention for children who are hard of hearing; the use of amplification (individual hearing aids and group amplification in educational settings) as recommended by an audiologist
- Speech and language intervention for individuals with more severe hearing impairment depending on the client's and family's preference and acceptance
- See the cited sources and *Hegde's PocketGuide to Treatment in Speech-Language Pathology* (3rd ed.) for details

Alpiner, J. G., & McCarthy, P. A. (2000). *Rehabilitative audiology: Children and adults* (3rd ed.). Philadelphia, PA: Lippincott Williams & Wilkins.

Bernthal, J. E., & Bankson, N. W. (2004). *Articulation and phonological disorders* (5th ed.). Boston, MA: Allyn and Bacon.

Elfenbein, J. L., Hardin-Jones, M. A., & Davis, J. M. (1994). Oral communication skills of children who are hard of hearing. *Journal of Speech-Language-Hearing Research, 37*, 216–226.

Hegde, M. N., & Maul, C. A. (2006). *Language disorders in children.* Boston, MA: Allyn and Bacon.

Martin, F. N., & Clark, J. G. (2003). *Introduction to audiology* (8th ed.). Boston, MA: Allyn and Bacon.

Northern, J. L. (1996). *Hearing disorders.* Boston, MA: Allyn and Bacon.

Paul, R. (1995). *Language disorders from infancy through adolescence.* St. Louis, MO: Mosby.

Peña-Brooks, A., & Hegde, M. N. (2007). *Articulation and phonological disorders in children.* Austin, TX: Pro-Ed.

Schow, R. L., & Nerbonne, M. A. (2002). *Introduction to audiologic rehabilitation* (4th ed.). Boston, MA: Allyn and Bacon.

Scott, D. M. (2002). Multicultural aspects of hearing disorders and audiology. In D. E. Battle, *Communication disorders in multicultural populations* (pp. 335–360) (3rd ed.). Boston: Butterworth-Heinemann.

Yoshinaga-Itano, C., & Downey, D. M. (1996). Development of school-aged deaf, hard of hearing, and normally hearing students' written language. *Votla Review, 98*, 3–7.

**Hearing Screening.** A mandatory procedure of quickly identifying who needs to be assessed by an audiologist and who does not; see Standard/Common Assessment Procedures on how to conduct a hearing screening.

**Hunter Syndrome.** To assess this syndrome, a variety of mucopolysaccharidosis syndrome, see Syndromes Associated With Communication Disorders.

**Huntington's Disease (HD).** Assessment of this degenerative neurological disease, also called *Huntington's chorea*, is a part of diagnosing a variety of subcortical dementia and a variety of dysarthria; the disease is associated with motor speech disorders and language impairment; see Dementia for general assessment procedures; also see Hyperkinetic Dysarthria under Dysarthria: Specific Types for an assessment of motor speech disorders; use the following information specific to HD.

### *Case History/Interview Focus*

- See **Case History** and **Interview** under Standard/Common Assessment Procedures
- Through the case history and interview, document the changes in cognition, general behavior, emotional responding, and communication skills as reported by the family members
- Ask the family members about the early signs of complaining, nagging, irritability, suspiciousness, and a false sense of superiority; take note that in later stages, the patient may be depressed with a suicidal tendency
- Because it is an autosomal dominant inheritance (affecting half the number of an affected person's offspring), explore in detail the familial incidence of the disease
- Obtain information on potential drug toxicity, arteriosclerotic diseases, and postencephalopathy

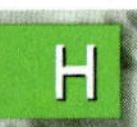


### *Ethnocultural Considerations*

- See **Case History** and **Interview** under Standard/Common Assessment Procedures
- Explore the family's dispositions and knowledge about degenerative diseases and their clinical management
- Assess the family's resources and the need for any support systems

### *Assessment of Huntington's Disease*

- Assess speech, language, memory, cognition (including orientation and confusion); take note that communication problems become evident somewhat later than the neurological symptoms; use procedures described under Dementia
- Assess motor speech disorders, especially hyperkinetic dysarthria, which are prominent communication disorders in clients with Huntington's disease; follow the procedures described under hyperkinetic dysarthria (see Dysarthria: Specific Types)
- Describe the neurological symptoms observed during the assessment (gait disturbances, chorea, tics, rigidity and slowness of movements)
- Describe the behavioral deviations noted during the assessment (e.g., fidgeting, confusion, or disorientation)
- Take note that mutism is a sign of the final stage of the disease

### *Standardized Tests*

- Consider administering a test of Dementia
- Consider administering a test of Dysarthrias

### *Related/Medical Assessment Data*

- Obtain the medical and neurodiagnostic reports that may shed light on potential neuropathology supportive of Huntington's disease

- Obtain information on psychiatric symptoms that are commonly associated with the disease
- Review the medical records for chorea and tic-like movement—the major neurological symptoms of the disease
- Integrate available medical, neurological, psychological-psychiatric, behavioral, and diagnostic medical laboratory findings with the results of the communication assessment

### *Standard/Common Assessment Procedures*

- Complete the Standard/Common Assessment Procedures
- Pay attention to the client's neurobehavioral symptoms; make a thorough orofacial examination

### *Diagnostic Criteria*

- Neuropsychiatric diagnosis of Huntington's disease with chorea as the dominant symptom
- Dementia and dysarthria

H

### *Differential Diagnosis*

- Distinguish Huntington's disease with its characteristic chorea, early signs of behavioral changes, and evidence of neuronal loss in the basal ganglia from related diseases that produce subcortical dementia (Parkinson's disease, supranuclear palsy, and Wilson's disease)
- See Dementia to make a differential diagnosis of diseases associated with subcortical dementias

### *Prognosis*

- Disease is progressive and irreversible
- Prognosis for implementing clinical management strategies that help control the behavioral symptoms of the client is good until the final stages
- Prognosis for family counseling on coping and the client's management strategies is good

### *Recommendations*

- Communication treatment in the initial stages; management of problems later
- Family counseling and management strategies
- See the cited sources and *Hegde's PocketGuide to Treatment in Speech-Language Pathology* (3rd ed.) for details

American Psychiatric Association (1994). *Diagnostic and statistical manual of mental disorders* (4th ed.). Washington, DC: Author.

Clark, C. M., & Trojanowski, J. Q. (2000). *Neurodegenerative dementias*. New York: McGraw-Hill.

Cummings, J. L., & Benson, D. F. (1983). *Dementia: A clinical approach*. Boston, MA: Butterworth.

Hegde, M. N. (2006). *A coursebook on aphasia and other neurogenic language disorders* (3rd ed.). Clifton Park, NY: Thomson Delmar Learning.

Jaques, A., & Jackson, G. A. (2000). *Understanding dementia* (3rd ed.). New York: Churchill Livingstone.

Simon, R. P., Aminoff, M. J., & Greenberg, D. A. (1999). *Clinical neurology* (4th ed.). Stamford, CT: Appleton & Lange.

Weiner, M. F. (1996). *The dementias: diagnosis, management, and research* (2nd ed.). Washington, DC: American Psychiatric Press.

**Hurler Syndrome.** To assess this syndrome, a variety of mucopolysaccharidosis syndrome, see Syndromes Associated with Communication Disorders.

**Hypernasality.** Excessive nasal resonance on nonnasal sounds; see Voice Disorders and Cleft Palate for assessment procedures; see also Dysarthria.

**Hypokinetic Agraphia.** Assess this handwriting problem by having the client write to dictation a paragraph or two or have the client copy a printed passage; take note of micrographic writing, which is writing with unusually small letters that get progressively smaller; needs to be assessed in some clients with neurodegenerative diseases including Parkinson's disease, although not a feature of clients with Alzheimer's disease.

**Hyponasality.** Reduced or absent nasal resonance in the production of nasal sounds; the same as denasality; see Voice Disorders and Cleft Palate for assessment procedures.

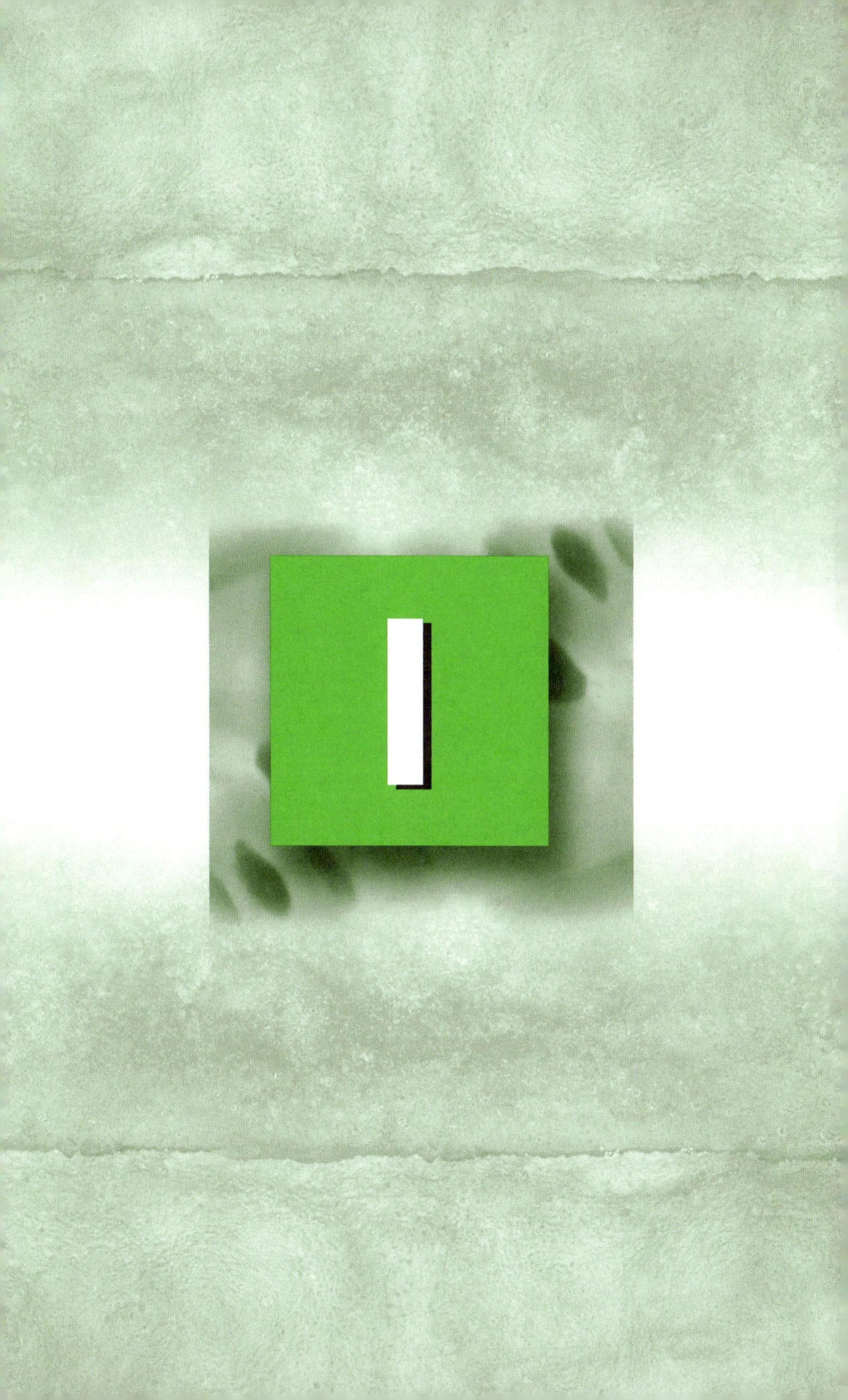
I

**Instruments for Aerodynamic Measures of Phonatory Functions.** Various instruments to measure aspects of respiratory functions that are relevant for voice and speech production; include the following:

- Aerophone II Voice Function Analyzer (Kay Elemetrics Corporation): A special hardware and software system used in a microcomputer to analyze various voice and speech characteristics and functions including airflow, air pressure, and sound pressure; includes a face mask for measuring aerodynamic variables; gives computer printouts for permanent record.
- Pneumotachograph: An instrument for measuring airflow; consists of a face mask with acoustic resistance, a pressure transducer, an amplifier, and a recording device; as the person speaks with the mask on, the instrument measures the rate of airflow through resistance and differential pressure variables.
- Phonatory Function Analyzer: A computerized instrument that measures, among other variables, airflow rate and total volume of expired air; see under Instruments for Voice and Speech Analysis.

I

**Instruments for Resonance Assessment.** Various instruments to measure resonance, especially nasal resonance including hypernasality and hyponasality; include the following:

- Nasal listening tube: A simple device that consists of a rubber tube with glass or plastic tips on each end; the client places one end on the nostril and the clinician places the other end in his or her ear; the clinician can judge nasal resonance or lack of it as the client produces sounds and words that contain nasal or oral sounds.
- Nasometer (Kay Elemetrics Corporation): A computerized instrument to measure nasal resonance; as the client speaks into two microphones that are separated by a nasal-oral separator, the instrument measures the relative nasal resonance; gives instantaneous feedback to the client.

**Instruments for Voice and Speech Analysis.** A variety of electronic and increasingly computerized instruments to assess various aspects of voice and speech; include the following:

- Visi-Pitch (Kay Elemetrics Corporation): A special hardware and software system used in a microcomputer to analyze various aspects of voice and speech including speaking fundamental frequency, the lowest and the highest frequencies, average loudness of a speech sample (relative intensity), minimum and maximum loudness, voice onset time, glottal attacks, and intonation and stress patterns; gives digital and oscilloscopic displays.
- Phonatory Functional Analyzer: A computerized instrument to measure aspects of phonation and airflow; measures phonation time, frequency, intensity, airflow rate, and total volume of expired air; with a face mask, can measure pitch in continuous speech; because it takes simultaneous measures of these variables, the interaction among them may be documented; the effects of changes induced in one variable may be documented; provides for computer printout of data for permanent record.
- Fundamental Frequency Indicator: An instrument to measure pitch; client holds a microphone to the larynx or under the nose and produces various vowels and syllables; gives readouts of habitual pitch, the best pitch, and the pitch range.

**Intellectual Disabilities.** Assessment of significant communication disorders that are associated with intellectual, social, and adaptive behaviors that are below normal during the developmental period requires a thorough knowledge of child development, including intellectual and social development of children; the developmental period extends up to age 18 years; assessment focus for speech-language pathologists is the communication disorders associated with intellectual disability; a comprehensive assessment is the responsibility of a team of specialists that includes, in addition to speech-language pathologists, psychologists and various special education specialists; see the cited sources at the end of this main entry and the companion volume, *Hegde's PocketGuide to Communication Disorders* for details on intellectual disability, its etiology and characteristics; generally, assessment procedures described under Language Disorders in Children and Articulation and Phonological Disorders are applicable with the following special considerations:



### *Assessment Objectives/General Guidelines*

- To assess and describe articulation and phonological disorders in children with intellectual disability
- To assess and describe language disorders
- To assess other communication problems including voice disorders and dysfluencies
- To screen hearing and request audiological assessment when the child fails the hearing screening
- To complete a team assessment with other specialists including psychologists and special education specialists
- To take note of any symptoms of a genetic syndrome to make appropriate referrals
- To suggest intervention strategies that include speech-language pathology services

### *Case History/Interview Focus*

- See **Case History** and **Interview** under Standard/Common Assessment Procedures
- Concentrate on the prenatal, natal, and postnatal factors that are known to be associated with intellectual disabilities
- Take a detailed case history of the child's speech, language, and motor development; ask parents about the first words, the rate at which the child learned new words, production of phrases and sentences, grammatical errors the parents have noticed in the child's speech, and the child's description of events, objects, or personal experiences (e.g., elaborated, brief, telegraphic)
- Get details on the child's academic status and placement in any special education programs, and areas in which the child is doing relatively better and areas in which the child has especial difficulty
- Obtain information on the familial prevalence of intellectual disabilities
- Get information on any associated clinical conditions, including physical, neurological, sensory, and emotional problems the child may have

### *Ethnocultural Considerations*

- See Ethnocultural Considerations in Assessment
- Because intellectual deficiency requires long-standing and expensive multidisciplinary educational as well as clinical services, explore in detail, the family's accessibility to services and the support they may need
- Select assessment procedures that are appropriate for the child from a minority group; be especially skeptic about the value of scores on standardized tests of intelligence

### *Assessment of Communication Disorders*

#### Assess Phonological Problems

- Record a speech and language sample (see Standard/Common Assessment Procedures)
- List the sounds misarticulated; classify them according to omissions (deletions), distortions, substitutions, and simplification of consonant clusters
- Make a phonological process analysis to identify patterns of misarticulations
- Use the additional procedures described under Articulation and Phonological Disorders



#### Assess Semantic Problems

- Assess word usage, vocabulary size, and variety of words used; ask parents about their estimate of the child's vocabulary size
- Use the procedures described under Language Disorders in Children
- Describe the classes of words that are especially difficult for the child

#### Assess Morphological Problems

- Use the recorded speech and language sample in assessing the production of morphological features
- Use client-specific procedures to sample morphological features that were not sampled in conversational speech; for example, show pictures of plural objects and ask the child to name them to evoke the regular or irregular plural morphemes; show action pictures and ask questions to evoke the present progressive "ing" or the auxiliary verbs
- Use the additional procedures described under Language Disorders in Children
- List the morphological features the child produced and those the child did not produce in obligatory contexts; calculate the percent correct response rate for assessed morphological features

#### Assess Syntactic Problems

- Use the recorded speech and language sample in assessing the production of syntactic features
- Take note of telegraphic speech (phrases and utterances with missing grammatical features), limited syntactic variety, repeated use of a few and simple sentence forms, lack of complex sentence forms in the sample, lack of questions or formal requests, and so forth

- Use the additional procedures described under Language Disorders in Children
- List the syntactic features the child produces and those the child does not

### Assess Pragmatic Problems

- Engage the child in conversational speech and take note of topic initiation, topic maintenance, and turn taking
- Make ambiguous statements to find out whether the child would request clarification
- Pretend that you did not understand when the child asks for clarification to assess appropriate responses to request for clarification
- Tell a story and then ask the child to retell it; ask the child to narrate a story; ask the child to tell you how he or she would play a certain game, fix a sandwich, or plan for a birthday party
- Use the additional procedures described under Language Disorders in Children
- List the pragmatic features the child produces and those the child does not; calculate the accuracy and frequency of the skills exhibited



### Assess Fluency Problems

- Note that the prevalence of stuttering in some children with certain kinds of intellectual disability (e.g., Down syndrome) is higher than it is in the general population
- Use the recorded speech and language sample in assessing fluency and dysfluency
- Use the additional procedures described under Stuttering
- List the types of dysfluencies the child produces
- List the total frequency of each dysfluency in the speech sample
- Count the number of spoken words in the sample
- Calculate the percent dysfluency (or stuttering) rate

### Screen Hearing

- Use the standard screening procedure; see Standard/Common Assessment Procedures
- Refer the child who fails the hearing screening to an audiologist for an audiological diagnosis

### Assess Language Comprehension Problems

- Observe the child for auditory language comprehension problems
- Use the procedures described under Language Disorders in Children

## *Standardized Tests*

- Use the selected standardized tests listed under Articulation and Phonological Disorders and Language Disorders in Children
- Be aware that children with intellectual impairment tend to perform less well on standardized tests than in conversational speech exhibited in natural settings
- Be especially careful in selecting standardized tests for children with varied ethnocultural backgrounds; try to use as many client-specific or criterion-referenced procedures as possible

### Related/Medical Assessment Data

- Obtain medical information of relevance
- Obtain audiological assessment data if hearing has been evaluated
- Obtain educational assessment data if available; get informal report from the child's teachers

### Standard/Common Assessment Procedures

- Complete the Standard/Common Assessment Procedures

### Diagnostic Criteria

- An independent diagnosis of intellectual disabilities by a psychologist is essential
- Significant intellectual and behavioral deficiencies are essential for the diagnosis
- Documentation of limited communication skills helps support the diagnosis of intellectual disability; however, from the standpoint of speech-language pathology services, limited communication skills are sufficient grounds to recommend treatment



### Differential Diagnosis

- Differentiate the different syndromes of intellectual disability; see Syndromes Associated with Communication Disorders
- Differentiate the communication disorders associated with intellectual disability with those associated with autism by describing the additional behavioral and emotional problems associated with autism; an independent diagnosis of autism will be helpful; see Autism for additional details
- Differentiate the communication disorders associated with intellectual disability with those associated with hearing impairment; a pattern of speech and voice disorders found in children and adults with hearing impairment will help distinguish the two sets of communication disorders; an independent diagnosis of hearing impairments will he helpful; see Hearing Impairment for additional details
- Differentiate the communication disorders associated with intellectual disability with those associated with specific language impairment; note that children with specific language impairment do not exhibit intellectual disability; any cognitive deficits found in children with specific language impairment will be subtle; see Language Disorders in Children for additional details

### Prognosis

- Varied across children; depends on the intellectual level of the child, family support, time at which intervention and rehabilitation efforts were initiated, the presence of additional complicating conditions (e.g., hearing loss or neuromotor problems), effectiveness of speech and language treatment offered
- Generally good prognosis for improved communication skills with effective, comprehensive, and sustained treatment

### Recommendations

- Early communication treatment
- Parent training in early language stimulation

- Coordination of communication treatment with academic programs in the case of school-age children
- Coordination of communication treatment with psychological services being received
- See the cited sources and the two companion volumes, *Hegde's PocketGuide for Communication Disorders* and *Hegde's PocketGuide for Treatment in Speech-Language Pathology* (3rd ed.)

American Association on Mental Retardation. [See the web site http://www.aamr.org for the definition and classification of mental retardation or intellectual disabilities and for various kinds of resources.]

American Psychiatric Association. (2000). *Diagnostic and statistical manual of mental retardation: Fourth Edition, text revision.* Washington, DC: Author.

Hegde, M. N., & Maul, C. M. (2006). *Language disorders in children: An evidence-based approach to assessment and treatment.* Boston, MA: Allyn and Bacon.

Nelson, N. W. (1998). *Childhood language disorders in context* (2nd ed.). Boston, MA: Allyn and Bacon.

Paul, R. (2001). *Language disorders from infancy through adolescence* (2nd ed.). St. Louis, MO: C. V. Mosby.

Reed, V. (2005). *An introduction to children with language disorders* (3rd ed.). Boston, MA: Allyn and Bacon.

**Interjudge Reliability.** Consistency with which two observers or clinicians measure the same phenomenon; clinically, the agreement between two clinicians who assess the same skill in the same individual; to assess interjudge reliability:

- Measure a skill from a client-specific procedure (e.g., tape-record a speech and language sample from the client); score the skills of interest (e.g., number of dysfluencies, production of morphological features, production of complex sentence forms, frequency of turn taking or topic initiation, correct production of phonemes)
- Submit the audiotape to another clinician to score the same skills evident in the same sample
- Compare your scores with those of the other clinician; if the two agree, then the measures have interjudge reliability

**Interview.** An assessment procedure in which the clinician and the client, as well as an informant, typically have face-to-face contact to discuss the presenting problem and its background; a technique of obtaining and offering information in professional settings; includes two major types:

- Case History/Opening Interview. Talking with the clients and their families and anyone else who can offer significant information on the client's health, behavior, and communication; designed to take a complete case history even if the client or the family has filled out a printed form; a part of all assessment efforts; concerned about the onset, development, and course of the presenting problem; the clients' and family members' view of the problem; health, behavior, and communication development information; previous assessment and treatment; this interview seeks to understand the presenting problem

- Postassessment/Closing Interview. Talking with the clients and their families at the end of an assessment session; designed to give the clients and the family members initial impressions gained from the just-completed assessment; may include a diagnosis, but typically includes a recommendation; an opportunity to answer the clients' or family members' questions about the problem and its treatment
- See Standard/Common Assessment Procedures.

**Intrajudge Reliability.** An essential feature of good assessment, intrajudge reliability is consistency in the result of a repeated measurement made by the same observer or clinician; in assessment, similar results obtained from repeated attempts at measuring communicative skills; with standardized tests, it is similar scores upon repeated administration of the same test by the same clinician; to establish intrajudge reliability:

- Readminister a standardized test to the same client and judge whether the two scores are similar; give at least a 1-week interval between the two administrations
- Take a second conversational speech sample (also with a break of one week) and analyze the skills of interest (e.g., number of dysfluencies, production of morphological features, production of complex sentence forms, frequency of turn taking or topic initiation, correct production of phonemes); judge whether the first and second measures are close; note that no two measures will be alike, but they should be close enough

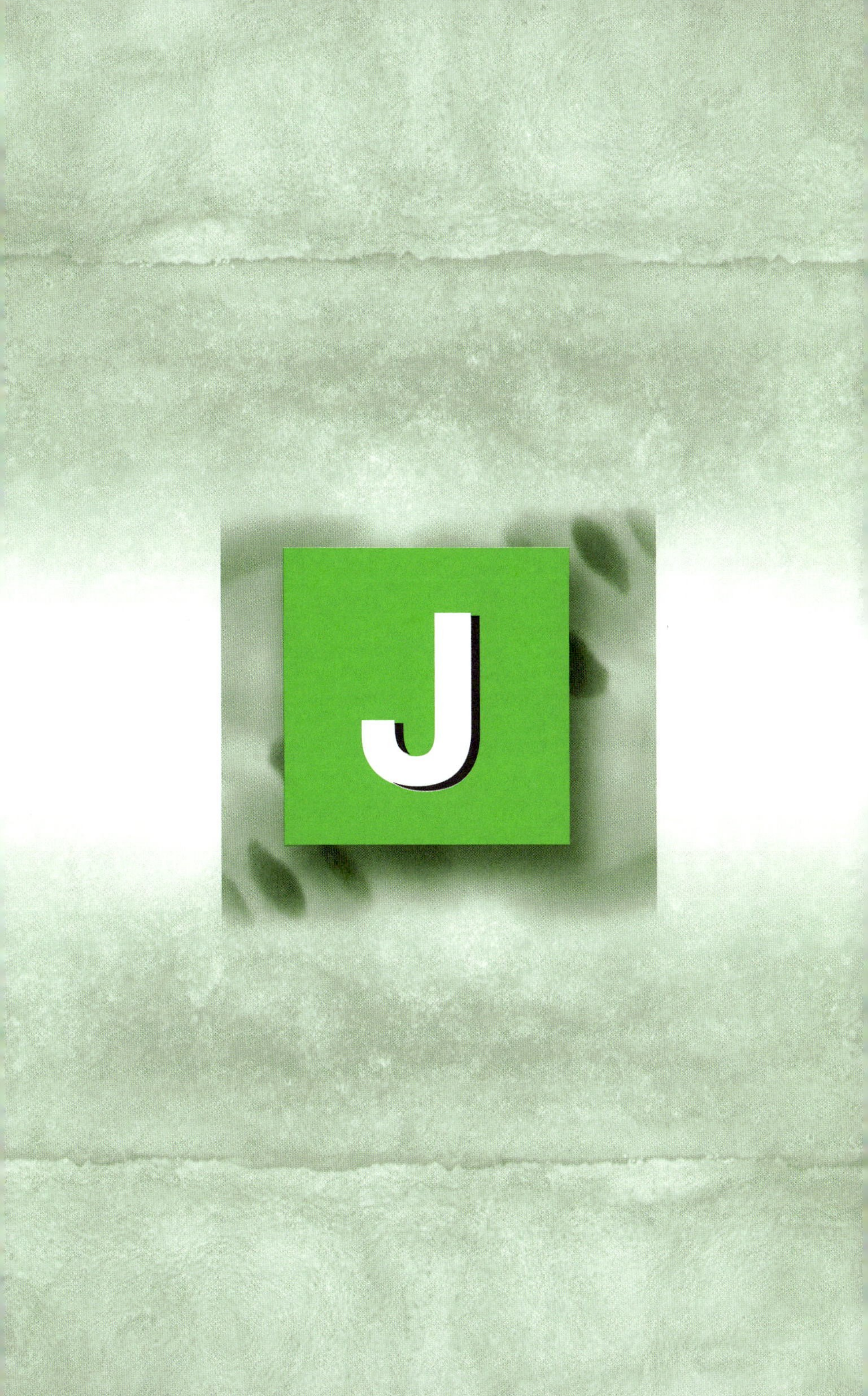
J

**Jargon.** Assessment of fluent but meaningless speech that contains invented words is a part of evaluating clients with aphasia and those with some psychiatric disorders (e.g., schizophrenia); assess jargon during the interview and throughout the assessment period by taking note of meaningless words the client creates and substitutes for regular words in the language the client cannot recall; see Aphasia for assessment details.

**Joint Attention.** Assessment of joint attention—two persons paying attention to the same event or object at the same time—is an element in the diagnosis of early communication skills of infants and young children; impaired joint attention is a sign of later language difficulties; to assess the lack of joint attention as an early sign of a communication disorder:

- Present stimulus objects or events (pictures, toys, actions) and look at them
- Observe whether the child immediately begins to look at the object or event
- If the child fails to look at the object or event, ask the child to look at it
- Take note of whether the child pays attention to the object or event you are paying attention to
- Repeat the procedure a few times with different objects or events

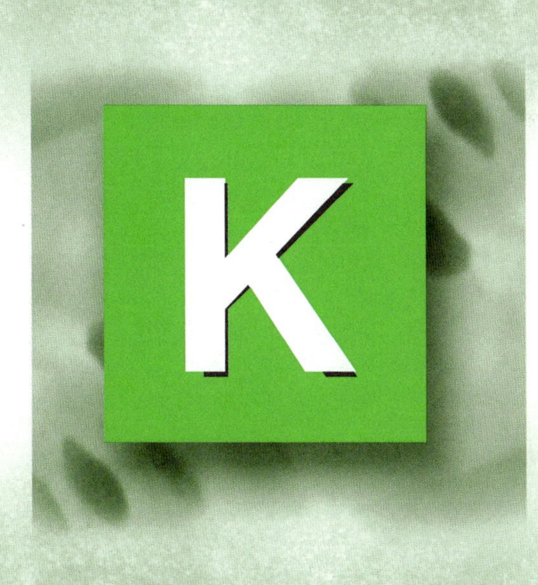
K

**Keratosis.** To assess lesions marked by an overgrowth of the horny layer of epidermis, see Voice Disorders; assess *hyperkeratosis* as a cause of voice disorder.

**Kinesthesia.** Assessment of impaired sensation of movement, found in certain neuromuscular disorders; may be a part of evaluating associated motor speech disorders.

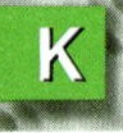

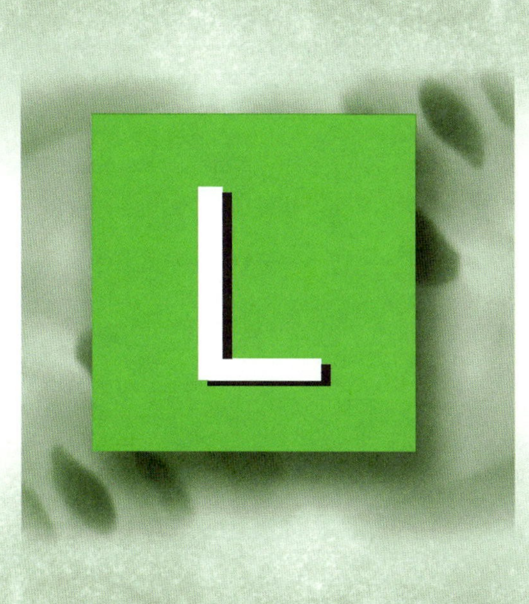
L

**Language Disorders in Adults.** Assessment of language problems in adults is often done in the context of neurological diseases or disorders that cause Aphasia, Dementia, Right Hemisphere Injury, and Traumatic Brain Injury; language disorders associated with these clinical conditions may include additional communication and behavioral deficits; for assessment procedures, see those main entries.

**Language Disorders in Children.** Assessment of limited or deficient language production skills with or without significant language comprehension problems in children requires an analysis of their semantic, phonological, syntactic, morphological, and pragmatic communication skills; differential assessment and diagnosis need to be made because language disorders are found in varied groups of children, some of whom have associated clinical conditions (e.g., autism or intellectual disabilities) and others present no other conditions; this section describes the assessment of language disorders in children with no other significant intellectual, behavioral, or psychiatric conditions; most of the assessment procedures described may also be used, with suitable modifications, to assess language disorders associated with such other clinical conditions as Intellectual Disabilities, Autism Spectrum Disorders, Hearing Impairment, and various Syndromes Associated With Communication Disorders.

### *Assessment Objectives/General Guidelines*

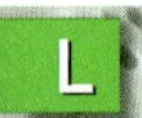


- To assess the extent and nature of the language delay or disorder
- To measure various aspects of existing language skills
- To assess language comprehension
- To assess or rule out the presence of associated clinical conditions (e.g., intellectual deficiency, hearing impairment, a genetic syndrome, or autism)
- To assess the family constellation and communication patterns
- To diagnose a language disorder
- To assess the social and educational demands made on the child
- To suggest potential treatment targets
- To make necessary referrals

### *Case History/Interview Focus*

- See **Case History** and **Interview** under Standard/Common Assessment Procedures
- Concentrate on language, speech, gestures, and the developmental sequence of communication
- Ask the parents or caregivers to compare the child's speech and language development with that of older siblings or peers of the child
- Seek information on the mother's health and disease conditions during pregnancy
- To help rule out associated clinical conditions, seek information from parents or other informants on intellectual disabilities, autism and other pervasive developmental disorders, hearing impairment or any other sensory limitations, any sign or a diagnosis of a genetic syndrome, and cerebral palsy or any other neurological impairment

- Request the parents or other informants to describe the language skills of the child and take verbatim notes of what they say

### *Ethnocultural Considerations*

- See Ethnocultural Considerations in Assessment
- Find out whether the child is a bidialectal English speaker or a speaker of another English dialect; the child may be an African American who speaks a dialect of American English (African American English or Black English) or a child who speaks an English dialect spoken elsewhere (e.g., Australia, South Africa, India, or New Zealand)
- Find out whether the child is bilingual; if so, find out which language is primary; also find out whether the secondary language is nominal or functional; some children may be nominally bilingual, but functionally monolingual English speakers; in which case, the assessment may be made in English unless the family members request a bilingual assessment
- If the child's primary language is other than English, arrange for an assessment in the child's primary as well as secondary language; get an interpreter if the assessment will be in a language you do not know
- Ask family members about family communication patterns; find out what language is predominantly spoken at home; in some cases, bilingual family members may code switch between languages, but the child's dominant language may still be English; in other cases, the child's dominant language may be English though the child and the family members may competently code switch between English and another family language; the family members may code switch, but still the child's and the family members' primary language may be other than English
- Do not administer a test to a child from an ethnocultural and linguistic minority group unless the standardization sample included children from that group
- For ethnoculturally diverse children, use alternative assessment formats, including Authentic Assessment, Client-Specific Procedures, Criterion-Referenced Assessment, Dynamic Assessment, and Portfolio Assessment; possibly, select elements from alternative assessment approaches that might suit an individual child
- Be skeptical about the validity of altering standardized test items in administering otherwise inappropriate tests to ethnoculturally diverse children who are not represented in the standardization sample
- Develop clinical resources on characteristics of the languages other than English that are spoken in your service area
- Always make an assessment of the family's cultural background as it relates to communication, disability, rehabilitation, and treatment
- Gauge the family's resources and needed support systems because treatment of language disorders can be a long and expensive enterprise; assess barriers to effective treatment and access to needed medical care

### *Screening*

- When a language disorder is not obvious, screen language to determine whether a more detailed assessment is needed
  - Evoke a brief conversation from the child

  - Take note of any deficiencies in the semantic, morphological, syntactic, and pragmatic aspects of the language
- Administer the latest version of one of the following standardized screening tests or measures:

| Test | Purpose |
|---|---|
| *Bankson Language Screening Test* (N. W. Bankson) | To screen semantic, morphological, and syntactic skills and auditory and visual perception (4 to 7 yrs) |
| *The Communication Screen* (N. Striffler & S. Willig) | To assess vocabulary and auditory comprehension skills (2.10 to 5.9 yrs) |
| *Denver Developmental Screening Test II* (W. K. Frankenburg & associates) | To assess language, personal-social, and motor development (2 wks to 6 yrs) |
| *Fluharty–2: Fluharty Preschool Speech and Language Screening Test-R* (N. B. Fluharty) | To screen basic speech and language skills (3 to 6.11 yrs) in about 10 minutes |
| *Joliet 3-minute Preschool Speech and Language Screen* (M. Kinzler) | To screen basic language skills (2 to 4 yrs) in less than 5 minutes |
| *Kindergarten Language Screening Test, Second Edition* (S. V. Gauthier & C. I. Madison) | To screen expressive and receptive language skills (3.6 to 6.11 yrs) in about 5 minutes |
| *Northwestern Syntax Screening Test* (L. Lee) | To screen syntactic, morphological, and semantic skills (3 to 8 years) |
| *Preschool Language Screening Test* (E. Hannah & J. Gardner) | To assess visual, motor, and auditory perceptual concepts (3 to 5.6 yrs) |
| *Speech-Ease Screening Inventory* (Speech-Ease) | To screen expressive and receptive language in about 7 to 10 minutes |



- Refer the child for a language assessment if the skills fall below expectations (based on either the conversational speech sample, the screening test, or both)

### *Assessment*

- Assess word production and usage (semantic skills)
  - Obtain parental reports on the types and number of words the child produces at home
  - Obtain parental reports on the production of single words and ascertain whether single word productions are the child's primary mode of communication
  - Ask the parents to list words the child produces, especially if the child produces only a limited number of words
  - Observe interactions between the child and the mother, father, another caregiver, or another family member and take note of the types and frequency of single word productions
  - Record a speech and language sample; engage the child in play-oriented interactions

        - Ask the child to name pictures (not point to them) as you show them
        - Have the child name objects and toys as you show them
        - Have the child tell a story by looking at pictures in storybooks
        - Ask the child to describe objects and their characteristics, and tell how to play the games you show the child or build structures with blocks
        - Have the child name actions depicted in pictures and ask the child what will happen next
        - Ask the child to narrate a personal experience; perhaps a birthday party the child recently had or a recent visit to the zoo
        - Tell a brief story and ask the child retell it
        - Present a puzzle that requires the child to ask questions or request and put it together with the child while encouraging as much speech as possible
    - While taking the language sample:
        - Take note of any unusual word usage
        - Take note of any overextension of words (e.g., use of the word *mother* to refer to all adult women or the use of the word *ball* to refer to all things round)
        - Take note of any underextensions (e.g., only the family Ford is a car and all other cars are not cars)
        - Take note of any signs of misunderstanding or misinterpretation of words
        - Take note of the use of general terms for more specific terms (*this, this thing, that, that thing*)
        - Classify words according to Semantic Relations; note that there is no conclusive evidence to suggest that theoretical and abstract semantic relations (e.g., nomination or agent of action) are empirically real for children

L

- Assess production of grammatical morphemes
    - Record an extended Speech and Language Sample (see Standard/Common Assessment Procedures)
    - Use all connected speech-language evoking procedures including picture descriptions, description of activities you and the child engage in, interaction between the child and family members, storytelling with the help of pictures, story retelling, narrating personal experiences (e.g., favorite vacation, movie, TV shows, friends, sports, other activities), and so forth; see Speech and Language Sample under Standard/Common Assessment Procedures for details
    - Design behavior-specific tasks to evoke production of particular grammatical morphemes; for example:
        - Ask the child to name pictures of single and multiple objects to assess the production of **plural morphemes** and ask "What is this?" and "What are these?" as you point to the single or multiple objects (e.g., show the picture of a single book and that of two or more books; show pictures of different kinds of objects); sample the production of all the allomorphic variations of the regular plural
        - Ask the child to name pictures that depict **irregular plural nouns** contrasted with their respective singular nouns (e.g., show pictures of

a child and several children, a man and several men, a woman and several women, and ask the child *Who is this?* and *Who are these?* as you point to the specific picture)

- Ask the child to describe actions depicted in the pictures to assess the production of the present **progressive *ing*** and the auxiliary verbs (e.g., ask *What is the boy doing?* or *What is the girl doing?* as you show and point to the pictures of a *boy running* and a *girl smiling*)
- Use the same action pictures to evoke grammatically complete sentences that would include a verbal **auxiliary** or a **copula** (e.g., ask *What is the boy doing? Say it in a complete sentence* to evoke the auxiliary *is* in *The boy is running;* or ask *Who is tall?* to evoke a copula in such sentences as *The giraffe is tall.*)
- Ask the child to say where an object is as you manipulate its location to assess the production of **prepositions** (e.g., ask the child *Where is the ball?* as you place it in a box, on the box, behind the box, beside the box, under the box); assess with multiple exemplars involving varied objects
- Ask the child to tell "Which is bigger?," "Which is smaller?," "Which is the smoothest?," and so forth to assess the production of **comparatives** and **superlatives**; to evoke verbal responses, show appropriate paired objects without naming them or without pointing to them
- Ask the child such questions as "Whose hat is this?," "Whose shoes are these?," and "Whose shirt is this?" as you show appropriate pictures to evoke the **possessive morpheme** in such responses as *man's hat, woman's shoes*, and *boy's shirt*; point to the relevant portion of the picture as you ask the question

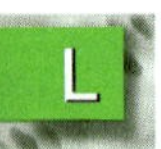

- Ask such questions as "What moves?" and "Who walks?" after demonstrating the movement of a car and walking by a puppet to evoke the production of **third person singular** in such responses as *car moves* and *puppet walks*
- Ask the child to complete such sentences as "This boy is . . . ('big')"; "This girl is . . . ('tall')"; "This ball is . . . ('red')" and so forth to assess the production of adjectives; show appropriate pictures to evoke responses
- Show relevant pictures and ask such questions as "Who is smiling?" or "Who is walking?" to evoke the production of such **pronouns** as "he" or "she" in phrases or sentences (e.g., *She is smiling* or *He is walking*)
- Show various pictures and tell the child a brief story and ask relevant questions to evoke the production of **regular past inflections** (e.g., tell the child that *The man is now yawning; he did the same yesterday; what did he do yesterday?* Or, *The man is now painting; he did the same yesterday; what did he do yesterday?*)

- Assess syntactic skills
  - Use the recorded speech and language sample to assess the production of syntactic structures
  - Administer one of the standardized tests of syntactic skills
  - Use the elicited imitation technique to assess the imitative production of sentences that the child did not produce in spontaneous speech

    - Write four to six sentences of a particular type (e.g., active declarative, passive, questions, requests, negations)
    - Model each of the sentences for the child to imitate
    - Record the child's response for a precise analysis of any missing or mismanaged elements
    - If time permits, administer each sentence on three trials to improve reliability; if time does not permit, make sure to repeat the procedure with three trials in establishing baselines before starting treatment
    - Calculate the percent correct imitation for each of the sentence types presented
    - Be aware that the correct imitation of a structure is not always an indication of correct spontaneous production
- Assess syntactic productions; calculate the percent correct use of major syntactic structures, elements of syntactic structures (such as adjectives), or those that are of special relevance to the child being evaluated; consider the following:
    - Noun phrases: A noun with one or more modifiers preceding it, often an adjective (e.g., *my shoes, big hat, that pencil*)
    - Verb phrases: Words or phrases that describe an action or state of being; consider the auxiliary and copular verbs as well (e.g., *he is running, that is nice*)
    - Prepositional phrases: A construction or preposition, a noun or pronoun, and a modifier (e.g., *the toys in the box are mixed up*)
    - Independent or main clause: A grammatically complete and correct sentence that can stand alone (e.g., *the lion growled*)
    - Subordinate clause: A construction that includes a subject and a predicate but cannot stand alone as grammatically correct (e.g., *because you are nice; though I like to play*); these can become complete sentences only when combined with independent clauses (*because you are nice, I like you; though I like to play, I have no time*)
    - Simple sentences: An independent clause with no subordinate clause (e.g., *I tried; she went*)
    - Declarative sentences: A construction that makes a statement (e.g., *this is a ball; the sun is shining*)
    - Compound sentences: A sentence with at least two independent clauses joined by a comma and a conjunction or with a semicolon; containing no subordinate clauses (e.g., *John is not as nice as Tom, but he can be nice on occasions; or, I went to see Jane; I found only her dog*)
    - Complex sentences: A sentence with one independent clause and one or more subordinate clauses (e.g., *I tried some small talk while we were in the elevator*)
    - Active sentences: Sentences in which the subject performs the actions of the verb (e.g., *Jenny hit the car*)
    - Passive sentences: Sentences in which the subject receives the action of the verb (e.g., *the car was hit by Jenny*)
    - Questions: Sentences that require more information or a yes/no answer

- Negatives: Sentences that reject or deny an affirmation (e.g., *that is a boy, not a girl; I don't like it; not for me, for him; not the car, but the puppet*)
- Requests: Sentences that ask others to perform certain actions (e.g., *please give me that car; please say yes; please hand me that*)
- Imperatives: Sentences that require others to perform certain actions; they are like commands (*look at me; stop that*)
- Use one of the computerized language sample analysis programs to evaluate the production of syntactic structures

- Assess conversational skills (pragmatic language skills)
  - Assess conversational repair. Assess skills of handling breakdown in communication; these include such skills as asking questions when messages are not clear and responding effectively to requests for clarification.
  - Assess the frequency with which the child makes requests for clarifications from a speaker
    - During conversational speech sampling, make several ambiguous or unclear statements (e.g., say *Give me the car* when you have displayed several toy cars; *Pick up the toy* when the child faces several toys)
    - Wait for the child to request clarification (e.g., the child may ask, *Which car?*, *Which one do you mean?*, or *I don't know which one*)
    - Count the frequency of such ambiguous statements you made and the number of acceptable requests for clarification the child made during the assessment session
    - To assess stimulability, model a request for clarification ("Ask me what do you mean?"; "Ask me which car")
    - Count the frequency of modeled requests for clarification and the frequency with which the child imitated your request
    - Do not give positive or corrective feedback for the presence or absence of requests for clarification
    - Calculate the percent correct requests for clarification (the total number of ambiguous statements made divided by the number of correct requests for clarification the child made multiplied by 100)
    - Repeat the procedures in a later session (e.g., at the beginning of reassessment when the child returns for treatment, during treatment when other language skills are being taught)
  - Assess the frequency with which the child responds appropriately to requests for clarification
    - During conversational speech sampling, play the role of a listener who does not fully understand the expressions of the child
    - Ask the child to repeat
    - Ask the child "What do you mean?"
    - Tell the child "I do not understand"
    - Negate a child's utterance so the child will clarify by assertion ("You did not go on the roller coaster 20 times, did you?"; the child might say "No, I went on it two times")

- Wait for a few seconds for the child to respond to your indication of lack of understanding
- Take note of adequate, inadequate, and lack of response
- Do not give differential feedback for inadequate clarifications, lack of clarifications, or acceptable clarifications
- Count the number of times you made requests for clarification and the number of times the child made a satisfactory clarification of his or her statements
- To assess stimulability, model clarified statements ("You mean you went on the roller coaster two times, right?")
- Rephrase the child's utterance into a question and say it with a rising intonation ("You went on the roller coaster 20 times?")
- Ask the child to say it differently
- Count the number of times the child imitated the modeled requests for clarification
- Calculate the percent correct compliance for requests for clarification and the percent correct imitation of modeled compliance for requests for clarification

- Assess topic initiation. Assess whether the child can introduce new topics of conversation; prompt the child if necessary, and take note of the opportunities given the child to introduce a topic and the actual number of times the child did introduce a topic for conversation.
  - During conversational speech sampling, arrange a variety of stimuli that could trigger new topics of conversation: objects, pictures, storybooks, topic cards (for children who can read), toys, structured play situations such as a kitchen, a doll house, and so forth
  - Introduce one of the stimulus items or situations and draw the child's attention to it (e.g., a picture of a family setting up a tent in a park)
  - Wait for the child to initiate conversation about the picture and the story
  - Count the number of times the child initiated a topic upon stimulus presentation
  - If the child does not initiate a topic, instruct the child to say something about the picture
  - Count the number of times the child initiated a topic when asked to say something
  - If the child still does not initiate a topic, prompt it by beginning the story ("They are setting up a . . .")
  - Count the number of times the child initiated topics upon specific verbal prompting
  - Accept statements that are remotely connected to the topic at hand; discount those that are irrelevant or inappropriate in your judgment
  - Do not give differential feedback for correct or incorrect responses and for no responses
  - Count the total number of stimulus presentations under each category (e.g., stimulus presentation and verbal prompting) and the total

number of appropriate topic initiations; calculate the percent correct topic initiations

- Repeat the measures on reassessment or at the beginning of treatment

- Assess topic maintenance. Assess whether the child can maintain conversation on a single topic for a duration that you judge is adequate; there are no specific standards on the duration, but there should be no abrupt termination of topics of conversation.
  - During conversational speech sampling, let the child select topics of interest for talking; prompt and suggest topics if necessary, but let the child lead you
  - Measure the duration (seconds or minutes) for which the child maintained the same topic of conversation; start a stopwatch as the child introduces a new topic, stop the clock as the child stops talking on that topic, or shifts to another topic
  - To assess the stimulability of topic maintenance skills, use such devices as *Tell me more, What about that?, What happened next?, Who said what?, Where was it?, When did that happen?;* measure the duration for which the child maintained a topic with such prompts
  - Do not give differential feedback to the child for topic maintenance or lack of it
  - Summarize the range of durations (the briefest and the longest) for which the child maintained topics
  - Calculate the typical duration (statistical mode, not the mean) for which the child maintained topics; for example, if the child talked on four topics, what was the most frequently observed duration for which the child maintained the topic?
  - Repeat the measures upon reassessment or before initiating treatment

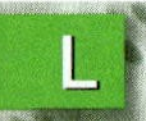

- Assess conversational turn taking. Assess whether the child can appropriately alternate between the roles of a speaker and that of a listener and whether the child interrupts you while you are talking and whether the child fails to talk when it is his or her turn.
  - During conversational speech sampling, observe the turn taking behavior because there will be plenty of opportunities for the two of you to exchange the listener and speaker roles; if judged adequate, there may be no need to spend additional time on this skill
  - If necessary, devote a few minutes of assessment time to measure turn-taking behaviors
  - Count the number of times the child interrupted your speech and thus took inappropriate turns
  - Count the number of times the child could have said something but did not (failure to take a turn when it is appropriate to take)
  - Count the number of times the child appropriately took conversational turns without special signals
  - To assess stimulability, count the number of times the child took turns when you signaled (e.g., when you give such verbal cues as *your turn* or nonverbal cues as a hand gesture to suggest *you speak*)

- Do not give differential feedback for correct or incorrect turn-taking behaviors
- Repeat the measures during reassessment or just before starting treatment on turn taking

- Assess eye contact. Assess whether the child maintained eye contact during conversation or whether the child was consistently looking away from you as he or she spoke; however, eye contact during conversation is potentially culturally determined; find out whether avoiding direct eye contact during conversation, especially with an authority figure (such as a clinician, teacher, or parents) is a cultural practice in the community to which the child belongs; assess this skill nonetheless, but interpret the clinical significance in light of what you find out about the cultural practice and whether the parents want the child to learn this skill
  - During conversational speech sampling, take note of lack of eye contact; if it is a significant problem, measure the durations for which the child maintained eye contact and the durations for which the child did not
  - To assess stimulability, instruct the child (e.g., *look at me as you talk to me*) to maintain eye contact and measure the duration for which the child maintains eye contact
  - Use clinical judgment in evaluating the measures because there are no specific guidelines on appropriate durations of eye contact in conversational exchanges; a persistent lack of eye contact during conversation is of clinical significance, interpreted again in light of the child's cultural background
  - Repeat the measures during reassessment or just before starting treatment
- Assess narrative skills. Assess this conversational skill as illustrated by a speaker's description of events (stories, episodes) and experiences in a logically consistent, cohesive, temporally sequenced manner.
  - During conversational speech sampling, observe and take note of narrative skills
  - Note that the overall narrative styles, amount of details and elaborations offered, use of emotional expression, and organization and sequencing of events may be influenced by the child's cultural background
  - Ask the child to describe such events as grocery shopping, eating in a restaurant, birthday parties, camping trips, vacations, playing certain games, and so forth to assess narrative skills
  - Read aloud or tell a story to the child and ask him or her to retell it
  - Retell the same story to the child and pause before important phrases or critical descriptions to assess whether the child will supply them
  - To assess stimulability, prompt phrases and descriptions as the child hesitates; observe whether the child picks up details and sequences
  - Tell a story with the help of pictures, and ask the child to retell it while looking at the pictures

        - Analyze the narratives for proper temporal sequence of events, inadequate character descriptions, misplaced story settings, missing details, sparse descriptions, abrupt ending, confused characters, and so forth
- Assess language comprehension
    - Observe the child's responses while taking a conversational speech sample to assess comprehension of your speech
    - Note irrelevant or inappropriate responses that suggest lack of comprehension
    - Note the response complexity level at which comprehension breaks down (e.g., correct comprehension of phrases but not sentences)
    - Give specific commands to assess comprehension; use or modify such strategies as the following:
        - Ask the child to point to a set of common pictures as you name them (e.g., *point to the car* or *point to the dog*); score the correct and incorrect responses
        - Ask the child to manipulate objects or toys (e.g., *put the block on the book* or *make the car go*); score the correct and incorrect responses
        - Ask the child to follow simple to progressively more complex commands (e.g., *please stand up*; *please shut that door*; and *please shut the door and open the drapes*); score the correct and incorrect responses
        - Ask the child to point to correct pictures that help assess the comprehension of grammatical morphemes and syntactic structures (e.g., *show me the boy is running*; *show me the girl is riding*; *show me two cups*; *show me the ball is in the box*; *show me the car is on the table*; *show me he is smiling*; *show me she is walking*); score the correct and incorrect responses

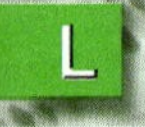


    - Assess the comprehension of abstract statements by asking the child to explain the meaning of proverbs you expect the child to have heard; note that proverbs and typical expressions are extremely culture-bound

### *Administer Selected Standardized Tests of Children's Language Skills*

- Use the Speech, Language, and Motor Development guidelines in assessing children
- If the child belongs to an ethnocultural minority group, use the guidelines on standardized test administration given under Ethnocultural Considerations in this main entry and also see the main entry, Ethnocultural Considerations in Assessment
- Be fully aware of the limitations of standardized tests, especially the limited sampling of skills (one or two opportunities given to produce a particular language structure); always supplement test results with an extended speech and language sample that affords multiple opportunities to produce various language structures
- Administer one or more of the following standardized tests or measures; administer the latest edition of tests that are known to be reliable and valid; use the following matrix to select the tests to be administered to a child:

| Tests of Child Language Skills | Purpose |
|---|---|
| *Assessment of Children's Language Comprehension* (R. Foster, J. J. Giddan, & J. Stark) | To assess comprehension of words and phrases (3 to 6.11 yrs) |
| *Bankson Language Test* (N. W. Bankson) | To assess production of semantic, syntactic, and morphological skills (4 to 8 yrs) |
| *Basic Language Concepts Test* (S. Englemann, D. Ross, & V. Bingham) | To assess basic language skills necessary to succeed in initial grades (4 to 6.6 yrs) |
| *Boehm Test of Basic Concepts* (A. E. Boehm) | To assess comprehension of basic semantic concepts (K to 2nd grade) |
| *Carrow Elicited Language Inventory* (E. Carrow-Woolfolk) | To assess imitative production of syntactic skills (3 to 7.11 yrs) |
| *Clinical Evaluation of Language Fundamentals—Fourth Edition* (E. Semel, E. Wiig, & W. Secord) | To assess production of semantic, syntactic, phonological, and memory skills (6 to 21.11 yrs) |
| *CELF—Preschool, Second Edition* (E. Semel, W. Secord, & E. Wiig) | To assess expressive, receptive, and pragmatic language skills (3 to 6 yrs) |
| *Comprehensive Receptive and Expressive Vocabulary Test* (G. Wallace & D. D. Hammill) | To assess expressive and receptive language skills by defining words and pointing (4 to 17.11 yrs) |
| *CSBC DP Infant Toddler Checklist and Easy Score* (A. Wetherby & B. Prizant) | To assess verbal/nonverbal skills of infants and toddlers (6.0 to 24 months) |
| *Evaluating Communicative Competence* (C. S. Simon) | To assess comprehension and production of pragmatic skills (9 to 17 yrs) |
| *Expressive One-Word Picture Vocabulary Test* (R. Brownell) | To assess one-word picture naming skills (2 to 10.11 yrs) |
| *Expressive Language Test* (R. Husingh, L. Bowers, C. LaGiudice, & J. Oman) | To test syntax, sequencing, categorizing, and describing (5 to 11.11 yrs) |
| *Expressive Vocabulary Test* (K . T. Williams) | To test labeling and synonyms (2.6 to adulthood) |
| *HELP Test—Elementary* (A. M. Lazzari) | To assess vocabulary, syntax, and definitions (6 to 11.11 yrs) |
| *Peabody Picture Vocabulary Test—Third Edition* (L. M. Dunn & L. M. Dunn) | To assess comprehension of single words (2.3 to 40.11 yrs) |
| *Preschool Language Scale—Fourth Edition* (I. R. Zimmerman, V. G. Steiner, & R. E. Pond) | To assess comprehension and production of language skills (birth to 6.11 yrs) |
| *Receptive One-Word Picture Vocabulary Test* (R. Brownell) | To assess receptive language skills through pointing task (2.11 to 11 yrs) |

*(continues)*

L

*(continued)*

| Tests of Child Language Skills | Purpose |
|---|---|
| *Sequenced Inventory of Communication Development—Revised* (D. L. Hedrick, E. M. Prather, & A. R. Tobin) | To assess comprehension and production of communication skills (4 months to 4 yrs) |
| *Structured Photographic Expressive Language Test—3* (J. Dawson & C. Stout) | To assess morphological and syntactic forms; includes alternative forms for African American English (4 to 9.11 yrs) |
| *Wiig Criterion-referenced Inventory of Language* (E. Wiig, 1990) | A criterion-referenced assessment tool for semantic, syntactic, morphological, and pragmatic skills (4 to 13 yrs) |
| *Test of Auditory Comprehension of Language—Revised* (E. Carrow-Woolfolk) | To assess comprehension of word categories, grammatical features, and syntactic constructions (3 to 9.11 yrs) |
| *Test for Examining Expressive Morphology* (K. G. Shipley, T. Stone, & M. Sue) | To assess production of morphological skills (3 to 8.11 yrs) |
| *Test of Early Language Development—Second Edition* (W. P. Hiresko, D. K. Reid, & D. D. Hammill) | To assess comprehension and production of semantic and syntactic structures (2.7 to 7.11 yrs) |
| *Test of Language Development—2 Primary* (P. L. Newcomer & D. D. Hammill) | To assess comprehension and production of words; articulation; and some grammatical features (4 to 8.11 yrs) |
| *Test of Language Development—2 Intermediate* (P. L. Newcomer & D. D. Hammill) | To test comprehension and production of words; articulation; and grammatical features (8.6 to 12.11 yrs) |
| *Test of Narrative Language* (R. B. Gillam & N. A. Pearson) | To assess narrative language skills (5 to 11.11 yrs) |
| *Test of Pragmatic Language* (D. Phelphs & T. Phelps-Gunn) | To assess social communication skills including abstract language (5.0 to 13.11 yrs) |
| *Test of Semantic Skills—Primary* (L. Bowers, R. Husingh, C. LaGiudice, & J. Oman) | To assess labeling, categorizing, and specifying attributes, definitions, and functions (4 to 8.11 yrs) |
| *Test of Word Finding* (D. J. German) | To assess single-word retrieval skills (6.6 to 12.11 yrs) |
| *Test of Word Finding in Discourse* (D. J. German) | To assess word-retrieval deficits in conversation (6:6 to 12.11 yrs) |
| *Test of Pragmatic Skills—Revised* (B. B. Schulman) | To assess verbal and nonverbal pragmatic skills (3 to 8.11 yrs) |
| *Token Test for Children* (F. DiSimoni) | To assess receptive understanding of temporal and spatial concepts (3 to 12 yrs) |

*(continues)*

*(continued)*

| Tests of Child Language Skills | Purpose |
|---|---|
| *Utah Test of Language Development—3* (M. J. Mecham) | To assess language production and comprehension (3 to 9.11 yrs) |
| *Wiig Criterion-Referenced Inventory of Language* (E. H. Wiig) | To make a criterion referenced assessment of semantic, syntactic, morphological, and pragmatic skills (4 to 13 yrs) |

## *Medical, Psychological, and Educational Assessment Data*

- Obtain any available medical data of importance in evaluating language disorders that might suggest a congenital disorder or genetic syndrome
- Obtain the results of the audiological evaluation if one was done to help rule out hearing impairment as the cause of language problems
- Obtain psychological data including the results of intelligence testing and cognitive functioning to help rule out intellectual disabilities as the associated clinical condition
- Obtain data on the child's educational achievement and assessment that might suggest learning disabilities and educational demands made on the child

## *Standard/Common Assessment Procedures*

- Complete the Standard/Common Assessment Procedures

## *Analysis of Results*

L

- Analyze the results of the comprehension assessment; identify the levels at which comprehension is adequate (e.g., correct comprehension of words or phrases)
- Identify the levels at which comprehension breaks down (e.g., poor comprehension of sentences; questions; two-element commands; requests)
- Estimate the level of comprehension of connected, spoken speech (e.g., 80% of words, phrases, or sentences comprehended)
- Analyze the kinds of words the child uses (e.g., nouns only; nouns and a few verbs; few or no adjectives); if possible, estimate the size of the child's vocabulary, especially if the child is producing mostly single words
- Calculate the Mean Length of Utterance (MLU)
- Calculate the length of the most frequently produced utterances (statistical mode, not the mean)
- Identify the shortest and the longest utterance
- List the grammatical morphemes the child produced with 100% accuracy in conversational speech and standardized tests
- List the grammatical morphemes the child failed to produce or produced at some inadequate level in either conversational speech or during standardized testing; quantify these observations (e.g., 0% production of past tense *ed* inflection; 10% accurate production of the present progressive *ing*)
- List the sentence types the child produced in conversational speech (e.g., simple, active, declarative; questions; negation; passive; requests; complex sentences; compound sentences; embedded sentences)

- List the sentence types the child did not produce in either conversational speech or during standardized testing
- Summarize the pragmatic features the child correctly used or managed (e.g., appropriate eye contact, acceptable turn taking, adequate topic initiation skills); to the extent possible, quantify these observations (e.g., appropriate topic initiation 80% of the opportunities given)
- Summarize the pragmatic features the child did not use or used inappropriately (e.g., lack of topic maintenance; poor narrative skills, inadequate response to request for clarification, lack of request for clarification); to the extent possible, quantify these observations (e.g., 100% failure in responding to requests for clarification)
- Summarize the child's phonological skills; make a thorough analysis as described under Articulation and Phonological Disorders if the data warrant
- Make a clinical judgment of voice; take note of voice problems, if any; conduct a voice assessment if the data warrant it; see Voice Disorders for assessment details
- Make a clinical judgment of fluency; conduct a fluency assessment if the data warrant it; see the main entry Fluency Disorders, especially Stuttering under that entry
- Use such computer software programs as Lingquest 1, Systematic Analysis of Language Transcripts, and Computerized Profiling

### *Diagnostic Criteria/Guidelines*



- Significantly limited or deficient language skills affecting all aspects of language (semantic, syntactic, morphological, and pragmatic skills)
- Diagnostic criteria specified in the school or clinic settings; most school districts have diagnostic criteria that are also meant to qualify the child for clinical or special educational services; use the criteria specific to your professional setting
- Absence of sensory deficits, intellectual deficiency, neuromotor problems, and psychiatric problems is essential to diagnose Specific Language Impairment
- If other clinical conditions exists, it may be the child's primary diagnosis (e.g., hearing impairment, autism, or intellectual impairment), although a diagnosis of language (and speech) disorders will be appropriate as well

### *Differential Diagnosis*

- Rule out the presence of associated clinical conditions
  - Differentiate specific language impairment from language disorders associated with autism
    - Take note of indifference to people and lack of interest in social communication
    - No imitation or echolalic speech
    - No interest in normal play or abnormal, stereotypic play
    - Idiosyncratic, irrelevant, and stereotypical speech
    - Stereotypical body movements
    - Preoccupation with objects and stimulus materials instead of conversation
    - Reluctance to be hugged, held, or touched
    - Preference to be left alone
    - Other features as ascertained from the parents; see Autism for details

- Differentiate specific language impairment from language disorders associated with hearing impairment
  - An audiological assessment report that documents the type and degree of hearing impairment
  - Significant phonological problems including the omission of final consonants, simplification of blends, and substitution of voiced consonants for voiceless consonants and vice versa
  - Greater difficulty in producing fricatives; distortions of various sounds
  - Hyper- and hyponasality; significant voice problems especially with deafness; abnormal flow of speech; and slower rate of speech
  - Other features ascertained from the parents; see Hearing Impairment for details
- Differentiate specific language impairment from language disorders associated with intellectual disabilities
  - An independent diagnosis of intellectual disabilities by a psychologist
  - A medical diagnosis of a genetic syndrome or associated medical conditions that cause intellectual disabilities (e.g., Down syndrome, prenatal lead poisoning, fetal alcohol syndrome, post-immunization encephalitis)
  - Poor academic performance, enrollment in special education programs
  - Note that generally simplified language associated with intellectual disabilities is similar to language disorders found in otherwise normal children who show specific language impairment
- Differentiate specific language impairment from language disorders associated with various kinds of brain injury
  - An independent diagnosis of brain injury and its cause (e.g., vehicular accident, falls, assault and gunshot, physical abuse)
  - Initial symptoms of coma (in some cases), confusion and posttraumatic amnesia; retrograde amnesia
  - Irritability, aggression, lethargy, anxiety, withdrawal, and other behavioral problems
  - Attention deficits and visual-spatial problems
  - Neuromotor dysfunctions including rigidity, tremors, spasticity, ataxia, or Apraxia
  - Mutism
  - Significant word retrieval problems



### *Prognosis*

- With systematic treatment, prognosis for improved language skills is good; the extent of improvement may vary depending on the child, family support, time of intervention, and the intensity and effectiveness of the intervention
- Most children with language disorders benefit from treatment
- Some deficits may continue into adolescent and adult years

### *Recommendations*

- Language intervention
- Parent training in language stimulation and maintenance activities at home
- Working with the child's teacher to coordinate treatment objectives and activities with academic goals and activities

- See the cited sources and the two companion volumes, *Hegde's PocketGuide to Communication Disorders* and *Hegde's PocketGuide to Treatment in Speech-Language Pathology* (3rd ed.) for details

Hart, B., & Risley, T. R. (1995). *The social world of children learning to talk.* Baltimore, MD: Paul H. Brookes.

Hegde, M. N., & Maul, C. A. (2006). *Language disorders in children.* Boston, MA: Allyn and Bacon.

Leonard, L. B. (1998). *Children with specific language impairment.* Cambridge, MA: MIT Press.

McCauley, R. J., & Fey, M. E. (2006) (Eds.). *Treatment of language disorders in children.* Baltimore, MD: Paul H. Brookes.

Nelson, N. W. (1998). *Childhood language disorders in context: Infancy through adolescence.* New York: McMillan.

Owens, R. E., Jr. (2004). Language Disorders: *A functional approach to assessment and treatment* (4th ed.). Boston, MA: Allyn and Bacon.

Paul, R. (2001). *Language disorders from infancy through adolescence* (2nd ed.). St. Louis, MO: C. V. Mosby.

Reed, V. (2005). *An introduction to children with language disorders* (3rd ed.). New York: Macmillan College Publishing Company.

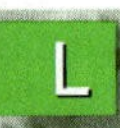

**Language Disorders in Infants and Toddlers.** Assessment of language (and speech) in infants and toddlers is essential to start an early language stimulation or formal professional treatment program when warranted; such early assessment and intervention will help prevent more serious problems later on; assessment of infants and toddlers should concentrate on all aspects of communication, including early speech development, nonverbal communication, physical and behavioral development; evidence of any intellectual or developmental disabilities; presence of a genetic syndrome; evidence of an autism spectrum disorder; hearing impairment or other sensory loss; most of these clinical conditions pose risks for more serious communication disorders later in the life of the child; assessment should also address family communication patterns—the parental interaction with the infant or toddler.

### *Assessment Objectives/General Guidelines*

- To make a family-centered communication assessment of infants and toddlers in both the clinic and home setting
- To begin assessment as early as possible and to repeat assessment throughout the childhood period
- To assess the family constellation, family communication patterns, family resources, and family strengths and limitations
- To work with other professionals and make interdisciplinary decisions regarding the assessment and how the outcome of the assessment will be used
- To suggest an early intervention program that may include both treatment in a clinical facility and interventional activities at home conducted by parents, other caregivers, and other family members (Individual Family Service Plans)
- Note that in assessing prematurely born children, the duration of prematurity (weeks by which the child was born prematurely) is subtracted from

the child's chronological age (CA) to derive the corrected gestational age (CGA) of the child; this correction is used throughout the first year

- Note that interdisciplinary assessment is the most useful in planning a family- and clinic-based intervention plan for the young child

### *Case History/Interview Focus*

- See **Case History** and **Interview** under Standard/Common Assessment Procedures
- Focus on family communication patterns, family strengths and weakness, early verbal and physical development of the infant, and family resources
- Gather information on the maternal health during pregnancy; seek information on various prenatal, natal, and postnatal factors that put the newborn at risk for later speech and language problems
- During the interview, get detailed information on the early signs of communication delay (e.g., lack of response to the mother's voice, lack of joint attention)
- Seek detailed information on the early motor and speech development of the child
- Get information on physical diseases; children who are often and seriously sick and hospitalized for extended durations may be vulnerable to speech and language delay

### *Ethnocultural Considerations*

- See Ethnocultural Considerations in Assessment
- Focus on cultural practices in child rearing; mother-child interactions; family communication patterns; culturally accepted roles for children in adult-child interactions
- Gauge the family members' sophistication in implementing a home language stimulation program if one were to be recommended; estimate the training needs
- Assess the family's resources and needed support system because an infant or toddler with communication deficits is likely to require long-term and expensive care not just to remediate the communication problems, but also to manage the associated problems

L

### *Assessment*

- Note that an infant or toddler needs a comprehensive interdisciplinary assessment and that some of the assessment areas described may be handled by other professionals (e.g., audiologists, medical professionals, child psychologists); the speech-language pathologist takes greater responsibility for communication assessment and perhaps feeding and oral motor development but contributes to assessing other areas as well
- Assess feeding and oral motor development
  - Assess suckling action (primitive form of sucking involving approximate lip closure, jaw movement, and extension and retraction of the tongue in the newborn; often in the newborn intensive care unit—NICU)
  - Assess sucking (negative intraoral air pressure, elevated tongue tip, firm lip closure, and more precise jaw movements)
  - Assess rooting (a reflexive turning toward tactile stimulation)

- Assess phasic bite reflex (bite and release movements when a nipple is placed in the mouth)
- Assess hearing and need for aural rehabilitation
  - Advocate an early assessment of hearing of an infant in the NICU
  - Refer the infant to an audiologist
  - Counsel the family members about hearing conservation and aural rehabilitation
- Assess general behavior and alertness
  - Assess the infant's physiological and attentional state in the NICU
    - Assess deep or light sleep states
    - Take note of drowsiness, alertness, and eye opening
    - Observe the infant's level of toleration of handling and the amount of stimulation the infant can take
    - Note frequent crying
    - Administer *Assessment of Preterm Infant Behavior* for this purpose (see Standardized Tests, Developmental Scales, or Screening Devices described later)
- Assess infant readiness for communication
  - Assess the infant's readiness for communication; observe whether the child is too sick to respond
  - Observe whether the baby has recovered from illness and is beginning to respond to environmental stimuli
  - Observe whether the baby begins to show reciprocal interaction with the environment
- Assess language comprehension and response to social stimuli
  - During the first six months, assess:
    - The baby's response to sound (alertness, diminished activity)
    - Response to familiar face (watching the face)
    - Response to familiar faces and mother's voice (becomes quiet, smiles)
    - Response to emotional tones (e.g., fear at hearing loud or angry voice)
    - Response to sight of food (anticipatory reaction)
    - Response to his or her name
    - Response to soft, affectionate, and pleasant speech directed to the baby (e.g., adult's smile, approach)
    - The child's comprehension of language and response to social stimuli at home by asking the parents about it
  - During six to 12 months of age, assess:
    - Response to names of family members (e.g., looking in certain directions, looking at the person whose name is called)
    - Response to strangers (e.g., signs of apprehension, moving away from the stranger)
    - Response to object names when the object is present (e.g., looking at it, reaching the object)
    - Response to sounds made by toys (e.g., looks at the object when sound is heard)
    - Response to "No" (e.g., cessation of activity; hesitancy; unpleasant facial expression)

- Response to scolding (e.g., frowning, crying, unpleasant facial expression)
- Response to action words (understands a few action words)
- Response to gestures (e.g., claps when clapping is modeled; touches body parts when this is modeled)
- Words the baby understands at home by asking the parents to list them

- During 12 to 18 months of age, assess:
  - Response to names of people and objects that are present (correct recognition of familiar names and objects)
  - Response to some names of objects and persons when the objects and persons are not present
  - Comprehension of possessor + possession (e.g., *Mommy's shoes*)
  - Response to simple commands
  - Response to varied gestures
  - Comprehension of language and social stimuli at home by asking the parents about it; note that parents tend to think that the baby understands everything though the research has not substantiated this
- During 18 to 24 months of age, assess:
  - Response to absent objects more precise and varied
  - Response to absent persons more precise and varied
  - Response to two-word combinations
  - Response to simple requests (e.g., can locate a missing object when requested)
  - Response to simple commands
  - Baby's comprehension of language structures at home by asking the parents or other caregivers about it
- During 24 to 36 months of age, assess:
  - Response to three-word sentences (correct comprehension of simple three-word sentences)
  - Response to commands (give two-, three-, and four-element commands to determine the level at which the child's comprehension breaks down).
  - Response to requests (give progressively more complex requests to determine the level at which the child's comprehension breaks down)
  - Ask questions involving *what, who*, and *where* and judge the appropriateness of responses to evaluate comprehension
  - The child's responses to language stimuli and social interactions at home by asking the parents and other caregivers about them

- Assess verbal communication
  - During the first six months, assess:
    - Normal crying
    - Vegetative sounds associated with feeding
    - Grunting and sighing
    - Vowel-like sounds
    - Sound vocalizations
    - Increased range of vocalizations
    - Differentiated facial expressions
    - Emergence of pleasure sounds (e.g., *mmmm*)

L

- Sounds the baby makes at home by asking the parents or caregivers to list them
- The emergence of marginal babbling (consonant-like sounds in babbling)

- During 6 to 12 months of age, assess:
  - The more frequent babbling (consonant-vowel syllable productions like *bababa* or *mamama*) emerging around 6 months of age
  - The addition of other sounds produced in the front of the mouth (e.g., /p/, /t/, /d/)
  - Turn taking in vocalization (e.g., the baby and a caregiver may vocalize in an alternating fashion)
  - Increased production of consonant-like sounds
  - Imitation of adult vocalizations or gestures
  - Point to things, which may begin during this stage
  - The emergence of social interaction and joint attention
  - The emergence of phonetically consistent forms—specific sounds in specific situations (e.g., one vowel sound to suggest a desire for an object and another sound to suggest disapproval)
  - Intonation in babbling or prosodic features, which tend to emerge around 6 months of age
  - Intentional communication between 9 and 10 months of age (e.g., specific gesturing or pointing; vocalizing while making eye contact)
  - The speech sounds, babbling, and other communicative behaviors the child exhibits at home by having the parents describe them

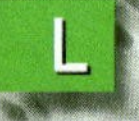

- During 12 to 18 months of age, assess:
  - Expanded repertoire of sounds produced
  - Increased use of gestures and vocalizations to obtain objects, draw attention, and regulate the behavior of caregivers
  - Production of first words
  - The speech sounds, meaningful vocalizations, and other communicative behaviors the child exhibits at home by having the parents describe them
- During 18 to 24 months of age, assess:
  - Expansion and differentiation of single word classes (nominals, action words, modifiers or adjectives)
  - More meaningful and consistent use of 10–15 words
  - Production of two-word phrases
  - Speech intelligibility, which should be at least 50% intelligible to caregivers
  - Unintelligible strings of syllables produced with a sentence-like intonation
  - Combination of intelligible and unintelligible syllables with a sentence intonation
  - Have the parents or caregivers describe words, phrases, gestures, and other communicative behaviors of the child
- During 24 to 36 months of age, assess:
  - Emergence of simple sentences
  - Three- and 4-word sentences; 5-word sentences toward the end of this period

- Production of questions (e.g., *What is that?* or *What you doing?*)
- Increased intelligibility of speech (up to 75%)
- Increased expressive vocabulary (at 24 months, just under 300 words; at 36 months, 900 to 1000 words)
- All aspects of language by taking a Speech and Language Sample (see Standard/Common Assessment Procedures), especially with the child at the end of this period; use informal play to evoke language productions
- Production of words, phrases, sentences, gestures, and other communicative behaviors of the child at home by having the parents or caregivers describe them

- Assess infant-caregiver interaction
  - Use the *Observation of Communication Interaction* by Klein and Briggs (1986) and the *Mother Infant Play Interaction Scale* by Walker and Thompson (1982); these instruments offer suggestions of the following kind
  - Observe and record the interaction between the baby and the mother (or another caregiver) at home (preferred); if in the clinical setting, arrange a natural interactive situation for the child and the mother; take note of the following:
    - How the mother handles and stimulates the baby; holding, cuddling, stroking, rocking, and so forth
    - How the mother expresses her affection for the baby; smiling and laughing in general and contingent smiling and laughing (reaction to similar behaviors in the child) in particular
    - How the mother plays with the child; quiet play or play with speech and vocalizations; the tone of speech and vocalization; presence or absence of contingent response to child's reactions
    - How the mother visually concentrates on the baby; take note whether the mother places or holds the infant at her eye level
    - The infant's mood and affect: take note of responsiveness and alertness or nonresponsiveness and disinterested disposition
    - How the mother responds contingently to the infant's behavior
    - How the mother modifies her interaction when the infant gives negative cues
- Assess play activities
  - Observe the child engaged in play with another child; make unobtrusive observations; take note of the child's pattern of interaction during play; observe whether the child:
    - Plays cooperatively with the other child or children
    - Engages in parallel play or isolated play
    - Indulges in constructive activities along or with other children
    - Engages in role playing and pretend play
    - Exhibits uncooperative or aggressive behaviors
    - Does not share toys
    - Does not talk much during play
    - Passively watches others play

## Standardized Tests, Developmental Scales, or Screening Devices

- Note that in assessing children under 3, few standardized instruments are available; most are developmental scales that help structure observations of the child to take note of the presence or absence of behaviors of interest
- Use the Speech, Language, and Motor Development guidelines in assessing infants and toddlers
- Consider using the following instruments:

| Instrument | Purpose |
|---|---|
| *Assessment of Preterm Infant Behavior* (H. Als, B. Lester, E. Tronick, & T. Brazelton) | To assess the infant's physiological and attentional state in the NICU |
| *Birth to Three Developmental Scale* (T. Bangs & S. Dodson) | To assess developmental delays |
| *Communication and Symbolic Behavior Scales* (A. M. Wetherby & B. Prizant) | To assess nonverbal and verbal communication in infants and children up to 6 yrs |
| *Early Language Milestone Scale* (J. Coplan) | To assess early communication skills (birth to 3 yrs) |
| *Language Development Survey* (L. Rescorla) | To screen language in toddlers |
| *Preschool Language Assessment* (M. Blank, S. A. Rose, & L. J. Berlin) | To assess language skills both formally and informally (3 to 5.11 yrs) |
| *Rossetti Infant-Toddler Language Scale* (L. Rossetti) | To assess communication and interaction in infants and toddlers |
| *Sequenced Inventory of Communication Development—Revised* (D. Hedrick, E. Prather, & A. Tobin) | To assess verbal and nonverbal communication in infants and children up to 4 yrs |
| *Preschool Language Scale* (I. Zimmerman, V. Steiner, & R. Pond) | To assess receptive and expressive language in infants and children up to 6.11 yrs |

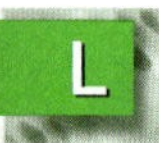


## Related/Medical Assessment Data

- Obtain medical information about the baby's illness, treatment plans, and prognosis
- Obtain psychological or behavioral assessment data describing the child's behavioral development
- Integrate communication and related assessment information with related/medical data

## Standard/Common Assessment Procedures

- Complete the Standard/Common Assessment Procedures

## Analysis of Results

- Analyze the results of assessment along with parent interview information
- List the infant's or toddler's strengths and limitations

- Describe the child's communication deficits
- Describe the family communication patterns, mother-child interactions, and problems in this area

### *Diagnostic Criteria/Guidelines*

- Note that in making an infant-toddler assessment, the examiner is more concerned with assessing the child in his or her family context than rendering a clinical diagnosis
- Deficiencies in preverbal, verbal, and nonverbal communication skills are essential to suggest a family and professional treatment plan

### *Prognosis*

- Generally good with early intervention and parent training
- With effective treatment and family involvement, speech and language skills of most young children improve significantly

### *Recommendations*

- Early intervention within the framework of a family service plan
- Parent training in language stimulation
- Both home-based and center-based intervention when warranted
- Periodic assessment
- More intensive center-based treatment if repeated assessment results suggest it
- See the cited sources and the two companion volumes, *Hegde's PocketGuide to Communication Disorders* and *Hegde's PocketGuide to Treatment in Speech-Language Pathology* (3rd ed.) for details



Billeaud, F. P. (2003). *Communication disorders in infants and toddlers* (3rd ed.). Boston, MA: Butterworth-Heinemann.

Gorski, P., Davidson, M., & Brazelton, T. (1979). Stages of behavioral organization in the high risk neonate: Theoretical and clinical considerations. *Seminars in Perinatology, 3,* 61.

Hegde, M. N., & Maul, C. (2006). *Language disorders in children: An evidence-based approach to assessment and treatment.* Boston, MA: Allyn and Bacon.

Klein, D., & Briggs, M. (1986). Observation of Communicative Interaction. DHS Publication No. MCJ 06351–01–0. Washington, DC: U.S. Government Printing Office.

Nelson, N. W. (1998). *Childhood language disorders in context* (2nd ed.). Boston, MA: Allyn and Bacon.

Paul, R. (2001). *Language disorders from infancy through adolescence* (2nd ed.). St. Louis, MO: C. V. Mosby.

Reed, V. (2005). *An introduction to children with language disorders* (2nd ed.). Boston, MA: Allyn and Bacon.

Rossetti, L. M. (2001). *Communication intervention birth to three* (2nd ed.). Clifton Park, NY: Thomson Delmar Learning.

Walker, L., & Thompson, E. (1982). Mother-infant play interaction scale. In S. Humenick-Smith (Ed.), *Analysis of current assessment strategies in the health care of young children and childbearing families* (pp. 56). Norwich, CT: Williams & Wilkins.

**Language Disorders in Older Students and Adolescents.** Assessment of language disorders in older students and adults poses some special challenges; although the situation in recent years has improved significantly, research information and clinical resources on language skills and disorders in older students and adolescents lag behind those available for younger children; unlike in children under 5 or 6 years of age, language skills in older students and adults change more gradually; disorders in their language may be more subtle; nonetheless, the clinician needs to assess semantic, morphological, syntactic, and pragmatic language problems in older students and adolescents; assessment should take note of problems that may have persisted from early childhood and those that are more specific to them; more specific problems that need to be assessed are due to a failure to acquire advanced skills of language and literacy; therefore, the assessment concerns include reading, writing, and advanced social and technical discourse; problems in critical and logical reasoning; mastery and expression of scientific, technical, literate, academic, logical, and discipline-specific terms; skills in word retrieval, word definitions, word relations, and skills in the use of figurative language need to be assessed; finally, production of advanced syntactic structures and pragmatic features also need to be assessed; for details on language and literacy disorders in older students and adolescents, see the sources cited at the end of this entry and the companion volume, *Hegde's PocketGuide to Communication Disorders*.

### *Assessment Objectives/General Guidelines*

L

- To evaluate the semantic, syntactic, morphological, and pragmatic aspects of both basic and advanced language skills, including abstract and academic language skills
- To evaluate reading and writing skills
- To relate communication skills to academic demands and performance
- To suggest treatment targets
- Note that adolescent language assessment may be more protracted than the assessment of language in a younger child because of the need to obtain writing samples, extended narratives, use of such abstract statements as proverbs, definition of terms, and so forth

### *Case History/Interview Focus*

- See **Case History** and **Interview** under Standard/Common Assessment Procedures
- Obtain information from parents, teachers, and peers about the adolescent's communication patterns
- Obtain information from teachers about the level of academic language the older student or adolescent is expected to master

### *Ethnocultural Considerations*

- See Ethnocultural Considerations in Assessment
- Pay special attention to the student's academic standing and social communication patterns
- Check whether the student is bilingual; if so, obtain information from teachers about the student's English proficiency to design appropriate assessment strategies

## Screening

- When a language disorder is not obvious, screen language to determine whether a more detailed assessment is needed
  - Evoke a brief conversation from the adolescent and take note of any language disorders; note that some language problems of the adolescent may be too subtle to be detected by brief conversational samples
  - Administer one of the following standardized screening tests or measures; note that only a few adolescent screening tests are available:

| Test | Purpose |
|---|---|
| *Adolescent Language Screening Test* (D. L. Morgan & A. M. Guilford) | To assess vocabulary, sentence construction, morphological features, and pragmatic aspects (11 to 17 yrs) |
| *Clinical Evaluation of Language Fundamentals—Revised Screening* (E. Semel, E. Wiig, & W. Secord) | To assess morphological, syntactic, and semantic features and auditory comprehension (5 to 16 yrs) |
| *Screening Test of Adolescent Language* (E. M. Prather, S. V. Breecher, M. L. Stafford, & E. M. Wallace) | To assess vocabulary, auditory memory span, language processing, and verbal expression (6 to 12 yrs) |

- Refer the older student or the adolescent who fails a screening test according to the test protocol for a language assessment



## Assessment

- Obtain an extended speech and language sample (see Standard/Common Assessment Procedures) for a typical analysis of language functions; note that you need especially structured tasks to assess many problems of the older student and the adolescent speaker
- Obtain a sample of conversation between the client and a peer, between the teacher and the client, and between the client and a family member or members
- Assess semantic skills
  - Assess difficulty in understanding and correctly using literate (academic, scholarly, learned) lexicon; make a list of such words as the following:

| | | | | | |
|---|---|---|---|---|---|
| assume | suppose | infer | interpret | hypothesize | define |
| compare | contrast | criticize | evaluate | summarize | predict |
| explain | describe | conclude | confirm | support (a statement) | discriminate |
| imply | concede | presume | guess | reject (a statement) | allude |
| fact | opinion | evidence | belief | contradictory | logical |
| rational | irrational | implicit | explicit | contrary | affirm |

    - Ask the client to define the terms on the list
    - Ask the client to contrast the meaning of terms:
        - Fact and opinion
        - Description and explanation
        - Inference and assumption
        - Suggestion and hypothesis
        - Belief and theory
        - Illusion and allusion
        - Since and because
        - Further and farther
        - Affect and effect
        - Alternate and alternative
        - Latter and later
        - Thought and feeling
    - Assess difficulty in understanding and correctly using figurative language; make a list of common proverbs, metaphors, and idioms and ask the client what they mean; for example:
        - A stitch in time saves nine
        - A penny earned is a penny saved
        - Put the cart before the horse
        - Put all your eggs in one basket
        - Don't kill the goose that lays the golden eggs
        - He is cold as ice
        - She is fit as a fiddle
        - Time is money
        - They wanted to bury the hatchet
        - Off the wall
        - Off the record
        - She looks like a million bucks
        - Skeleton in the closet
    - Assess word retrieval problems in conversational speech; take note of false starts, pauses, revisions, repetitions, beating around the bush, use of general versus specific words that suggest word retrieval problems; take note of words that are retrieved with difficulty
    - Assess deficient word definition skills; in addition to having the client define literate words, obtain a list of words from the teacher or the client's textbooks; ask the client to define them
    - Assess word relation problems by having the client define and contrast synonyms and antonyms; analyze a writing sample to see whether the same words are overused (instead of words with similar meanings)
    - Assess difficulty in using precise terms during conversation and narrative tasks; take note of the frequency with which such expressions as "this," "that," "you know what I mean," "this thing," and "that stuff" are used; infer the precise words that were not produced
- Assess syntactic skills
    - Use the speech and language sample, narratives, writing samples, and several behavior-specific tasks to make a syntactic skills analysis

- Assess sentence lengths in C-units (*communication units*) or T-units (*terminal units*); note that:
  - Both C-units and T-units contain an independent clause and such modifiers as a dependent clause
  - C-units may be incomplete sentences (e.g., *Very much* in response to *Did you like the food?*), whereas T-units have to be complete sentences
  - You should count the number of words per unit and calculate both the mean and the mode (the most frequently observed length)
- Assess the use of low-frequency structures; take note of low-frequency structures that the client used and those that he or she did not use; examples of low-frequency syntactic structures include:
  - Correct production of passive sentences (e.g., *The examination was thoughtfully constructed to make sure that most students would pass it*)
  - Correct production of the modal auxiliary verb (e.g., *They should have studied harder*)
  - Correct production of the perfect aspect (e.g., *He had been spending money recklessly*)
  - Correct production of the appositives (e.g., *John Laughlin, the famous comedian, left the audience laughing hysterically*)
  - Correct production of elaborated subjects (e.g., *National parks such as Yellowstone, Yosemite, Grand Canyon, and Bryce Canyon are treasures of the American West*)
  - Correct postmodications (e.g. *The next person to pull the handle could win the jackpot*)
- Assess the use of complex sentences containing subordinate clauses; use the C- and T-units for this analysis; take note of the clause structures the client used and those the client did not; calculate the number of clauses used in utterances; for instance:
  - *I saw only lions and snakes* contains 1 T-unit (one main clause)
  - *That was a person who knew everything but did not know anything* has three T-units (the main clause *that was a person* and the two subordinate clauses *who knew everything* and *but did not know anything)*
- Assess the use of more precise (hence shorter) expressions instead of wordy, vague, and roundabout expressions
- Assess the use of cohesion devices or connectives (e.g., such expressions as *therefore, as a result of, consequently, subsequently, because of*); take note of the contexts of in which such devices should have been used but the client did not
- Assess agreement (e.g., noun-verb agreement) in both connected speech and writing samples
- Assess the use of ambiguous pronouns; take note of the pronouns that the client did not use or used infrequently
- Take note of all other syntactic and morphological errors, some of which may have persisted from early childhood

- Assess pragmatic skills
  - Use the speech and language sample and narratives
  - Assess the use of correct register, which is language appropriate to the context, situation, and conversational partner; use the role-playing technique to see whether the student switches from one kind of register to the other
    - You play the role of a peer and talk to the student
    - You play the role of a teacher and talk to the student
    - You play the role of a parent and talk to the student
    - If practical, obtain speech samples from the home and classroom; observe the speech as the client interacts with a peer; obtain a teacher's report
  - Take note of inappropriate use of gestures in conversation
  - Systematically introduce several topics and judge the acceptability of topic maintenance; take note of abrupt shifts the student implements in conversational topics
  - Request the older student or adolescent to clarify certain statements; request more information; ask the student to say it differently; ask the student to explain it; judge whether the client modifies statements or just repeats; judge the amount of new information the client adds
  - Ask the client to narrate a story or retell a story he or she reads; judge event sequencing, details of narration, correct representation of the characters, and appropriate inference of feelings and thoughts of the characters
  - Count the frequency of maze behavior (false starts, too many hesitations, interjected extraneous statements, frequent revisions, repetitions and other kinds of dysfluencies, and repeated but unsuccessful attempts to express the same ideas)
  - Take note of irrelevant or extraneous comments throughout the interview and assessment periods
  - Throughout the interview, make vague and nonspecific statements to assess whether the student asks for clarification; and take note of the number of requests for clarification; assess whether the student can vary the type of request for clarification (e.g., *What do you mean? I am not sure I understand you! Explain it to me, please! I didn't get it*)
  - Assess the frequency with which the client asks you to repeat simple information or uncomplicated questions that might suggest poor listening skills
- Assess reading and writing skills
  - Ask the client to read aloud a printed passage that is at his or her grade level; follow the student's reading on a copy of the passage being read aloud; analyze the reading errors; take note of:
    - Misreading of words
    - Generally struggled reading (lack of fluency in oral reading) characterized by pauses, frequent back-and-forth movements, revisions, exasperation at difficult words, giving up on certain words
    - Dysfluencies in oral reading; repetition of words or phrases, interjecting extraneous comments, and prolonging certain sounds

    - The overall rhythm of reading, which may be normal or impaired because of the struggled reading
  - Ask questions about the read material to assess reading comprehension; take note of correct and incorrect answers to your questions
  - Dictate a passage for the student to write; ask the student to spontaneously write something to reflect his or her experience; ask the student to copy a brief printed passage; ask the student to bring an extended writing assignment he or she may have submitted to the teacher and analyze the various writing samples for problems in writing:
    - Spelling errors, poor formation of letters, general organization and neatness, and overall quality of handwriting
    - Analyze errors in punctuation; judge the accuracy of the use of the comma, semicolon, period, dash, quotation marks, and parenthetical constructions
    - Analyze the writing sample for its content; in the case of the extended piece of writing (e.g., an essay submitted to the teacher) judge the adequacy, depth, appropriateness, and details of information offered
    - Analyze errors of syntax in the written samples; identify wrong or incomplete sentences; judge whether the writing is restricted to just a few syntactic constructions, lacking in variety
    - Judge the appropriateness of the language to the topic of writing; take note of technical word usage, pro and con arguments elaborated, conclusions offered, and support for views advocated
    - Analyze the written passage for cohesion and correct use of words that indicate cohesion
    - Count the use of low-frequency syntactic structures (e.g., such noun phrase postmodifications as *an aircraft called the airbus, Mr. Johnson the teacher*, or *the woman who does not work here*; such passive sentences as *the man was hit by the train*)



### *Medical, Psychological, and Educational Assessment Data*

- Obtain any available medical data of importance in evaluating language disorders
- Obtain the results of the audiological evaluation
- Obtain the psychological data including the results of intelligence testing and cognitive functioning
- Obtain data on the adolescent's educational achievement and assessment that might suggest learning disabilities
- Obtain writing samples from the adolescent's teachers for further analysis if warranted
- Examine the adolescent's textbooks to select words and phrases that might be included in additional assessments

### *Standard/Common Assessment Procedures*

- Complete the Standard/Common Assessment Procedures

### *Standardized Tests of Adolescent Language Skills*

- Administer one or more of the following standardized tests or measures
- Consider the student's ethnocultural background before you select a test

- If ethnoculturally appropriate tests are not available for a given student, use the assessment outline given before, expand if necessary, and make a client-specific or criterion-referenced type of assessment where you note the presence and absence of skills necessary to succeed academically and socially

| Test | Purpose |
|---|---|
| *Adapted Sequenced Inventory of Communication Development for Adolescents and Adults with Severe Handicap* (S. E. McClennen) | To assess communication skills in severely handicapped individuals with sensory and neuromotor involvement (adolescent to adulthood) |
| *Bilingual Syntax Measure II* (M. K. Burt & H. C. Dulay) | To assess expressive syntactic skills in English and Spanish (3rd to 12th grade) |
| *Clinical Evaluation of Language Fundamentals—Third Edition* (E. Semel, E. Wiig, & W. Secord) | To assess semantic and syntactic skills (5 to 16 yrs) |
| *Evaluating Communicative Competence* (C. S. Simon) | To assess language processing, metalinguistic skills, and pragmatic aspects (9 to 17 yrs) |
| *Fullerton Language Test for Adolescents* (A. R. Thorum) | To assess morphological skills, oral commands, syntactic skills, and idioms (11 yrs to adult) |
| *Rhode Island Test of Language Structure* (E. Engen & T. Engen) | To assess receptive syntax, especially in hearing-impaired children and adolescents (3 to 20 yrs) |
| *Test of Adolescent Language—3* (D. D. Hammill, V. L. Brown, S. C. Larsen, & J. L. Weiderholt) | To assess language, reading, writing, and auditory comprehension skills (12 to 24.11 yrs) |
| *Test of Adolescent/Adult Word Finding* (D. J. German) | To assess naming, nouns, verbs, sentence completion, description, and categories (12 to 80 yrs) |
| *Test of Language Competence—Expanded Edition* (E. Wiig & W. Secord) | To assess metalinguistics, multiple meanings, inferences, figurative language, and conversational skills (2.9 to 18.11 yrs) |
| *Test of Word Knowledge: Two levels* (E. Wiig & W. Secord) | To assess definitions or words, antonyms, synonyms, and multiple meanings (5 to 8 & 8 to 17.11 yrs) |
| *The Word Test: Adolescent* (L. Zachman & associates) | To test concrete and abstract word definition skills (12 to 17 yrs) |

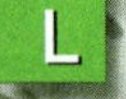


### Analysis of Results

- Analyze the speech and language sample for semantic, syntactic, morphological, and pragmatic problems as suggested in the detailed outline

- Analyze the literacy skills as suggested in the outline
- List the deficiencies and strengths of the client
- Relate your assessment data to educational demands and curricular materials

### *Diagnostic Criteria/Guidelines*

- Significant deficiencies in advanced language skills
- Limitations or problems in literacy skills, academic language, and abstract language

### *Differential Diagnosis*

- Distinguish between persistence of early childhood problems from additional language problems due to a failure to acquire more advanced features of language

### *Prognosis*

- Prognosis generally good for improved advanced language skills
- The extent of improvement may depend on the adolescent, family support, time of intervention, and intensity of intervention
- Most adolescents with language disorders benefit from treatment

### *Recommendations*

- Language intervention to strengthen the advanced features of language
- Working with the adolescent's teachers to coordinate treatment activities with academic activities
- Integrating literacy skills to language treatment programs
- Home intervention programs implemented by family members or other primary caretakers
- See the following cited sources and *Hegde's PocketGuide to Treatment in Speech Language Pathology* (3rd ed.) for details

Hegde, M. N., & Maul, C. A. (2006). *Language disorders in children: An evidence-based approach to assessment and treatment.* Boston, MA: Allyn and Bacon.

Larson, V. L., & McKinley, N. L. (2003). *Communication solutions for older students: Assessment and intervention strategies.* Eau Claire, WI: Thinking Publications.

Nippold, M. A. (1993). Developmental markers in adolescent language: Syntax, semantics, and pragmatics. *Language, Speech, and Hearing Services in Schools, 24,* 21–28.

Nippold, M. A. (2007). *Later language development: School-age children, adolescents, and young adults* (3rd ed.). Austin, TX: Pro-Ed.

Paul, R. (2001). *Language disorders from infancy through adolescence* (2nd ed.). St. Louis, MO: C. V. Mosby.

Reed, V. (2005). *An introduction to children with language disorders* (3rd ed.). Boston, MA: Allyn and Bacon.

Ripich, D. N., & Creaghead, N. A. (1994). *School discourse problems* (2nd ed.). San Diego, CA: Singular Publishing Group.

**Language Sampling.** See Speech and Language Sampling under Standard/Common Assessment Procedures.

L

**Laryngectomy.** Assessment of clients with laryngectomy is done with a view to provide an alternative means of communication because of the loss of all or part of the diseased or damaged larynx to surgical treatment; assessment should take into consideration not only the loss of the natural source of sound to produce speech but also the changes in the anatomy of the laryngeal area, which creates a need to breathe through a surgically created stoma (hole) in the neck; for details on the diseases and trauma that necessitate the surgical removal of the larynx and associated details, see the sources cited at the end of this entry and the companion volume, *Hegde's PocketGuide to Communication Disorders*.

### Assessment Objectives/General Guidelines

- To counsel the client about available options for communication after laryngectomy
- To help select the best methods of communication for the client by getting the entire family involved in the process
- To make periodic assessment to evaluate the need for change in the rehabilitation program
- Note that no form of alaryngeal speech can be rejected without careful consideration and assessment of candidacy with trial therapy

### Case History/Interview Focus

- See **Case History** and **Interview** under Standard/Common Assessment Procedures
- Focus on the patient's surgical and medical treatment, rehabilitation, and family communication patterns and preferences

### Ethnocultural Considerations

- See Ethnocultural Considerations in Assessment

### Alaryngeal Speech Options

- Electronic larynxes: Relatively small, battery-powered units that contain a vibrator that produces a tone when turned on; sound may be carried into the mouth by a tube or the unit may be held against the neck to transmit the sound via skin into the mouth; sound is articulated into speech; many varieties on the market
  - Advantages include ease of use, volume and pitch controls, sufficient loudness of speech produced, and good speech intelligibility when well trained
  - Disadvantages include electronic noise; an unnatural electronic vocal quality; problems in using on tender, swollen, or scarred neck tissue; need for good articulation skills; and repair costs
- Esophageal speech: Speech produced by supplying air into the esophagus, creating vibration in the pharyngeal-esophageal (P-E) segment, and articulating the sound into speech
  - Advantages include more natural sound and lack of a handheld mechanical device
  - Disadvantages include difficulty in learning it, low pitch for women, low intensity of speech produced, and some people are not candidates for secondary anatomical variations

- Tracheoesophageal speech: Speech produced with a voice prosthesis inserted into a small fistula or puncture made through the tracheal wall into the esophagus in a surgical procedure called tracheoesophageal fistulization or puncture (TEF/TEP); during exhalation, air from the lungs is directed into the prosthesis by occluding the stoma with a finger or one-way speaking valve; air then passes through the prosthesis and into the esophagus; sound is produced as the air passes through the vibrating P-E segment; sound is then articulated
  - Advantages include a more natural air supply into the esophagus (compared to the laryngectomy without TEF/TEP), rapid learning of speech, and newly designed prostheses require less maintenance and can last several months
  - Disadvantages include the small risk involved in additional surgical procedure (TEF/TEP), stenosis of the fistula or stoma, aspiration of the prosthesis, maintenance and cleaning of the fistula site and prosthesis, prosthesis failure, and not all clients are candidates for secondary anatomical variations

## Assessment

- Note that a main assessment task is to familiarize the client with the available options for alaryngeal communication, to determine the candidacy for a particular type of alaryngeal speech by trying different methods, and then to select one for more intensive therapy
- Visit the client prior to surgery and describe the effects of surgery on communication and the options for alternative modes of communication; if possible, assist the client in acquiring an intra-oral electronic larynx for use immediately after surgery and provide some basic training
  - Note that clients may or may not be in a favorable disposition to appreciate all you say
  - Provide sufficient positive information on the possibilities of developing new forms of communication
  - Let the client know that it is possible to resume work, and lead a normal life with few exceptions
  - Tell them to be client with themselves after surgery
  - Offer information about financial assistance
  - Let them know about the support groups
  - Have a rehabilitated laryngectomized person visit the client or family only if they welcome your suggestion
  - Have the client and family meet other members of the professional team
  - Get the family members involved in this preoperative counseling session
  - Counsel the family about taking care of the client immediately after he or she returns home
  - Leave printed information about surgery, postoperative care, and methods of alaryngeal communication with the client and family
- After surgery, begin a more detailed discussion and demonstration of alaryngeal modes of communication and the available options to the client and family members
  - Show, describe, and demonstrate the use of an electronic larynx for both neck placement and intra-oral use

- Describe and demonstrate esophageal speech
- Describe and demonstrate tracheoesophageal speech if this is an option for them
- Describe the availability, cost, and maintenance of different devices
- Briefly mention some of the advantages and disadvantages of different approaches; do not overemphasize the limitations of a particular approach or device at this time so that the client does not prematurely rule out an option or options
- Tell the client that initially he or she may use one method (e.g., a pneumatic device) and later another method (e.g., an electronic larynx or esophageal speech)
- Let the client try the different options to the extent the physical condition permits (e.g., an intra-oral electronic larynx or an electrolarynx with an intra-oral adapter may be easier to try at this initial phase; neck tenderness may prevent a trial of other alternatives requiring neck placement).
- Give the client and family members as much printed information as available
- If the client has already undergone TEP, remove catheter or fistula dilator, measure the fistula, select an appropriate size and style prosthesis, initiate speech training with the prosthesis in place, and educate the client regarding maintenance and care of the prosthesis and fistula site



- Assess the client's preference
  - During the demonstration of options, note the client's reactions
  - Note the hand dexterity, skill in handling the device, and initial success
  - Do not let the client get discouraged about his or her initial failure in using a particular device or method; emphasize that practice is the key to success and what seems difficult initially may be easier later on, especially as the client recovers from surgery
  - Ask about his or her preferences and find out why
  - Ask family members about their preferences although the client's success with a method may be most important
- Assess candidacy for an electronic larynx
  - Assess how well and how efficiently the client uses the device
  - Show, describe, and demonstrate the use of an electric larynx; demonstrate both intra-oral and neck placement
    - Place the device on the neck or in the mouth
    - Articulate speech sounds
    - Note how well the client handles the unit
    - Note the presence or absence of manual dexterity in manipulating the switches of the unit
  - Note the rate of learning (fast, slow, or little progress over several trials)
  - Try units from different manufacturers to find out whether one of them better suits the client
  - Let the client express concerns and ask all questions
  - Ask the client about preferences and reasons for preferences
  - Discuss the problems noted and positively reinforce any sign of success

- Assess candidacy for esophageal speech
  - Note that assessing candidacy for esophageal speech takes time because to see initial success that helps select the method, persistent efforts often are needed
  - Note that the following factors suggest success with esophageal speech, although individual differences may override some or all of them; in efficient learning of esophageal speech:
    - Younger clients are more successful than older clients; after age 60, the success rate may be 50%
    - Hearing loss is a negative factor
    - Integrity of tongue strength and mobility is a necessary factor (for both air injection and articulation of sounds)
    - Structural and functional integrity of the esophagus (no rupture or stricture) is essential
    - P-E segment should neither be too lax nor too tensed
    - Oral and pharyngeal tissue damage due to radiation may make it a more difficult task
    - Combination of total glossectomy and laryngectomy is detrimental, requiring surgical and prosthetic rehabilitation
  - Try the injection (positive pressure) and inhalation (negative pressure) methods; note that most clinicians prefer the injection method
    - Describe, explain, and demonstrate each method
    - Give sufficient practice before making a judgment about its suitability
    - Ask the client to be patient and persistent
    - Take note of problems and discuss them with the client
    - Encourage any sign of success
    - Note that the injection method is inappropriate for clients with glossectomy
    - Note that for clients with glossectomy, inhalation (not injection) is the only method of producing esophageal speech

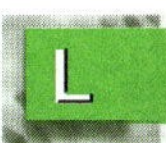


- Assess candidacy for tracheoesophageal speech
  - Note that tracheoesophageal speech requires additional surgery (TEF/TEP) and the use of a voice prosthesis
  - Assess the presence of pharyngoesophageal spasm which will prevent success with TEF/TEP; have a physician administer an insufflation test; use such a standard procedure as the Blom-Singer insufflation test kit:
    - Note that a failed insufflation test indicates too much tension, constriction, or spasm in the P-E segment which indicates the segment to be a poor source of vibration
    - Failed attempts at esophageal speech may also reveal an inadequate P-E segment for voice production
    - Note that a radiological assessment may be needed to confirm tension and spasm of the P-E segment
  - Note that the surgeon may recommend Botox injections, pharyngeal constrictor myotomy, or the pharyngeal plexus block (neurectomy) for those who fail the insufflation test

        - Myotomy involves the unilateral cutting of the laryngeal constrictors (inferior and middle pharyngeal constrictor muscles) to reduce constriction and spasm
        - Botox injections involve injecting botulinum toxin into the pharyngeal constrictor muscles to reduce constriction and spasm, and the injection needs to be repeated periodically
        - Pharyngeal plexus block involves sectioning the nerves that supply the pharyngeal constrictor muscles, especially the middle constrictor, to reduce spasm and tension
        - Note that if an insufflation test is done prior to TEF/TEP, myotomy or neurectomy may be performed along with TEF/TEP
    - Visual acuity and manual dexterity in removing and inserting the voice prosthesis
    - Adequate depth and diameter of the stoma to use the voice prosthesis
    - Mental and emotional stability
    - Understanding of the care and use of the voice prosthesis
- Select a method of alaryngeal speech for systematic training
    - Consider all initial selections tentative
    - Be prepared to reassess, select another mode of alaryngeal communication, and retrain the client

### *Related/Medical Assessment Data*

- Integrate medical, surgical, and general health data into your assessment data in selecting the method of the alaryngeal mode of communication

### *Standard/Common Assessment Procedures*

- Complete the Standard/Common Assessment Procedures

### *Prognosis*

- Prognosis for survival varies across clients; many variables including the general health of the client, extent of cancerous growth, recurrence of cancer, and the effectiveness of surgical treatment
- Significant hearing loss with no amplification negatively affects the learning and maintenance of alaryngeal speech
- Prolonged and intense radiation therapy may retard the progress of alaryngeal communication rehabilitation
- Prognosis for learning one or the other form of communication is good for most if not all clients

### *Recommendations*

- Communication treatment with an optimal method of alaryngeal speech determined through assessment and trial therapy
- Periodic assessment preceding and following additional surgical or medical treatment
- See the following cited sources and the companion volume, *Hegde's PocketGuide to Treatment in Speech-Language Pathology* (3rd ed.) for details

Boone, D. R., McFarlane, S. C., & Von Berg, S. L. (2005). *The voice and voice therapy* (7th ed.). Boston, MA: Allyn and Bacon.

Case, J. L. (2002). *Clinical management of voice disorders* (4th ed.). Austin, TX: Pro-Ed.

Casper, J. K., & Colton, R. H. (1998). *Clinical manual for laryngectomy and head and neck cancer rehabilitation* (2nd ed.). Clifton Park, NY: Thomson Delmar Learning.

Doyle, P. C., & Keith, R. L. (2005). *Contemporary issues in the treatment and rehabilitation of head and neck cancer*. Austin, TX: Pro-Ed.

**Laurence-Moon-Bardet-Biedl Syndrome.** To assess this syndrome, also known as the *Laurence-Moon syndrome*, see Syndromes Associated With Communication Disorders.

**Laurence-Moon-Biedl Syndrome.** To assess this syndrome, also known as the same as *Laurence-Moon syndrome*, see Syndromes Associated With Communication Disorders.

**Left Neglect.** Assessment of left neglect is important in clients with brain injury, especially right brain injury

- Have the client read a printed page and see whether the client ignores the material on the left half of the page
- Observe the client or interview the family members or health care staff to assess any evidence of left neglect (e.g., uncombed left side of the head; not using the pockets on the left side of the body, bumping into things on the left side)
- Ask the client to draw a human face or the face of a clock to see whether the client neglects to draw the left side of the image
- See Right Hemisphere Syndrome for details

L

**Literacy and Literacy Skills.** Assessment and treatment of literacy skills and literacy problems in school-age children are part of the professional responsibility of speech-language pathologists; because most if not all literacy skills are language based, these skills may be evaluated in the context of speech and language assessment; speech-language pathologists have historically assessed reading and writing skills in adult clients with aphasia; it is only in recent years that clinicians have extended their expertise to literacy skills in children; speech-language pathologists have an opportunity to help improve the academic success of students they assess and treat because of the close relationship that exists between oral language skills and literacy skills; it is better to complete a speech and language evaluation before embarking on a literacy evaluation; if practical, literacy and speech-language evaluations may be integrated.

### *Assessment Objectives/General Guidelines*

- To assess the emergent literacy, reading, and writing skills in children, typically during the speech and language assessment
- To help make an independent assessment of literacy skills in collaboration with the teacher and other special education specialists
- To identify literacy skills that may be integrated with speech and language treatment
- To identify literacy skills that may need more intensive and dedicated treatment or instruction
- To help design a home literacy program based on the assessment results; to offer suggestions to parents on stimulating and encouraging literacy skills in their children

## Case History/Interview Focus

- During the interview, concentrate on the family members' literacy skills, literacy-related values they hold, and their reading and writing habits
- Explore the literacy resources available to the child at home (e.g., availability of books, a work area, and such facilities to read and write as a suitable chair and desk)
- Find out whether the parents regularly read aloud to the child and help teach reading and writing skills to the child

## Ethnocultural Considerations

- Pay special attention to the home environment and literacy resources available to minority families
- Explore the support systems the parents may need (e.g., access to a public library; bookstores that offer story reading sessions for children; organizations that may supply free books for children)
- During assessment, select reading materials that are at the child's grade and culturally appropriate for the child's background

## Screening

- During speech and language assessment, screen emergent and literacy skills
  - Ask the child to count, recite a nursery rhyme, or sing a song
  - Ask the child to name a few printed letters of the alphabet
  - Show a printed sentence and ask the child to show a word and a letter
  - Show logos and signs commonly seen in the child's environment and ask whether the child can say what they mean (e.g., fast food restaurant logo, stop sign, exit and enter signs, bathroom signs for men and women)
- During speech and language assessment, screen literacy skills at the early elementary levels
  - Ask the child to identify all the letters of the alphabet
  - Ask the child to read a grade-appropriate passage and ask questions to assess comprehension of the read material
  - Ask the child to print the letters of the alphabet
  - Ask the child to write a few sentences taken from the child's grade book
- During the speech and language assessment, screen later literacy skills
  - Ask the child to write two or three paragraphs
  - Ask the child to read aloud a passage from a book at the child's grade level and ask questions about reading comprehension

## Assessment of Literacy Skills

- Assess emergent literacy skills in preschool children
  - Evaluate the child's print awareness
    - Ask the parents whether the child has shown an early interest in printing the letters of the alphabet
    - Ask the parents whether the child likes to be read to aloud
    - Ask the parents whether the child pretends to "read" a storybook by looking at the pictures
    - Show a collection of commonly encountered logos and signs and ask the child to tell what they mean (e.g., a stop sign or signs in supermarkets)

        - Display a few children's books the child can have easy access to; see whether the child would pick up a book and look into it
        - Ask the child to count numbers
        - Ask the child to recite the alphabet, nursery rhymes, days of the week, or names of the months
        - Show a few printed sentences and ask the child to point to a word and a sentence
        - Hand a book to the child and ask the child to show the front and the back of the book
        - Hand a book upside down to the child and see whether the child would turn it around for correct orientation
        - Ask the child to point to the beginning and the end of a story in a simple storybook
        - Name the letters of the alphabet and ask the child to point to each (e.g., *Can you find the letter s? The letter b?*)
- Assess reading and writing at the early elementary level
    - Evaluate the child's letter identification skills
        - Ask the child to name all the letters of the alphabet in a systematic manner (A through Z)
        - Ask the child to name a few letters presented in a random manner
        - Ask the child to make the kind of sound a letter represents (while pointing to different printed letters, ask, "How does this sound?")
    - Evaluate the child's early reading skills
        - Assess whether the child can sound out letters to read simple words
        - Assess the child's oral reading skills; have the child read a passage from the child's grade level; count the misreading of words, hesitations in reading, and omission of words
        - Assess fluency in reading by counting the number of words read per minute
        - Take note of excessively struggled reading
        - Assess comprehension of orally or silently read material; ask questions about the material and judge the level of comprehension
    - Evaluate the child's elementary writing skills
        - Have the child draw simple drawings
        - Have the child spontaneously write a brief passage; copy a small passage from the child's grade-level book
        - If the child cannot write or copy a passage, ask the child to print all the letters of the alphabet
        - If the child cannot print the letters of the alphabet, ask the child to trace the letters
        - Assess the smoothness with which the child draws a figure; judge the adequacy of the details provided and the orientation of the drawing
        - Analyze the writing errors; judge whether the child plans a piece of writing or rushes to write only to cross out, erase, start all over, and so forth
- Assess reading and writing at the more advanced level
    - Assess more advanced reading skills

        - Ask the child to read aloud a longer and more complex piece of printed material, selected from the child's grade level
        - Take note of the reading errors
        - Ask questions about the read material to assess the child's comprehension
        - Ask the child to distinguish between literary genres (e.g., an essay, a poem, a novel, nonfiction)
        - Ask the child about the different purposes of texts or pieces of writing (e.g., inform, entertain, persuade)
    - Assess more advanced writing skills
        - Have the child write a brief essay on a topic of his or her choice; it may be a personal narrative (e.g., a vacation experience, a book recently read)
        - Obtain an essay or writing assignment the child may have completed and submitted to the teacher
        - Analyze the writing mechanics, including the child's word usage, spelling, letter formation, capitalization, and punctuation
        - Analyze the overall organization and neatness of the writing
        - Analyze the sentence structures, their correctness and variety
        - Analyze the logical sequence (e.g., a good introduction and conclusion), cohesiveness, adequacy of the narrative content and its detail, paragraph transitions, and so forth
- Assess abstract language skills
    - Ask the child to define selected terms that you find in the child's textbook
    - Ask the child to give examples of concepts described in his or her grade level books
    - Ask the child the meaning of selected proverbs, idioms, and slang
    - Ask the child to define selected synonyms and antonyms sampled from the child's book or graded for appropriateness for the child's grade
    - Ask the child to describe how he or she would plan for a camping trip
    - Tell a story and ask the child to retell it
    - Ask the child about the moral of the story
- Assess phonological awareness
    - Take note that although much has been written about phonological awareness, no experimental evidence suggests that such skills as phoneme manipulation and segmentation need to be taught before children can learn to read or write; if preferred, however, assess such phonological awareness skills as:
        - Isolating a phoneme within a word (e.g., *What is the first sound in the word cat? What is the last sound in the word man?*)
        - Recognizing the same phoneme in different words (e.g., *Loss, toss, and moss—What sound do all these words end with?*)
        - Segmenting phonemes (e.g., *How many sounds are in the word mat?*)
        - Deleting a phoneme from a word (e.g., *Say soup. Now say it without the s sound*)
        - Substituting one phoneme for another in a word (e.g., *Say mad. Now say it again, but change the* **/m/** *to* **/b/**)

### *Medical, Psychological, and Educational Assessment Data*

- Obtain information on any evidence of brain injury or neuromotor problems that may affect literacy skills
- Obtain information on any emotional or psychiatric problems (e.g., autism spectrum disorders) that may complicate the learning of literacy skills
- Obtain audiological assessment reports in case of a child with hearing impairment
- Obtain psychological reports to rule out intellectual deficiencies, or if they do exist, take them into consideration in the analysis of literacy assessment data

### *Standard/Common Assessment Procedures*

- Complete the Standard/Common Assessment Procedures

### *Standardized Tests of Literacy Skills*

- Administer one or more of the following literacy skills; check the availability of other tests not listed
- If the standardized tests are inappropriate for a child with a varied ethnocultural background, use a criterion-referenced or client-specific assessment outline of the kind described earlier to make a nonbiased assessment of the child's skills

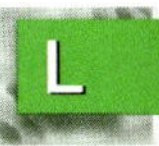


| Test | Purpose |
|---|---|
| *Comprehensive Test of Phonological Processing* (R. K. Wagner, J. K. Torgesen, & C. Rashotte) | To assess phoneme manipulation skills including sound deletion, segmentation, and blending (5 yrs to adult) |
| *Gray Diagnostic Reading Test* (B. R. Bryant, J. L. Widerholt, & D. P. Bryant) | To assess letter-word identification, reading, and phonological awareness skills (6 to 13.11 yrs) |
| *Phonological Awareness Test* (C. Robertson & W. Slater) | To assess various phoneme manipulation and other phonological awareness skills (5 to 9 yrs) |
| *Test of Early Written Language* (W. P. Hersko, S. R. Herron, & P. K. Peak) | To assess emergent literacy skills; includes narrative writing task (3 to 10.11 yrs) |
| *Test of Reading Comprehension* (V. L. Brown, D. D. Hammill, & J. L. Widerholt) | To assess comprehension of general vocabulary and syntactic similarities (17.11 yrs to adult) |
| *Test of Written Expression* (R. McGhee, B. R. Bryant, S. C. Larsen, & D. M. Rivera) | To assess writing skills including essay writing (6.6 to 14.11 yrs) |
| *Test of Written English* (V. Anderson & S. Thompson) | To assess written expression and paragraph writing (6 to 17.11 yrs) |
| *Woodcock Language Proficiency Battery* (R. W. Woodcock) | To assess oral language, writing, and reading; has English and Spanish forms (2 yrs to adult) |

### Analysis of Results

- Summarize the tasks presented and the problems noted for each level separately
- Integrate the literacy assessment results with speech and language assessment data

### Diagnostic Criteria/Guidelines

- Literacy problems in school-age children may be diagnosed if the child's reading and writing skills do not meet the standards set for each grade level
- Preschool children may be diagnosed to be at risk for later reading and writing problems if they do not exhibit emergent literacy skills
- Significant oral speech and language problems almost always suggest a valid diagnosis of some literacy problems

### Differential Diagnosis

- Literacy skill deficiencies in otherwise normal children should be distinguished from such deficiencies that are due to associated clinical conditions
- Children with neuromotor problems (e.g., those with cerebral palsy) may have handwriting problems; such problems need special considerations in teaching and training approaches
- Children with hearing impairment also may have reading and writing problems that need to be distinguished from literacy problems without sensory disabilities

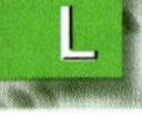


- Children with autism may have reading and writing problems that need to be distinguished from literacy problems in otherwise normal children
- Children with traumatic brain injury and (rarely) aphasia also may have reading and writing problems
- In most such cases, a differential diagnosis is made on the basis of an independent diagnosis of the associated clinical condition and its symptom complex

### Prognosis

- Prognosis for improved literacy skills with effective teaching is good for most if not all children who have difficulties in reading and writing
- Most reading and writing problems may be due to ineffective instruction, therefore, improved instruction and integration of literacy skill training with speech and language training may improve prognosis for most children

### Recommendations

- Integration of literacy skill training into speech and language training
- Independent literacy training if the speech-language pathologist's time permits
- Working with the regular classroom teachers to support literacy skills in their students by collaborative work
- Selecting speech-language treatment goals that enrich or enhance literacy skills
- Working with the family to promote literacy skills in their children by implementing a home literacy stimulation program

Catts, H. W., & Kamhi, A. (1999). *Language and reading disabilities.* Boston, MA: Allyn and Bacon.

Hegde, M. N., & Maul, C. A. (2006). *Language disorders in children: An evidence-based approach to assessment and treatment.* Boston, MA: Allyn and Bacon.

Kaminski, R. A., & Good, R. H. (1996). Toward a technology for assessing basic literacy skills. *School Psychology Review, 25,* 215–227.

Snow, C. E., Burns, S., & Griffin, P. (Eds.) (1998). *Preventing reading difficulties in young children*. Washington, DC: National Academy Press.

Snow, C. E., Scarborough, H. S., & Burns, M. S. (1999). What speech-language pathologists need to know about early reading. *Topics in Language Disorders, 20*(1), 48–58.

Whitehurst, C. G., & Lonigan, C. J. (1998). Child development and emergent literacy. *Child Development, 69*(3), 848–872.

L

# M

**Magnetic Resonance Imaging (MRI).** A group of basic and newer neurodiagnostic imaging methods to diagnose lesions in the brain; the basic method does not introduce radioactive material into the body, nor does it expose the structures to X-ray.

- In the basic MRI:
  - The patient's head is placed in a magnetic field; the hydrogen atoms in the brain align themselves with the magnetic field
  - An electromagnet pulse is then introduced; this briefly disturbs the alignment, but the hydrogen atoms quickly realign when the pulse is stopped; this realignment produces electromagnetic signals called *resonant frequency*
  - The computer constructs an image of the structure by the *resonant frequencies* generated by the cells (hence the name, *magnetic resonance imaging*)
- The method produces images that are clearer than those produced by CT scans and detects smaller lesions missed by the latter; this method has evolved into several newer procedures that include the following:
  - In the **functional MRI**
    - A contrast material is injected into the client (unlike in the basic method)
    - Cerebral blood flow variations related to the different areas of brain activation are detected
    - Currently more of a research tool than a clinical diagnostic procedure
  - In the **diffusion-weighted MRI**
    - Images are constructed by detecting the microscopic motion of water protons in the brain tissue
    - Cerebral ischemia in stroke patients is better detected than in some of the other methods
    - Cerebral edema due to stroke versus other reasons may be distinguished
  - In the **profusion-weighted MRI**
    - Images are constructed based on blood flow variations
    - Diffusion-weighted and profusion-weighted images can be compared to better understand brain damage in stroke (and other) patients
  - In the **MRI spectroscopy**
    - The traditional MRI is used in conjunction with this procedure
    - Images are created by detecting the biochemical composition of tissue being scanned
    - Neuronal loss due to Alzheimer's disease may be shown by detecting chemical changes across scanned tissue

**Maximum Phonation Duration (MPD).** Assessment of maximum phonation duration, also known as maximum phonation time (MPT), is important in the diagnosis of various disorders; reduced maximum phonation durations may be found in clients with voice disorders and those with dysarthria; consonants /s/ and /z/ and the vowel /a/ have been used to assess this task; to assess MPD or MPT:

- Ask the client to phonate /s/ and /z/ for as long as possible; the duration of /z/ values measured in seconds may be lower than the duration of /s/ values in vocal pathology; normally, the two values are close to each other

- Ask the client to prolong the vowel /a/; compare the patient's duration against the norms
  - For young males, the range is 22.6 to 34.6
  - For young females, the range is 15.2 to 26. 5
  - For elderly males, the range is 13.0 to 18.1
  - For elderly females, the range is 10.0 to 15.4
- Interpret the norms flexibly; they are not to be interpreted rigidly because of the wide ranges

**Mean Length of Utterance (MLU).** The average length of utterances measured in morphemes; an index of language acquisition or performance of children; needs 50 utterances that are consecutive and intelligible; the following guidelines have been suggested by Brown (1973) and Chapman (1981):

- Transcribe each intelligible utterance on a separate line; discard unintelligible segments
- Count each word as one
- Count a bound morpheme as one (e.g., the plural *s* morpheme)
- Count contracted morphemes as one (the result is two morphemes because the word and the contraction are both counted; e.g., *he's* is counted as two)
- Count all grammatical morphemes as one (e.g., *ing, ed*)
- Count all words repeated for emphasis
- Count compound words (e.g., *birthday*) as one
- Do not count fillers (e.g., such interjections as *mm*)
- Divide the total number of morphemes by the total number of utterances to obtain the MLU

Brown, R. (1973). *A first language: The early stages.* Cambridge, MA: Harvard University Press.

Chapman, R. (1981). Exploring children's communicative intents. In J. Miller (Ed.), *Assessing language production in children* (pp. 111–138). Boston, MA: Allyn and Bacon.

**Mental Retardation.** To assess communication disorders associated with mental retardation, see Intellectual Disabilities.

**Mixed Dysarthria.** To assess this variety of motor speech disorders, see Dysarthria: Specific Types.

**Mixed Transcortical Aphasia.** To assess this type of aphasia, which has both transcortical motor and transcortical sensory features, see Aphasia and Aphasia: Specific Types.

**Mohr Syndrome.** To assess this syndrome, also known as the *oro-facial-digital syndrome type II*, see Syndromes Associated With Communication Disorders.

**Motor Agraphia.** To assess writing disorders seen in adults who have had normal writing skills but have them now impaired because of neurological problems, see Agraphia and Aphasia.

**Motor Aphasia.** The same as Broca's aphasia; see Aphasia: Specific Types for assessment procedures.

**Motor Speech Disorders.** Assessment of motor speech disorders involves an evaluation of communication disorders and associated clinical manifestations; requires an understanding of the neuropathology that creates a variety of speech, voice, resonance, and prosodic disorders; essentially, motor control of speech muscles or motor programming of speech movements may be impaired; for assessment procedures, see the main entries for Apraxia of Speech and Dysarthrias; see also Apraxia of Speech in Adults and Apraxia of Speech in Children; see also Dysarthria: Specific Types for ataxic dysarthria, flaccid dysarthria, hyperkinetic dysarthria, hypokinetic dysarthria, mixed dysarthria, spastic dysarthria, and unilateral upper motor neuron dysarthria.

**Multi-infarct Dementia (MID).** A form of Dementia due to multiple strokes; now considered a subtype of *vascular dementia*; for assessment procedures, see Vascular Dementia; for etiology and symptomatology, see the companion volume, *Hegde's PocketGuide to Communication Disorders*.

**Mutational Falsetto.** To assess this high-pitched voice, which is a continuation of prepubertal voice after attaining puberty, see Voice Disorders.

**Mutism.** Assessment of mutism requires a knowledge of various clinical conditions that lead to, or are associated with, lack of oral speech; assessment of mutism may be a part of evaluating various kinds of neurological diseases that cause dysarthria and dementia that may terminate in mutism; mutism may also be a voice disorder; it may be classified a psychiatric disorder in some cases; see the companion volume, *Hegde's PocketGuide to Communication Disorders* for the etiology and symptomatology of mutism; assess mutism with the following procedures:



- Assess selective mutism: Assess this psychiatric variety of mutism
  - Ask the family members whether the client is heard talking in certain situations while refusing to talk in other situations
  - Find out whether the mutism has lasted at least one month
  - During assessment, observe the client's effective communication with gestures and facial expressions
  - Observe limited verbalizations that may be characterized by monotonous or altered voice
  - To apply the diagnostic criteria specified in the *Diagnostic and Statistical Manual of the American Psychiatric Association*
    - Is mutism evident for more than a month? In case of children, does it persist after the first month in school?
    - Is the mutism situation-specific?
    - Does the mutism cause impairment in social or personal communication? In the case of children, does it negatively affect academic performance?
    - Can shyness, embarrassment in social situations, ethnocultural differences, bilingual status, gender differences, or lack of knowledge on topics of conversation be ruled out as the cause of mutism?
  - Diagnose mutism if the answer is *yes* to all of these questions
- Assess mutism associated with other disorders: In such cases, do not treat mutism as *selective* or as a separate diagnostic category but as a symptom of

various neurological and neurodegenerative disorders in their final stages; assess mutism in:

- Dementia; because mutism in clients with dementia is found in the last stage, it does not pose a diagnostic challenge; a diagnosis of dementia will have been well established by the time a client loses all speech; the clients will have lost neuromotor control over their vocal mechanism; such mutism is involuntary (versus *selective mutism*); see Dementia
- AIDS, especially when dementia sets in, is associated with mutism in the final stages; here, too, the diagnosis of AIDS and the subsequent dementia will have been well established; see AIDS Dementia Complex
- Various types of dysarthria; assess mutism in clients who have flaccid dysarthria, hypokinetic dysarthria, hyperkinetic dysarthria, or spastic dysarthria; see Dysarthria: Specific Types for assessing communication disorders in clients with this type of motor speech disorder
- Apraxia of speech; mutism is associated with severe apraxia of speech where the neuromotor speech programming is affected; diagnosis of mutism in such cases is contingent on the diagnosis of a severe form of Apraxia of Speech
- Transient mutism; this may be diagnosed in the acute stage of aphasia in adults; a history of stroke or other neurological event is associated with this type of mutism; because it is transient, it does not pose a diagnostic challenge; see Aphasia
- More lasting mutism may be assessed in clients with severe aphasia and apraxia of speech; once again, the primary diagnosis will be a combination of aphasia (perhaps global aphasia) and apraxia
- Mutism in children may be diagnosed with a history of aphasia (more common than in adults with aphasia)
- Various other conditions, including diffuse cortical damage (as in persistent vegetative state); seizure disorders; surgical removal of corpus callosum to control otherwise uncontrollable epilepsy; bilateral lesions in the orbito-mesial frontal cortex, limbic system, and reticular formation; clients with *locked-in syndrome*; toxic drug influences (especially the drugs given after liver and heart transplant)
- Take note that when mutism is associated with neuromotor disorders, assessment of such problems as orofacial weakness, paralysis, rigidity, hypokinesia, or hyperkinetic movements will be necessary
- Take note that mutism may be more common in bilingual children than in monolingual children; during assessment, pay special attention to the bilingual status of the child and take a detailed case history relative to learning two languages and mutism in one or both languages
- See the following cited sources and the companion volume, *Hegde's PocketGuide to Communication Disorders*.

American Psychiatric Association. (2000). *Diagnostic and statistical manual of mental retardation: Fourth Edition, text revision.* Washington, DC: Author.

Duffy, J. R. (2005). *Motor speech disorders: Substrates, differential diagnosis, and management*. St. Louis, MO: Elsevier Mosby.

M

McInnes, A., & Manassis, K. (2005). When silence is not golden: An integrated approach to selective mutism. *Seminars in Speech and Language, 26*(3), 201–210.

Toppelberg, C. O., Tabors, P., Coggins, A., Lum, K., & Burger, C. (2005). Differential diagnosis of selective mutism in bilingual children. *Journal of the American Academy of Child and Adolescent Psychiatry, 44*(6), 592–595.

Wintgens, A. (2005). Selective mutism in children. *Child Language Teaching and Therapy, 21*(2), 214–216.

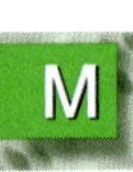

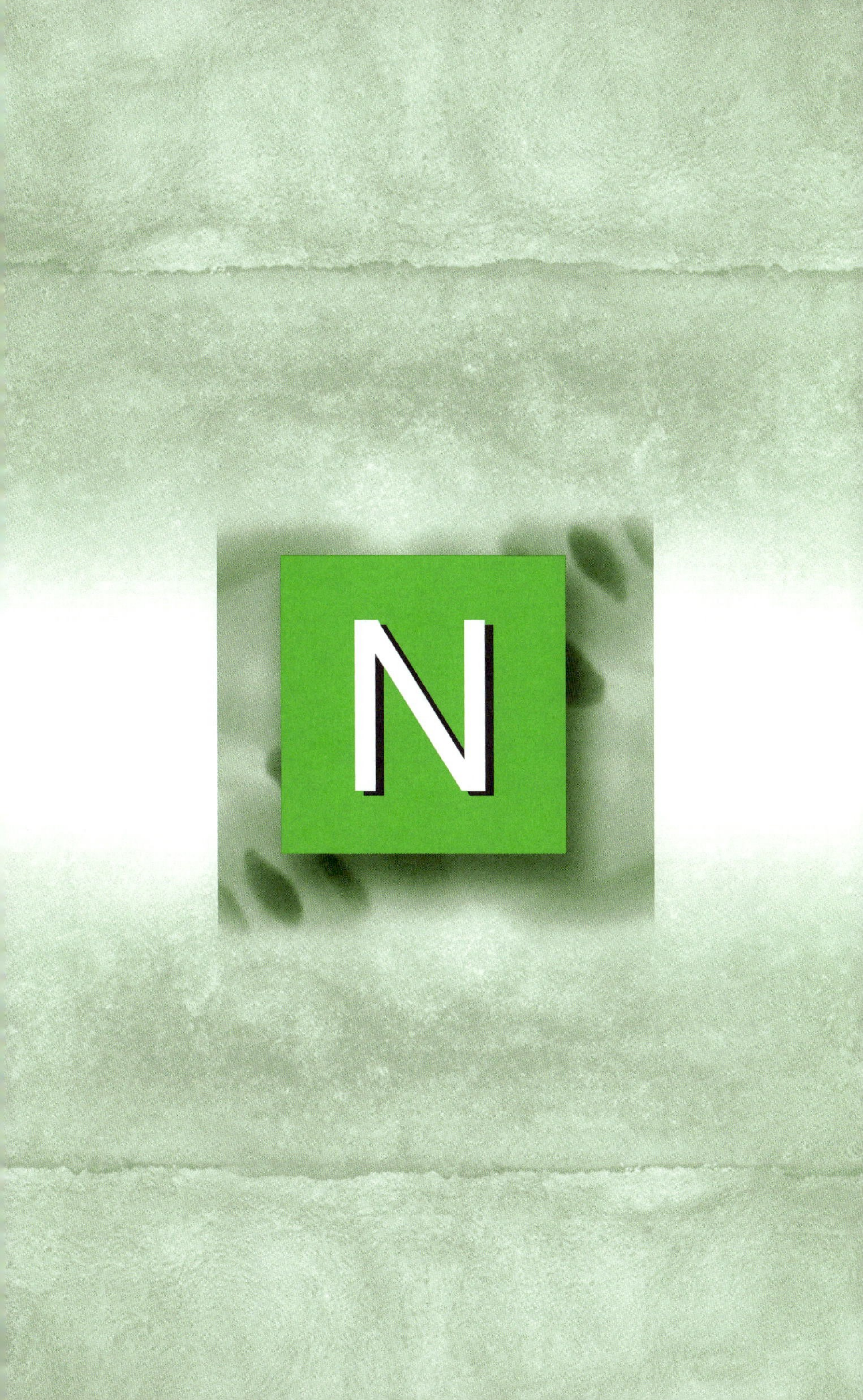
N

**Narrative Skills.** Assessment of narrative skills is important in the diagnosis of language disorders; various kinds of narrative tasks may be designed to evaluate a client's skills in narrating events and experiences in a sequential, chronologically correct, and logically consistent manner.

- Assess the following kinds of narratives
  - Personal narratives. Ask the client to describe at least three personal experiences in detail; if the client has problems selecting personal experiences to narrate, suggest a few (e.g., a favorite vacation the client took, a funny experience at work or school, a personal hobby or game the client enjoys)
  - Script narratives. Ask the client to describe selected routine events in life; ask the client to describe at least three events; suggest events as needed (e.g., how to make a sandwich, how to get to a certain place, how to organize a birthday or anniversary party, how to build a deck or some other structure)
  - Fictional narratives. Ask the client to tell three small stories he or she may have read or heard; may be the theme of a movie; tell a story to the client and ask the person to retell it
- Record and analyze the narratives
  - Tape-record the narratives for later analysis
  - Analyze the narratives for their logical sequence, sufficiency of details provided, correct characterizations of people involved in the narrative event, cohesion of story or narrative elements, and introduction, build-up of information, conclusion, and other matters of organization
- For additional assessment procedures, see Language Disorders in Children; see also Aphasia

**Nasal Emission.** Assessment of audible escape of air through the nose during speech production is important in clients with cleft palate and flaccid dysarthria; assessment of nonnasal speech sound productions, especially of voiceless plosives and fricatives, is especially important; frequently, hypernasality needs to be assessed as well as the two conditions that may coexist; see Cleft Palate for assessment procedures.

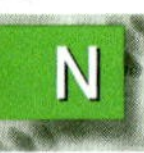


**Nasendoscope.** A mechanical device used to examine internal organs illuminated by a fiberoptic tube inserted through the nose; see Endoscopy.

**Neglect.** To assess neglect in clients with brain injury, especially *left neglect* associated with injury to the right side of the brain, see Right Hemisphere Syndrome; assess neglect in clients with left hemisphere lesions, although the symptoms are less common than those found in people with right hemisphere lesions; generally, assess by:

- Observing whether the client bumps into things on the left (or the right) visual field; ask the family members or care givers whether this is a problem they have observed at home or at a health care facility
- Asking the client to read a passage and taking note of whether the person ignores one side of the printed material (typically the left side of the page) while complaining that what is read does not make sense
- Having the client draw such simple objects as the face of a clock or human faces to evaluate whether the person omits details on one or the other side, often the left side

**Neurodiagnostic Techniques.** A variety of medical instrumental procedures designed to diagnose neural pathology; see alphabetical listing for the following neurodiagnostic techniques:

- B-Mode Carotid Imaging
- Carotid Phonoangiography
- Cerebral Angiography
- Computerized Axial Tomography
- Electroencephalogram (EEG)
- Magnetic Resonance Imaging (MRI)
- Positron Emission Tomography (PET)
- Single-Photon Emission Computed Tomography (SPECT)

**Neurogenic Stuttering.** Assessment of fluency disorders in children and adults requires a differential diagnosis of cluttering, stuttering of early childhood onset, and neurogenic stuttering; neurogenic stuttering is typically diagnosed in adults with known neuropathology; see Neurogenic Stuttering under Fluency Disorders for assessment procedures.

**Nonfluent Aphasias.** Assessment of nonfluent aphasia requires a differentiation from various types of fluent aphasia and among the varieties of fluent aphasias; relatively intact fluency of speech (whether the speech is totally meaningful or not), or even hyperfluency, is contrasted with relatively effortful, nonfluent speech to make the diagnosis; see Aphasia for general assessment procedures; see Aphasia: Specific Types for procedures to assess the following major nonfluent aphasias: Broca's aphasia, transcortical motor aphasia, and global aphasia; also see Fluent Aphasias to make differential diagnoses.

**Nonpenetrating (Closed-Head) Injury.** To assess this type of head injury in a client, examine the medical records to ascertain that the meninges of the brain remained intact, although the skull may or may not have been fractured or lacerated; for assessment targets and procedures in clients with closed-head injury, see Traumatic Brain Injury.



**Nonverbal Oral Apraxia.** Assessment of difficulty in executing nonspeech oral movements is important in clients with neurological disorders who are thought to have a motor programming or planning deficit; see Apraxia and Apraxia of Speech for assessment details.

- To assess nonverbal oral apraxia, have the client perform various oral movements:
  - Examine the client's medical records to substantiate lesions in the cerebral structures including the frontal and central opercula and anterior portions of the insula
  - Ask the client to lick lips, whistle, clear throat, smile, move the tongue around in the mouth or stick it out, puff the cheeks out, and so forth
  - Observe the same movements that are adequately performed spontaneously
  - Observe whether it co-occurs with apraxia of speech as it frequently does

**Nuclear Agenesis (or Aplasia).** To assess this syndrome, also known as the *Moebius syndrome*, see Syndromes Associated With Communication Disorders.

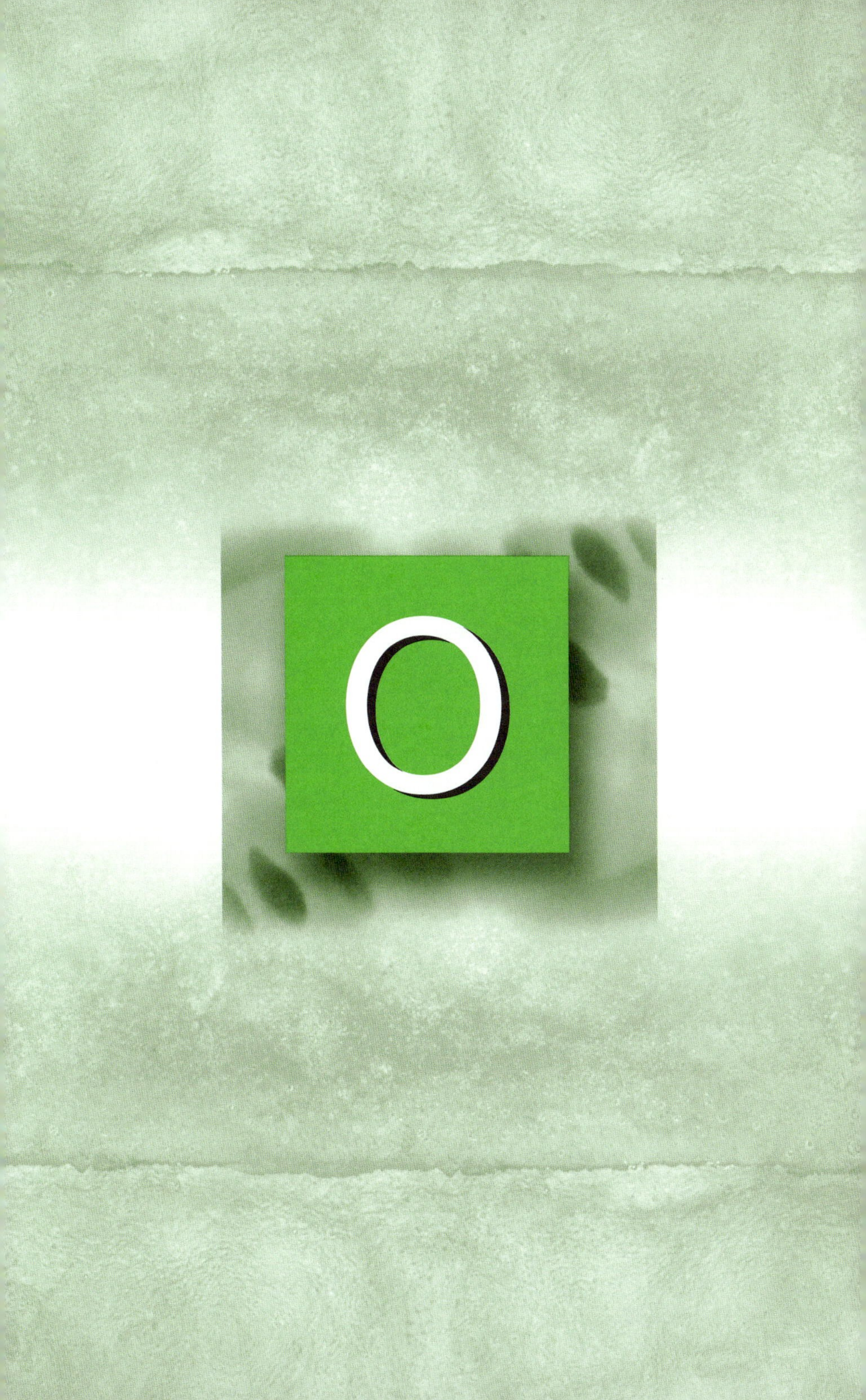
O

**Occipital Alexia.** To assess this type of reading disorders, see Alexia.

**Oculo-Auriculo-Vertebral Dysplasia.** To assess this syndrome, also known as the *Goldenhar syndrome*, see Syndromes Associated With Communication Disorders.

**Open-Head Injury.** To assess the communication disorders associated with this type of head injury; see Penetrating Head Injury under the main entry, Traumatic Brain Injury.

**Orofacial Examination.** An important part of assessment to evaluate the structural and functional integrity of the orofacial structures; especially important when neuromotor or neurophysiological problems are suspected; see Standard/Common Assessment Procedures for assessment details.

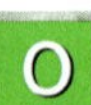

P

**Palilalia.** Assess compulsive repetition of words and phrases, sometimes with progressively faster rate and decreasing loudness in clients with many neurological diseases including Parkinson's disease, Pick's disease, Alzheimer's disease, and traumatic lesions of the basal ganglia, multiple sclerosis, posttraumatic encephalopathy, and progressive supranuclear palsy; to assess:

- Observe the client's repetition of words and phrases that you say when you do not request imitation
- Assess whether each repetition occurs multiple times
- Take note of whether the repetitions increase in rate as multiple repetitions are exhibited
- Observe whether the vocal intensity decreases as the compulsive repetitions increase
- Have the client read aloud a passage and compare the number of repetitions in oral reading versus conversational speech; document a lower frequency of repetitions in oral reading than in conversational speech

**Paraphasias.** To assess unintended word or sound substitutions, often found in clients with aphasia, see Aphasia.

**Parietal-Temporal Alexia.** To assess the reading difficulties associated with parieto-temporal lesions, also known as alexia with agraphia, see Alexia.

**Parkinsonism.** It is important to assess symptoms similar to those found in Parkinson's disease but without the etiology of that disease; assess parkinsonian symptoms in:

- Clients with Alzheimer's disease, vascular disease, drug-induced neuromotor problems, Lewy body dementia, and Pick's disease
- See Parkinson's Disease for assessment details

**Parkinson's Disease.** Assessment concerns in clients with Parkinson's disease include such neurological symptoms as tremor and rigidity; psychiatric symptoms including depression; visuospatial disturbances and writing problems; soft, monotonous, and rapid speech; and crowded word productions without the usual pauses between phrases; symptoms of dementia need to be assessed when there is evidence of it; see Dementia for general assessment procedures; symptoms of dysarthria need to be assessed because hypokinetic dysarthria is associated with it; see Dysarthria and Hypokinetic Dysarthria under Dysarthria: Specific Types for assessment procedures; consider the following that are specific to Parkinson's disease:

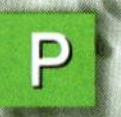


### *Case History/Interview Focus*

- See **Case History** and **Interview** under Standard/Common Assessment Procedures
- Obtain a detailed case history on changes in the client's cognition, general behavior, emotional responding, and communication skills
- Obtain information on the onset and progression of such early neurological symptoms as slowness of movements, rigidity, tremors, pill-rolling movement of fingers, gait and postural problems, and so forth
- Review the medical records about any neurodiagnostic evidence of postencephalitic or arteriosclerotic diseases, degeneration of brainstem nuclei, and so forth

## Ethnocultural Considerations

- See Ethnocultural Considerations in Assessment
- Assess the family's resources, access to neurological and other medical treatment and rehabilitation, and the support systems the family may need

## Assessment

- Assess speech, language, memory, cognition (including orientation and confusion)
- Take note of reported sleep disturbances, confusion, hallucinations, and delirium
- Assess micrographia, writing with increasingly small letters, which is a unique writing problem clients with Parkinson's disease exhibit
- Check whether the client has better preserved language compared to clients with other forms of dementia to support a diagnosis of Parkinson's type of dementia; follow the procedures described under Dementia
- Assess such symptoms as reduced stress, monopitch, reduced loudness, palilalia, short rushes of speech, increased and variable rate of speech, phoneme repetitions, and other symptoms of hypokinetic dysarthria; see Dysarthria: Specific Types

## Standardized Tests

- Consider using standardized tests described under Dementia and Dysarthrias

## Related/Medical Assessment Data

- Integrate available medical, neurological, psychological, behavioral, and diagnostic medical laboratory findings with the results of the communication assessment

## Standard/Common Assessment Procedures

- Complete the Standard/Common Assessment Procedures

## Diagnostic Criteria

- Medical and neurological evidence of Parkinson's disease with its characteristic neurobehavioral symptoms
- Dementia and Dysarthrias that are characteristic of Parkinson's disease

## Differential Diagnosis

- Differentiate Parkinson's disease from such other diseases as Huntington's Disease, Wilson's Disease, and Supranuclear Palsy that are associated with subcortical dementia
- See **Differential Diagnosis** under Dementia

## Prognosis

- More favorable for clients with tremor
- Degenerative, irreversible disease

## Recommendations

- Communication treatment in the early stages
- Management and coping strategies for the client and family members in later stages
- Family counseling and management strategies

- See the following cited sources and *Hegde's PocketGuide to Treatment in Speech-Language Pathology* (3rd ed.) for details

Cummings, J. L., & Benson, D. F. (1983). *Dementia: A clinical approach.* Boston, MA: Butterworth.

Hegde, M. N. (2006). *A coursebook on aphasia and other neurogenic language disorders* (3rd ed.). Clifton Park, NY: Thomson Delmar Learning.

Murray, L. L. (2000). Spoken language production in Huntington's and Parkinson's diseases. *Journal of Speech, Language, and Hearing Research, 43*(6), 1350–1366.

Rajput, A. H. (2001). Epidemiology and clinical genetics of Parkinson's disease. In C. M. Clark & J. Q. Trojanowski (Eds.), *Neurodegenerative dementias* (pp. 177–192). New York: McGraw-Hill.

Simuni, T., & Hurtig, H. I. (2001). Parkinson's disease: Clinical picture. In C. M. Clark & J. Q. Trojanowski (Eds.), *Neurodegenerative dementias* (pp. 193–203). New York: McGraw-Hill.

**Penetrating (Open-Head) Injury.** This kind of head injury is diagnosed when there is evidence of a perforated or fractured skull and torn Meninges; see Traumatic Brain Injury for assessment procedures.

**Perseveration.** Assess this tendency to repeatedly give the same wrong response to stimuli in clients with brain injury; during assessment, note that clients with traumatic brain injury or stroke who are asked to name a picture may give a wrong response, realize the mistake, and yet repeatedly give the same wrong response.

**Phonemic Paraphasia.** Assess this aspect of language disorders found in clients with Aphasia; during the interview, conversational speech sampling, and testing periods, take note of the client's substitution of one phoneme in the intended word with another phoneme (e.g., saying *loman* for *woman*); also take note of an unnecessary phoneme the client may add to a word (e.g., saying *wolman* for *woman*).

**Phonological Awareness.** Assessment of phonological awareness has been emphasized in recent years as a means to suggest intervention for literacy skills in children and to suggest a need for phonological treatment; a child who lacks phonological awareness—the knowledge that syllables and words are created from sounds and sound combinations—is likely to have reading and writing problems; although phonological awareness is correlated with phonological as well as literacy problems, there is no convincing experimental evidence that teaching phonological awareness will help improve articulation or literacy skills; however, clinicians who wish to assess the various subskills of phonological awareness may consider the following:

- Rhyming. Assess whether the child can identify rhyming words
  - Present words that sound alike or rhyme and ask the child to identify them
  - Present a word and ask the child to suggest words that rhyme with what is presented
  - Present a set of rhyming and non-rhyming words and ask the child to sort them out

P

- Alliteration. Assess whether the child can identify alliteration (beginning and ending sounds in words)
  - Present words that begin and end with different sounds
  - Ask the child to identify the sounds that begin and end those words
- Phoneme isolation. Assess whether the child can identify sounds in different positions in a word
  - Present selected words
  - Ask the child whether a specific sound occurs in the beginning, end, or middle of a word
- Sound blending. Assess whether the child can blend two or more sounds that are temporally separated by a few seconds into a word
  - Orally present sounds within selected words with brief pauses between sounds (e.g., *c-a-t; m-a-n*)
  - Ask the child what word the sounds make
- Syllable identification. Assess whether the child can identify the number of syllables
  - Orally present selected words
  - Ask the child to identify the number of syllables in each word presented through clapping, finger tapping, or by verbally stating
- Sound segmentation. Assess whether the child can break down words into their individual sounds
  - Present oral or printed words (depending on whether the child can read or not)
  - Ask the child to tell the number of phonemes in each word
  - Ask the child to tell whether the same sound occurs in multiple words
  - Ask the child to say a word without a sound specified (e.g., *Say drag; now say it without the* /d/)
  - Ask the child to change a sound in a word by substituting it with a requested sound (e.g., *Say time; now change the t sound to an l sound and say the word*)
- See also Literacy Skills for assessment of related skills

**Phonological Disorders.** Assessment of phonological disorders requires an analysis of patterns in multiple misarticulations that significantly affect the intelligibility of speech; contrasted with an assessment of errors of articulation that may lack a pattern; see Phonological Processes for patterns and Articulation and Phonological Disorders for a description of disorders and their assessment.



**Phonological Processes.** Assessment of phonological processes requires a knowledge of phonological rules that help organize multiple errors of articulation into different and distinct patterns; presumably, each pattern is governed by a phonological rule; each process is a specific way in which a child simplifies adult productions of speech sounds; major processes and their assessment procedures include the following:

### *Assessment of Phonological Processes: General Guidelines*

- Record an extended speech sample that is representative of the child's conversational speech; see Articulation and Phonological Disorders as well as

Standard/Common Assessment Procedures on taking a speech and language sample

- Analyze the errors of articulation; take note of each phoneme error
- Group the errors according to the phonological processes; take note that the processes are sometimes named and described differently in different sources; use one consistent and well-defined set of processes to make an analysis; note that most phonological processes are normal up to a chronological age point and disorders beyond that point; some patterns are more common than others; some have greater effect on intelligibility than others; assess the following major phonological processes in a child with multiple misarticulation; note that a child may not exhibit all of the processes described

### Analyze the Phonological Processes

- Assimilation processes: Assess whether one sound in a word leads to a change in another sound in the same word; in many cases, assimilative errors are similar to substitution errors; in assimilation, the influence of one sound on another is the main source of error; such an influence is not a factor in simple substitutions.
  - Alveolar assimilation: Production of an alveolar sound instead of a velar
    - *dot* for *goat*
    - *tot* for *coat*
  - Coalescence: Production of a single sound instead of two adjacent sounds
    - *fip* for *sweep*
    - *pip* for *beep*
  - Devoicing: Production of a voiceless consonant instead of a voiced consonant
    - *back* for *bag*
    - *sip* for *zip*
  - Diminutization: Addition of [i] or a consonant and [i]
    - *eggi* for *egg*
    - *nodi* for *no*
  - Epenthesis: Insertion of a vowel (an error of addition); often between two consonants in a consonantal cluster
    - *bə lu* for *blue*
    - *sə mile* for *smile*

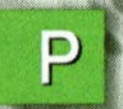

  - Labial assimilation: Production of a labial consonant instead of a nonlabial consonant in a word that contains another labial
    - *beab* for *bead*
    - *bop* for *top*
  - Metathesis: Production of sounds in their reversed order within a word
    - *peek* for *keep*
    - *likstip* for *lipstick*
  - Nasal assimilation: Production of a nasal consonant instead of an oral consonant in a word that contains a nasal
    - *nam* for *lamb*
    - *nun* for *fun*
  - Prevocalic voicing (voicing assimilation): Voiced production of voiceless consonants when they precede a vowel (prevocalic position)

        - *bea* for *pea*
        - *Dom* for *Tom*
    - Reduplication (doubling): Repetition of a syllable within a word
        - *wawa* for *water*
        - *kaka* for *cat*
    - Velar assimilation: Production of a velar consonant instead of a nonvelar consonant in a word that contains a velar
        - *keak* for *teak*
        - *guck* for *duck*
- Substitution processes (simplification processes): Similar to *substitutions* in the traditional analysis, substitution processes involve replacement of one sound with another sound.
    - Affrication: Production of an affricate instead of a fricative or stop
        - *chun* for *sun*
        - *chu* for *shoe*
    - Apicalization: Production of an apical (tongue tip) consonant instead of a labial consonant
        - *dee* for *bee*
        - *tee* for *pea*
    - Backing: Production of more posteriorly placed consonants instead of more anteriorly placed consonants (velar consonants in place of alveolar consonants)
        - *boak* for *boat*
        - *hoop* for *soup*
    - Deaffrication: Production of a fricative instead of an affricate
        - *pez* for *page*
        - *ship* for *chip*
    - Denasalization: Production of an oral sound with a similar place of articulation (homorganic sound) instead of a nasal sound
        - *by* for *my*
        - *dame* for *name*
    - Depalatalization: Production of an alveolar fricative instead of a palatal fricative or affricate
        - *su* for *shoe*
        - *wats* for *watch* (diacritic under ts) ◡
    - Final consonant devoicing: Production of an unvoiced final consonant instead of a voiced final consonant
        - *bet* for *bed*
        - *bik* for *big*
    - Fronting: Production of more anteriorly placed consonants instead of more posteriorly placed consonants (e.g., alveolar consonants instead of velar consonants)
        - *tee* for *key*
        - *su* for *shoe*
    - Gliding: Production of a glide (w, j) instead of a liquid (l, r)
        - *pwey* for *play*
        - *yewo* for *yellow*

P

  - Glottal replacement: Production of a glottal stop (ʔ) instead of other consonants
    - *tuʔ* for *tooth*
    - *bæʔ* for *bat*
  - Labialization: Production of a labial consonant in place of a lingual consonant
    - *fum* for *thumb*
    - *vase* for *days*
  - Stopping: Production of stop consonants in place of other sounds (often fricatives)
    - *teat* for *seat*
    - *doup* for *soup*
  - Vocalization (vowelization): Production of vowels in place of liquids or nasals
    - *fawo* for *flower*
    - *dippo* for *zipper*
- Deletion processes (structure processes): Similar to *deletions* in the traditional analysis, deletion processes involve the elimination of certain sounds in syllables and words.
  - Cluster reduction or cluster simplification: Omission (deletion) of one or more consonants in a cluster of consonants
    - *bes* for *best*
    - *seep* for *sleep*
  - Consonant deletion: Omission of an intervocalic consonant
    - *mai* for *mommy*
    - *dai* for *Dotty*
  - Initial consonant deletion: Omission of word-initial consonants
    - *at* for *pot*
    - *oop* for *soup*
  - Final consonant deletion: Omission of a consonant at the end of a word or syllable
    - *kæ* for *cat*
    - *pu* for *pool*
  - Unstressed (weak) syllable deletion: Omission of a syllable, usually an unstressed syllable
    - *nana* for *banana*
    - *tephone* for *telephone*



### *Administer a Phonological Process Assessment Instrument*

| Test | Purpose |
|---|---|
| *Assessment of Link Between Phonology and Articulation—Revised* (R. J. Lowe) | To assess 15 phonological processes through short sentences and with picture stimuli |
| *Assessment of Phonological Processes—Revised* (B. W. Hodson) | To assess 40 phonological processes in 7 categories with objects, pictures, and body parts |

*(continues)*

(continued)

| Test | Purpose |
|---|---|
| *Bankson-Bernthal Test of Phonology* (N. W. Bankson & J. E. Bernthal) | To assess consonant productions, phonological error patterns, and intelligibility |
| *Compton-Hutton Phonological Assessment* (A. J. Compton & J. S. Hutton) | To assess sound productions in initial and final word positions to identify phonological error patterns |
| *Computerized Articulation and Phonology Evaluation System* (J. Masterson & B. Bernhardt, 2001) | To assess phonological processes through color photographs |
| *Computerized Profiling* (S. Long & M. Fey) | To assess phonological processes with an IBM-compatible or Macintosh computer |
| *Hodson Assessment of Phonological Processes* (B. Hodson) | To identify priorities in the treatment of unintelligible children; not a traditional test of phonological processes |
| *Khan-Lewis Phonological Analysis* (L. Khan & N. Lewis) | To assess 15 phonological processes with 44 words from the Goldman-Fristoe Test of Articulation |
| *Macintosh Interactive System for Phonological Analysis* (J. Masterson & F. Pagan) | To assess 27 phonological processes or rules with a Macintosh computer |
| *Natural Process Analysis* (L. Shriberg & J. Kwiatkowski) | To assess 8 natural phonological processes with a 90-word spontaneous speech sample |
| *Phonological Process Analysis* (F. Weiner) | To assess 16 phonological processes with 136 picture stimuli |

- Analyze the conversational speech sample and the results of the assessment instrument to describe the processes the child exhibits

### *Apply the Diagnostic Criteria for Phonological Process Assessment*

- Note that phonological processes are normal in children up to a certain age; a process is abnormal or in need of treatment only when it persists beyond a certain age; use the following guidelines to assess processes that are clinically significant in a child:

P

| Processes Disappearing by Age 3 | Processes Persisting after Age 3 |
|---|---|
| Unstressed syllable deletion | Cluster reduction |
| Final consonant deletion | Epenthesis |
| Consonant assimilation | Gliding |
| Reduplication | Vocalization |
| Velar fronting | Stopping |
| Diminutization | Depalatization |
| Prevocalic voicing | Final devoicing |

### *Recommendations*

- Treatment to eliminate phonological processes that persist beyond their normal course
- See Articulation and Phonological Disorders for additional details

Bernthal, J. E., & Bankson, N. W. (2004). *Articulation and phonological disorders* (5th ed.). Boston, MA: Allyn and Bacon.

Lowe, R. J. (1994). *Phonology: Assessment and intervention applications in speech pathology*. Baltimore, MD: Williams & Wilkins.

Peña-Brooks, A., & Hegde, M. N. (2007). *Assessment and treatment of articulation and phonological disorders in children* (2nd ed.). Austin, TX: Pro-Ed.

Smit, A. B. (2004). *Articulation and phonology: Resource guide for school-age children and adults*. Clifton Park, NY: Thomson Delmar Learning.

Stoel-Gammon, C., & Dunn, C. (1985). *Normal and disordered phonology in children*. Austin, TX: Pro-Ed.

Williams, A. L. (2003). *Speech disorders: Resource guide for preschool children*. Clifton Park, NY: Thomson Delmar Learning.

**Pick's Disease.** Assessment and diagnosis of Pick's disease has undergone some changes in recent years; Pick's disease, a progressive neurological disease associated with a gradual decrease in the tissue mass in the frontotemporal regions of the brain is currently considered a part of frontotemporal dementia; this type of dementia includes variants other than Pick's disease, but they all share a common feature of frontotemporal atrophy; assessment of dementia associated with Pick's disease or other variants of frontotemporal pathology is described under Dementia; in addition, see Frontotemporal Dementia for certain unique assessment considerations that apply to Pick's disease as well.

**Positron Emission Tomography (PET).** A neurodiagnostic procedure based on computed tomography; measures the differential metabolic rates in different areas of the brain; useful in diagnosing neuropathology associated with communication disorders, including aphasia; in this procedure:

- The client is injected with a radioactive substance that spreads throughout the brain
- The scanning machine scans the amount of radioactivity in the brain
- The scanning machine detects differences in the amount of radioactivity in different scanned regions
- The results suggest different rates of cerebral metabolism; a lower-than-normal metabolic rate suggests neuropathology



**Posterior Isolation Syndrome.** To assess this type of aphasia, also known as *transcortical sensory aphasia*, see Aphasia: Specific Types.

**Pragmatic Language Skills.** Assessment of pragmatic language skills, also called conversational speech skills, is essential to diagnose language disorders in both children and adults; several specific aspects of conversation need to be assessed to make a comprehensive analysis of a client's communication skills; for details, see Language Disorders in Children.

- Assess topic initiation: Hold a 20-minute conversation with the client; introduce only a few topics of conversation and note whether the client initiates new conversational topics when you give a brief break or when prompted (e.g., *What else do you want to talk about? Is there something else you want to talk about?*)
- Assess topic maintenance: Hold a 20-minute conversation with the client and evaluate whether the client can talk on the same topic for an extended duration of time; the duration is highly variable and will depend on the topic as well as social appropriateness; make clinical judgments
- Assess conversational turn taking: Hold a 20-minute conversation with the client and note how many times the person talked when yielded and how many times the person failed to take a turn when it was his or her turn to talk; prompt, by saying "It is you turn now," "I want you to talk now," and so forth to see whether turn taking improves; take note of the frequency with which the client interrupted you while you were talking; make clinical judgments about the adequacy of turn taking skills
- Assess eye contact: Judge the appropriate durations for which the client maintained eye contact with you as you hold a conversation; note that this skill is culturally determined and may not be a significant pragmatic language skill in some cultures
- Assess conversational repair strategies: During conversation, make ambiguous, unclear, or mumbled statements to assess whether the client will ask for clarification; frequently make requests for clarification by such statements as "I don't understand," "I am not sure," and "What was that?" to evaluate whether the client will modify the statements; count the number of times the client should have requested clarifications and the number of times the client actually did; similarly, count the number of times the client should have modified his or her statements and the number of times the client actually did
- Assess narrative skills: Tell or read aloud a story to the client and ask it to be retold; ask the client to silently read a story and retell it; ask the client to tell a story he or she knows; ask the client to narrate an experience (e.g. vacation trip, how to make a sandwich, how to work with a computer, how to build something); analyze for cohesion, logical sequence, characterization, story details, and accuracy of sequence and information offered

**Primary Progressive Aphasia.** Assessment procedures used to evaluate the typical types of aphasia are appropriate to assess this atypical form of aphasia, also know as *progressive dysarthria* or *progressive anarthria*; it may even be considered *apraxia with dysarthria*; the typical forms of aphasia are not progressive, a distinguishing point; to assess progressive aphasia:



- Review medical, neurological, and neurodiagnostic procedures for evidence of any degenerative neurological diseases of insidious onset (e.g., Pick's disease and frontotemporal dementia)
- Assess initial aphasic-like symptoms (hence the name, *primary progressive aphasia*)
- Repeat the assessment to note any progression of symptoms
- Contrast this with the typical types of aphasia, which have a relatively sudden onset

- Use additional assessment procedures described under Aphasia and Apraxia of Speech

**Prognosis.** A professional judgment made about the future course of a disorder or disease under specified conditions; a conditional statement of best judgment given certain facts; a predictive statement about what might happen under different circumstances; highly dependent on individual variables; in making prognostic statements:

- Consider the appropriateness of making only probabilistic statements, not statements of certainty; let the clients and their family members know that the statements are matters of judgments based on what is known; qualify statements with factors that affect the outcome of a disorder
- Take such factors as the physiological course of an underlying disease and general health of the client, especially older clients with communicative disorders, into consideration
- Qualify prognostic statements in light of the severity of the disorder and what is known about its natural course over time
- Specify that prognostic statements change depending on the conditions or events that will follow a diagnosis; prognosis may be very different with treatment versus prognosis without intervention
- Impress on the clients and their families that generally, prognosis for improved communication skills is good for most clients (unless they are in the more advanced stages of dementia), but that the degree of progress will depend on the intensity of treatment, cooperation of the client and family members, the client's motivation to work hard in and outside the clinical setting, duration of the treatment, adequate follow-up, and additional treatment

**Progressive Supranuclear Palsy (PSP).** To assess the communication disorders associated with this somewhat rare degenerative disease of the brainstem, basal ganglia, and cerebellum, during assessment:

- Take note of the early-stage symptoms that may resemble those of Parkinson's disease
- Observe the characteristic paralysis of the upward gaze (ophthalmoplegia)
- Observe the characteristic neurological symptoms, including the gait and balance problems, frequent falling, and neck rigidity
- Assess various kinds of dysarthrias that are associated with the disease; mixed dysarthria and dysphagia may be found in early stages; hypokinetic and spastic dysarthria also may be evident and in need of assessment; see Dysarthria for details on assessment procedures
- Assess such other communication problems as palilalia associated with frontal atrophy, aphonia, and slowly developing Dementia.

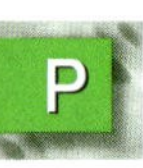


**Prosopagnosia.** To assess difficulty in recognizing familiar faces, although the voice of a person may help recognize the face, see Right Hemisphere Syndrome with which it is most frequently associated.

**Psychiatric Problems Associated With Communication Disorders.** Assessment of several communication disorders needs a basic knowledge of psychiatric and neurological problems; many clients with dementia and neurodegenerative diseases present specific psychiatric symptoms along with communication, behavioral, cognitive, and motor symptoms; some other clients present communication disorders that are entirely psychiatric in nature; these include stuttering due to malingering or faking, certain forms of mutism, a type of aphonia, and a type of dementia; see the companion volume, *Hegde's PocketGuide to Communication Disorders*, for additional information; to assess psychiatric problems related to communication disorders, see the sources cited at the end of this main entry and consider the following:

***Abulia.*** Assessment of abulia, an extreme lack of motivation to do anything, may be relevant in individuals who lack motivation to talk as well, leading to a form of mutism called *akinetic mutism*; even though it may be considered a psychiatric disorder, it has a neurological basis; to assess abulia:

- Review the case history and medical diagnostic reports for possible neurological involvement; the client may have emerged from a mute state; check history for evidence of recovery from strokes and trauma
- Check the client's level of consciousness; clients who are abulic and do not talk are alert and attentive; other clients who do not talk may be unresponsive or may appear drowsy
- Rule out peripheral neuromotor disorders because abulia is not due to them
- Check evidence for frontal lobe damage, the most frequent cause of abulia
- Look for apathy; indifference; extremely limited amount of aphonic, whispered talking; and possibly, limited speech with very soft voice

***Aphonia—Functional.*** Assessment of aphonia without a neurological basis, also called *functional aphonia* or *psychogenic aphonia*, is essential to distinguish loss of voice in clients who have an organic basis for their lack of vocal fold adduction and vibration (e.g., bilateral vocal fold paralysis with a wide-open glottis); functional aphonia is treated as a psychiatric or behavioral disorder; to assess:

- Obtain first a medical evaluation that clears the client of organic pathology leading to a lack of voice (e.g., bilateral paralysis of the vocal folds due to neurological diseases)
- Identify possible stress factors in life surrounding the onset of aphonia through a careful and detailed interview
- Look for any evidence of psychiatric symptoms in the past
- Investigate potential advantages the client may be gaining from lack of voice (positive reinforcement); the client may be complimented on effective whispering and gesturing, with which they communicate well
- Investigate whether aphonia is an avoidance reaction resulting in negative reinforcement (e.g., an excuse from oral presentations in school or at work)
- During the interview, make some jokes to assess phonation accompanying laughter
- Take note of phonation during throat clearing; ask the client to demonstrate his or her throat clearing
- Take note of phonation during coughing; ask the client to demonstrate his or her coughing

P

***Delusions and Hallucinations.*** Assessment of delusional speech may be important in several types of communication disorders; although *delusional* *disorder* is a specific psychiatric problem, many clients with neurodegenerative diseases and dementia may exhibit coexisting delusional beliefs; assess delusions, hallucinations, or both in:

- Clients with Alzheimer's Disease; assess their delusions of persecution
- Clients with frontotemporal dementia; assess their delusions without persecutory thoughts; they may not experience auditory hallucinations
- Clients with Parkinson's Disease; assess their visual hallucinations, which are more common than auditory hallucinations; to assess, these clients need to be probed because they are not likely to report them; check whether antiparkinsonian drugs have aggravated the symptoms
- Clients with Huntington's disease; assess persecutory delusions and hallucinations
- Clients with progressive supranuclear palsy; assess their frightening visual hallucinations and delusions
- Clients with AIDS Dementia Complex; assess their hallucinations and delusions
- Clients with Creutzfeldt-Jakob disease; assess their hallucinations and delusions
- Clients with dementia caused by repeated head injury (as in professional boxers); assess their delusions of persecution

***Euphoria and Mania.*** Assessment of exaggerated feeling of well-being may be necessary in:

- Clients who have frontotemporal dementia; assess their abnormally elevated mood, excessive jocularity, exaggerated self-esteem, which may all alternate with depression
- Clients with Huntington's disease; assess their euphoric-like false sense of superiority
- Clients with AIDS Dementia Complex; assess their mania (as well as its opposite, depression)
- Clients with Creutzfeldt-Jakob disease; assess their euphoria (as well as its opposite, depression)
- Clients with vascular dementia; assess their frequent mood swings, which include euphoria
- Clients with dementia caused by repeated head injury (as in professional boxers); assess their euphoria (and depression)

P

***Depression.*** Although depression in some clients may be mistakenly diagnosed as dementia (see Pseudodementia under this entry), many forms of dementia and neurodegenerative diseases have depression as one of the symptoms; in such cases, assess depression along with other symptoms; although a diagnosis of depression is not the responsibility of speech-language pathologists, it is essential to take note of depression that will have an effect on assessment results (client may be disinterested or uncooperative during assessment)

- Take note of depression in clients with most forms of dementia, including clients with AIDS Dementia Complex
- Take note of depression in clients who are in their early stages of neurodegenerative diseases and are not yet showing serious signs of dementia (e.g., clients with Alzheimer's disease, Huntington's disease, Parkinson's disease)

- Observe such classic symptoms of depression as apathy, lack of interest in any activity, lack of pleasure in activities that were once pleasurable, a feeling of hopelessness and dejection, a gloomy and pessimistic outlook on life, feeling of sadness, verbalization of all of these negative feelings, difficulty concentrating on assessment tasks, loss of memory, and psychomotor retardation (slowness in performing actions)
- Ask the family members or caregivers about symptoms of depression; in addition, obtain information on lack of appetite, libido, sleeplessness, restlessness, or agitation
- Interpret the assessment results in light of the client's depression; the client's social and communication skills (or potential for them) may be underrated because of depression

***Factitious Disorders.*** Assessment of communication disorders that are factitious may be an occasional diagnostic challenge faced by speech-language pathologists; factitious disorders—those that are simply invented by the client—typically take the form of physical diseases that require hospitalization and sometime serious and painful treatment, but may occasionally take the form of stuttering or a voice disorder; in diagnosing a factitious disorder:

- Evaluate the motivation of the symptoms; about the only motivation one can find will be the desire to play the role of a sick person
- Assess potential gain from the disorder; there usually is no gain, there might actually be much pain, because the client will have convinced at least some medical professionals to perform extensive and painful procedures on himself or herself; some clients have been unnecessarily amputated because of their insistence
- Examine the case history for frequent travel to various hospitals, specialists in varied and distant places, and never-cured illnesses that keep appearing in the client
- Examine the case history or interview the family members to document potential self-inflicted injuries or self-induced diseases (e.g., injecting harmful substances into oneself, ingesting anticoagulants to induce serious bleeding)
- Take note of the tone in which the client reports his or her problems; usually it is done with a dramatic flare, a sense of triumph at having a mysterious or difficult-to-treat disorder
- Take note that in some clients the symptoms are predominantly psychological or psychiatric (e.g., memory loss, depression, anxiety) and in other clients the symptoms are those of serious physical diseases; the latter is sometimes called the *Munchausen syndrome*, characterized by an intention to get hospitalized and stay in the hospital
- See the next section on Malingering for a differential diagnosis

P

***Malingering.*** Assessment of malingering can be challenging because a symptom complex is being faked (feigned) by a client to gain a certain advantage; the clinician not only has to scrutinize the symptoms and the conditions of their onset, but also the motivation of the client for exhibiting the symptoms; the conscious and well-planned symptoms may resemble a variety of disorders; speech-language pathologists occasionally see malingered stuttering; voice disorders, especially mutism; cognitive dysfunction, especially faked memory loss, that is disproportionate with the extent of traumatic brain injury; movement disorders with no neurological basis; and hearing loss; more common in medical and psychiatric practice are the malingered chronic pain and various forms of physical and mental disability (related to auto accidents and occupations); also seen with varying frequency are functional visual loss (malingered blindness), epileptic-type seizures, and various simulated physical illnesses; to assess malingering:

- Scrutinize the total symptom complex carefully; though the person consciously faking a disorder has studied it, he or she is still not an expert in it
- Note any features of the client that are at odds with the known characteristics of the disorder; for instance:
  - A person who feigns stuttering may continue to stutter under delayed auditory feedback (DAF); masking noise may fail to reduce stuttering; may stutter even when the person slows the speech down; note that a subvariety of feigned stuttering is ictal stuttering, which is stuttering in individuals who have been feigning epileptic seizures with no neurological basis
  - A person who fakes a hearing loss may turn toward the direction of a sound that is suddenly presented; may carefully avoid dangerous sound signals in the environment that are not supposed to be heard (e.g., may carefully avoid traffic without seeing it); on occasion, may follow a command quickly given at normal vocal intensity; a pure tone audiogram may not fit any pattern of conductive loss, sensorineural loss, or mixed loss; an otologist will have ruled out auditory pathology
  - A person who feigns mutism may very well articulate whispered speech all the time, thus avoiding most of the handicaps of not being able to speak; on occasion, while whispering, a normal voice may be heard although it is quickly shut off; a normal voice may be heard when the person coughs; family members may have heard the normal voice under an emergency (e.g., a client who shouts *fire!* and then remains voiceless); there will be no vocal pathology to account for the disorder
- To diagnose malingering, the clinician should not observe the symptoms that are incongruent with what is well established about the disorder, but also take into consideration the following:
  - Positive reinforcement the person may be gaining from the disorder; the clinician should establish a potential for monetary gain from the disorder; typically, when legal issues are entangled with the feigned disorder, some gain or positive reinforcement is at least suspect (e.g., a factory worker who is suing his or her employer for a hearing loss that appears to be feigned)
  - Negative reinforcement derived from the disorder; an army captain who needs to shout orders to soldiers, but has suddenly gone mute on the battleground, may quickly be removed from the dangerous battlefield and placed in a distant and safe hospital; thus, the avoidance of a stressful combat zone provides quick and effective negative reinforcement for the feigned disorder
  - Noncooperation with assessment or noncompliance during clinical examination, along with all other signs, also suggest malingering; the client:
    - May be unwilling to be assessed (possibly because of the fear of detection)

        - May refuse to participate in assessment tasks or participates reluctantly
        - May claim inability to perform a requested task (a person who feigns stuttering may claim he or she cannot read aloud any more; a person who fakes mutism may claim inability to cough when requested, but may do so reflexively)
        - May feign misunderstanding of instructions given during assessment, often to explain their own noncompliance or wrong responses
        - May fail to follow through suggestions (e.g., a person who feigns stuttering may not comply with a request to bring a taped speech sample from home)
        - May not keep assessment or treatment appointments
    - Additional supportive evidence to diagnose malingering may come from the presence of other psychiatric disorders (personality disorder, hypochondria, pathological lying, and so forth) that may have been diagnosed in the past
    - Note that traditionally, malingering is explained as a *conversion reaction*, a Freudian term that means that a repressed and unconscious sexual or other kind of socially unacceptable conflict has surfaced in disguise as the symptom the client presents; there is very little experimental support for this *psychopathological* explanation of behavior disorders
    - Differentiate malingering from factitious disorders from a lack of obvious gain or positive reinforcement that characterizes the latter, contrasted with definite gain and positive reinforcement inherent to the former; individuals with factitious disorders may even suffer pain, but those who malinger avoid pain at all cost and may even avoid recommended treatment; people with factitious disorders seek treatment repeatedly, even though many specialists have refused to offer it because of ethical reasons (not being able to medically and ethically justify the treatment)

***Mutism—Selective.*** Assess this psychiatric variety of mutism that some clients experience; note that mutism may be found in the final stage of dementia associated with neurodegenerative diseases; see also Mutism as a main entry; to assess:

- Ask the family members whether the client is heard talking in certain situations while refusing to talk in other situations
- Find out whether mutism has lasted at least one month
- During assessment, observe the client's effective communication with gestures and facial expressions
- Observe the limited verbalizations that may be characterized by monotonous or altered voice
- To apply the diagnostic criteria specified in the *Diagnostic and Statistical Manual of the American Psychiatric Association*:
    - Is mutism evident for more than a month? In the case of children, does it persist after the first month in school?
    - Is mutism situation-specific?
    - Does mutism cause impairment in social or personal communication? In the case of children, does it negatively affect academic performance?

  - Can shyness, embarrassment in social situations, ethnocultural differences, bilingual status, gender differences, or lack of knowledge on topics of conversation be ruled out as the cause of mutism?
- Diagnose mutism if the answer is *yes* to all of these questions

**Pseudodementia.** Assessment of dementia may be complicated by the presence of depression which often gives the false impression of true dementia; pseudodementia, which is dementia-like symptoms in depressed clients who are *not* demented, need a careful assessment; speech-language pathologists may encounter this diagnostic difficulty when assessing clients who are depressed without dementia but appear to be demented versus those who have dementia of various kinds but are also depressed; both groups will present communication deficits that the speech-language pathologist will need to evaluate; in assessing pseudodementia:

- Review the medical and psychiatric evaluation reports on the client
- Look for evidence of depression, which is the main reason why some clients are diagnosed with dementia even though they are not actually demented
- Take note of apathy, limited speech, low vocal intensity, a generally sad disposition, and forcing oneself to perform the assessment tasks—all of which suggest depression (not necessarily dementia)
- Take note of more rapid progression of apparent cognitive impairment than what is found in generally slowly progressing dementia associated with neurodegenerative diseases
- Assess visual memory tasks, on which depressed clients with symptoms of dementia may do better than clients with neurodegenerative dementia
- Take note of a history of psychiatric problems in clients with depression
- Work closely with the clinical psychologists or psychiatrists in the diagnosis of depression, dementia, and associated communication problems

**Schizophrenia.** Assessment of aberrant speech patterns associated with schizophrenia, a serious form of mental or psychiatric disorder, may be a concern to speech-language pathologists working in psychiatric, neurological, or general medical settings; most likely a diagnosis of schizophrenia will have been made by a psychiatrist or psychologist; if not, the speech-language pathologist's careful assessment of communication patterns will help support a diagnosis of schizophrenia because aberrant communication is a diagnostic sign of this psychotic disorder; to assess schizophrenic speech and language:

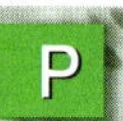


- Interview the client and record a conversational speech sample; observe the client as he or she verbally interacts with health care staff, family members, and friends who visit
- Have the client describe pictures, narrate personal experiences, or retell stories
- Ask the client about his or her difficulties, why the person is in the hospital, and what seems to be the problem; inquire about hobbies, interests, family, and friends
- Analyze the speech samples and look for the following kinds of speech and language problems:

- Frequent and abrupt changes in the topic of discussion or conversation; speaking on topics or ideas that are remotely or loosely related to the point of discussion
- Irrelevant answers to questions and irrelevant comments
- Meaningless repetition of words and phrases
- *Word salad*, or meaningless, incoherent, and unusual word combinations
- Incoherent, disorganized, illogical, and vague speech; alternatively, the speech may be excessively concrete
- For the most part, a general poverty of speech with little expressive speech with brief answers that are empty and devoid of content; alternatively, excessively detailed verbosity
- Inappropriate stress patterns in sentences and continuous speech
- Rapidly deteriorating prosodic features of speech (abnormal melody and pitch of the voice)
- Poor eye contact and impaired gestures and body language (take note of these during the interview and conversation with the client)
- Expression of delusional thoughts (e.g., the idea that some people are planning to harm him or her)
- Expression of speech that suggests hallucinations (e.g., the claim that the person is hearing voices or seeing nonexistent objects or persons)

- Take note of additional features that are supportive of schizophrenia
  - A lack of affect and feelings associated with speech and its variable content
  - A general flattening of affect, with markedly reduced emotional expressions
  - Alternatively, a tendency to express emotions that are incongruent with the situation, stimuli, questions asked, or one's own experiences (e.g., the person may laugh while narrating a sad experience)
  - Some memory and intellectual impairment, although individuals with schizophrenia are not thought to be seriously intellectually impaired; during remission, they may still be somewhat eccentric, but do not show significant intellectual or memory impairments
  - A tendency to simply sit for long periods with no interest in doing anything
  - A tendency to be confused and disoriented
  - A lack of insight into one's own condition
- Take into consideration the client's culture, age, and gender in assessing deviations in emotional expression, eye contact, gestures, and body language
- Take into consideration the client's religious beliefs in evaluating what might otherwise be considered hallucinations (e.g., hearing God's voice)

American Psychiatric Association (1994). *Diagnostic and statistical manual of mental disorders* (4th ed.). Washington, DC: Author.

Bianchini, K. J., Greve, K. W., & Love, J. M. (2003). Definite malingered neurocognitive dysfunction in moderate/severe traumatic brain injury. *Clinical Neuropsychology, 17*(4), 574–580.

Duffy, J. R. (2005). *Motor speech disorders: Substrates, differential diagnosis, and management.* St. Louis, MO: Elsevier Mosby. *[see Chapter 14 on Acquired psychogenic and neurogenic speech disorders]*

Gorman, W. F. (1982). Defining malingering. *Journal of Forensic Science, 27*(2), 401–407.

Hinson, V. K., & Haren, W. B. (2006). Psychogenic movement disorders. *Lancet Neurology, 5*(8), 695–700.

Lauter, H., & Dames, S. (1991). Depressive disorders and dementia: The clinical review. *Acta Psychiatrica Scandinavica Supplementum*, 366, 40–46.

Seery, C. H. (2005). Differential diagnosis of stuttering for forensic purposes. *American Journal of Speech-Language Pathology, 14*(4), 284–297.

Speedie, L., Rabins, P., Pearlson, G., & Moberg, P. (1990). Confrontation naming deficits in dementia of depression. *Journal of Neuropsychiatry and Clinical Neuroscience, 2*(1), 59–63.

Turner, M. (1999). Malingering, hysteria, and the factitious disorders. *Cognitive Neuropsychiatry, 4*(3), 193–201.

Vossler, D. G., Haltiner, A. M., Schepp, S. K., & associates (2004). Ictal stuttering: a sign suggestive of psychogenic nonepileptic seizures. *Neurology, 63*(3), 516–519.

Zapotocky, H. G. (1998). Problems of differential diagnosis between depressive pseudodementia and Alzheimer's disease. *Journal of Neurological Transmission Supplement, 53*, 91–95.

**Pure Agraphia.** To assess this form of writing problem without an associated reading difficulty, see Agraphia.

**Pure Alexia.** To assess this writing problem, also known as *alexia without agraphia*, see Alexia.

P

R

**Receptive Aphasia.** To assess this type of aphasia, which is the same as Wernicke's aphasia, see Aphasia: Specific Types.

**Reliability.** Consistency with which the same event is repeatedly measured; consistency of scores or values on standardized tests across repeated testing; a criterion for selecting assessment procedures, especially standardized tests; select a test that reports adequate reliability of at least one kind; most reliability measures are expressed in terms of a correlational coefficient; the higher the correlational coefficient, the greater the reliability.

- Alternate form reliability: Consistency of measures when two forms of the same test are administered to the same persons; also known as parallel form reliability; needs two versions of the same test that sample the same behaviors.
- Test-retest reliability: Consistency of measures when the same test is administered to the same persons twice; the two sets of scores are correlated; high positive correlation between the two sets of scores suggests stability of scores over time.
- Split-half reliability. A measure of internal consistency of a test; the responses to the items on the first half of the test or those given to the even-numbered items are correlated with responses given to the items on the second half or the odd-numbered items; to derive this kind of reliability, the first and the second half of a test should measure the same skill; generally overestimates reliability because it does not measure stability of scores over time.

**Right Hemisphere Syndrome.** Assessment of individuals with right brain injury requires more than an evaluation of communication deficits; to make a comprehensive diagnosis of deficits that have an effect on communication and its treatment, the clinician needs to assess the affective, attentional, and perceptual characteristics of clients with right hemisphere damage; the clinician needs to take into account the various neurological conditions and causes associated with right brain injury; for details on the epidemiology, etiology, and symptomatology of right hemisphere syndrome, see the sources cited at the end of this entry and the companion volume, *Hegde's PocketGuide to Communication Disorders*.

### *Assessment Objectives/General Guidelines*

- To evaluate the perceptual and attentional deficits associated with right hemisphere syndrome
- To assess communication disorders associated with the syndrome
- To support or justify a diagnosis of right hemisphere syndrome
- To identify the strengths and deficits that help plan not only a communication treatment program but also a general rehabilitation program

R

### *Case History/Interview Focus*

- See **Case History** and **Interview** under Standard/Common Assessment Procedures
- Review the case history and the medical records that may document the onset and recovery from stroke, traumatic brain injury, brain tumors, or other clinical conditions
- During the interview, interpret the client's information on his or her problems with caution because most clients with right hemisphere syndrome tend to deny their illness or specific symptoms

- Seek information on the client's difficulties from the family members or other caregivers to obtain a valid picture of the client's symptoms
- Note that some family members or even health care workers may not have noticed the subtle language problems of the client
- Note that some family members may think the client is confused

## *Ethnocultural Considerations*

- See Ethnocultural Considerations in Assessment
- In assessing attention and perceptual skills, select stimuli that are appropriate to the client's ethnocultural background; if standardized tests are not appropriate, design client-specific stimulus materials
- Assess the family communication patterns and their resources; take note of the support system the family may need

## *Assessment: Perceptual and Attentional Deficits*

- Assess left-sided neglect and attentional deficits
- Administer standardized tests, observe the client during the interview and assessment, and seek information from the family members
- Use client-specific materials whenever possible; most perceptual and attentional deficits may be tested by devising various kinds of clinical tasks
  - Draw small circles, dots, squares, or lines on a sheet of paper, randomly spaced, and ask the client to cross out all of them; note that the client with left neglect will cross out only the stimuli on the right half of the page
  - Draw horizontal lines on a sheet of paper and ask the client to draw vertical lines through all of them to divide them into two equal halves; note that a client with left neglect will divide the line such that the left portion will be larger than the right side
  - Observe the client for evidence of neglect (e.g., the client may forget to comb the hair on the left side of the head)
  - Ask the client to describe his or her problems on the left side of the body; note that the client may deny the existence of a paralyzed left limb
  - Ask the family about evidence of neglect (e.g., bumping into things or persons on the left)
  - Interview hospital staff about evidence of neglect
  - Touch both arms simultaneously and ask the client to report the sensation; note that the client may report sensation on only the right side (even if the left has no sensory problems)
  - Ask the client to write a paragraph or copy a paragraph; note the distribution or organization of writing on the page for evidence of neglect
  - Ask the client to cross out a specific letter when the target letters are printed along with the nontarget letters on a sheet of paper; count the number of correctly crossed out letters and their location for evidence of inattention, neglect, or both
  - Show objects or pictures of objects that the client has regularly used in the past to assess a failure to recognize such objects (e.g., show a pen to a writer, a picture of a hammer to a carpenter, or a picture of a tractor to a farmer and ask *What is this?*)

- Continue to take note of neglect as you assess such other skills as reading and writing
- Assess disorientation
  - Ask such questions as "Where are you now?" and "Where is your home?" "What is the name of this place?" "When did you get here?" to assess spatial orientation
  - Ask questions about the time, date, month, and year to assess orientation to time
  - Ask the client to name his or her doctor, nurse, or health care staff to assess orientation to people in the client's environment
  - Ask the client "Who is she?" or "Who is he?" while pointing to staff that is taking his or her care to assess facial recognition of people in the surrounding area
- Assess constructional impairment
  - Ask the client to copy a block design of the kind found in nonverbal intelligence tests
  - Arrange a matchstick figure on the desk and ask the client to copy it
  - Ask the client to draw or copy the face of a clock; note the crowding of all numbers on the right half of the circle
  - Ask the client to copy printed figures and designs; note the omission of details, especially details on the left side of the figures or designs
- Assess affective deficits
  - Observe the client for evidence of difficulty in expressing emotions (e.g., does the client show facial expressions consistent with verbal expressions?)
  - Demonstrate different facial expressions of emotions and ask the client to identify them (e.g., identifying a happy or a sad face)
  - Show pictures of faces that clearly depict contrasting emotions and ask the client to name the emotional experience
  - Show pictures that express contrasting emotions and ask the client to match them with appropriate printed words (e.g., *happy* or *sad*)
  - Print a few isolated sentences and ask the client what they mean to assess his or her difficulty in deciphering emotional meaning without context (e.g., show sentences like *The man was angry* or *She is feeling sad*)
  - Observe the client as you look for evidence of difficulty in using prosodic features to surmise emotional expression
- Assess denial of illness
  - Ask various questions about the client's problems and evaluate the responses for evidence of denial (e.g., *Do you have problems of writing now? Why are you here in the hospital? What kinds of tasks are difficult for you now?* and *Do you have a problem moving your left hand?*) and take note of the answers that might suggest denial of obvious problems
  - Interview the family members about the client's denial of physical or behavioral problems
  - Judge the client's level of motivation for assessment or treatment; low motivation may suggest denial
  - Observe whether the client makes attempts at self-correction; lack of such attempts may suggest denial

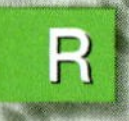

- Assess impaired inference
  - Tell a brief story and ask the client to describe its moral or message and its implied meaning
  - Tell a few proverbs and ask the client to say what each means (e.g., *What does it mean to say that "a stitch in time saves nine"?*)
  - Tell a few metaphors and ask the client to say what each means (e.g., *What does it mean when you say "the problem was nipped in the bud"?*)
  - Tell a joke without its punch line and ask the client to complete it
  - Show pictures that show absurdities and ask the client what is wrong with them and why (e.g., the picture of a cat chasing a dog)
  - Place a variety of objects on the table and ask the client to classify them according to similarities and differences; take note of any errors to evaluate difficulty in abstraction and inferencing
- Assess impaired reasoning, planning, organizing, and problem-solving skills
  - Ask the client to describe how he or she would plan a shopping trip
  - Ask the client to describe how he or she would plan a brief vacation
  - Ask the client to describe the steps involved in organizing a birthday party
  - Ask the client to describe how he or she would plan a meal for a few guests
- Assess problems in logical reasoning
  - Present a series of logical and absurd statements and ask the client to sort them
  - Ask the client to explain why a statement is absurd
  - Use other assessment data (e.g., those related to impaired inference, discourse cohesion, and sequencing events in storytelling) to make judgments about logical reasoning skills
- Assess other behavioral deficits
  - Ask the family members or hospital staff about signs of depression (e.g., lack of interest in food or visitors)
  - Obtain psychological or psychiatric reports on depression and other behavioral problems
  - Interview family members or caretakers about impulsive and uninhibited behavior (e.g., emotional outbursts or inappropriate jokes); observe and take note of these behaviors during the interview and assessment
  - Observe the client's speed of responses, concentration on various assessment tasks, and distractibility

### *Assessment: Communication Disorders*

- Take a conversational speech sample
- Assess prosodic problems
  - Take note of any prosodic deviations (e.g., rate variations, monopitch and monoloudness, and equal or inappropriate stress patterns)
  - Take note of hypermelodic speech
  - Ask the client to imitate an intonational pattern of a modeled sentence; take note of any deviations in intonational patterns including variations in stress and pitch

   - Note the expression of emotionality in speech
- Assess inappropriate and anomalous speech
   - Record all inappropriate responses to questions, anomalous responses, and meaningless or irrelevant comments
   - Document inappropriate humor
   - Take note of rambling speech
   - Take note of potential for obvious confabulation
   - Question the family members and other caregivers about inappropriate and anomalous speech, off-color jokes, confabulations, and rambling and meaningless speech
- Assess problems in distinguishing significant from irrelevant information
   - Tell or read a story aloud and ask the client to retell it
   - Take note of any insignificant details retold and missing important details
   - Take note of any missing background information in story retelling or in narrating events and experiences
- Assess problems in comprehending implied meanings
   - Use the same or similar tasks involved in assessing impaired inference
   - Take note of the degree to which the client states or summarizes literal versus implied and unstated meanings, conclusions, and consequences
- Assess problems in integrating information
   - Present a short story in which the sentences are written on separate cards
   - Ask questions about the story
   - Use the procedures described under Assess Impaired Inference and Assess Impaired Reasoning, Planning, Organizing, and Problem-Solving Skills to evaluate the integration of information
   - Evaluate the continuity, cohesion, and logical sequencing of events evident in discourse that might suggest problems in integrating and sequencing information
- Assess problems in pragmatic speech and language skills
   - Evaluate eye contact during discourse
   - Take note of the number of times the client interrupts you
   - Take note of the number of times the client fails to yield to you when you try to speak
   - Take note of excessive talking
   - Initiate a topic of conversation and assess whether the client maintained it for a reasonable amount of time
   - Take note of any irrelevant, tangential, or inappropriate comments, jokes, and interruptions
   - Note how often the client complies with requests for clarification of statements he or she makes
   - Make some ambiguous statements and note how often the client asks for clarification
- Assess auditory comprehension of language
   - Assess auditory comprehension of speech during the interview
   - Assess comprehension of emotional tone of speech directed to the client
- Assess word retrieval problems
   - Take note of any naming difficulties the client exhibits

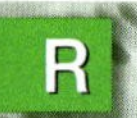

   - Take note of any other word retrieval problems as evidenced by pauses and word substitutions that suggest word retrieval problems
- Assess reading and writing problems
   - Obtain as much detailed information as possible on premorbid reading and writing skills and interests and involvement in these activities
   - Make a more detailed assessment of literacy skills only if they are important to the client
   - Reanalyze the assessment data pertaining to neglect and attention to evaluate their role in reading and writing deficits (e.g., ignoring the left side of the printed page while reading and drawing only the right side of a picture)
   - Have the client read a paragraph or two; take note of the tendency to read only the right half of the page while complaining what is read does not make sense; ask questions about the material to assess reading comprehension
   - Assess functional reading skills including reading a medical prescription, restaurant menu, and daily newspaper
   - Ask the client to write a paragraph and analyze it for errors (e.g., repetition of letters, poor letter formation, confused spacing, crowding of the letters on the right side, failure to provide a left margin)
   - Assess functional writing skills by having the client write as you dictate a message and a set of directions
- Assess dysarthria
   - Assess the production of speech sounds from the speech sample; analyze the pattern of errors
   - Take note of any phonatory deviations that might be present

## Standardized Tests

- Administer selected subtests of a test of aphasia; in addition, consider administering one or more of the following tests:

| Test | Purpose |
|---|---|
| *Behavioral Inattention Test* (B. A. Wilson, J. Cockburn, & P. Halligan) | To assess unilateral visual neglect |
| *The Bells Test* (L. Gautheir, F. Dehaut, & Y. Jonette) | To assess selective attention by crossing out only the bells on a printed page that contain other stimuli |
| *Burns Brief Inventory of Communication and Cognition* (M. Burns) | To assess visuospatial skills, expressive and receptive prosody, inference, and metaphoric language |
| *Mini Inventory of Right Brain Injury* (P. A. Pimental & N. A. Kingbury) | To assess visual-perceptual skills, higher language function, affect, and general behavior |
| *Rehabilitation Institute of Chicago Clinical Management of Right Hemisphere Dysfunction* (A. Halper, L. R. Cherny, & M. S. Burns) | To test visual and perceptual skills and pragmatic language skills; the test also provides an interview and client-caregiver observation schedule |

*(continues)*

R

*(continued)*

| Test | Purpose |
|---|---|
| *Revised Token Test* (M. M. McNeil & T. E. Prescott) | To assess auditory comprehension of spoken commands through token manipulations |
| *Right Hemisphere Language Battery* (K. L. Bryan) | To assess comprehension of metaphors, implied meanings, humor, and other language functions |
| *Test of Visual Field Attention* (CoolSprings Software) | To assess visual attention by presenting stimuli on a computer screen |
| *Test of Visual Neglect* (M. L. Albert) | To assess visual neglect by crossing out lines drawn on a sheet |

## *Related/Medical Assessment Data*

- Integrate available medical, neurological, psychological, behavioral, and diagnostic medical laboratory findings with the results of the communication assessment

## *Standard/Common Assessment Procedures*

- Complete the Standard/Common Assessment Procedures

## *Diagnostic Criteria*

- History and medical evidence consistent with right hemisphere injury, especially strokes, tumors, or head trauma
- More pronounced perceptual and affective disorders than specific language disorders
- More pronounced communication disorders than specific loss of language functions

## *Differential Diagnosis*

- Differentiate right hemisphere syndrome from aphasia typically caused by left hemisphere pathologies
- Use the following grid to distinguish between right hemisphere syndrome and aphasia:

### Right Hemisphere Syndrome or Aphasia?

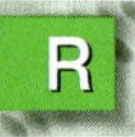


| Right Hemisphere Syndrome | Aphasia |
|---|---|
| Only mild problems in naming, fluency, auditory comprehension, reading, and writing | Significant or dominant problems in naming, fluency, auditory comprehension, reading, and writing |
| Left-sided neglect | No left-sided neglect |
| Denial of illness | No denial of illness |
| Speech is often irrelevant, excessive, rambling | Speech is generally relevant |
| Often lack of affect | Generally normal affect |

*(continues)*

(continued)

| Right Hemisphere Syndrome | Aphasia |
|---|---|
| Possibly, impaired recognition of familiar faces | Intact recognition of familiar faces |
| Rotation and left-sided neglect in drawings | Simplification of drawings |
| More prominent prosodic defect | Less prominent prosodic defect |
| Inappropriate humor | Appropriate humor |
| May retell only nonessential, isolated details (no integration) | May retell the essence of a story |
| Understands only literal meanings | May understand implied meanings |
| Pragmatic impairments more striking (lack of eye contact, impaired topic maintenance, etc.) | Pragmatic impairments less striking |
| Though possessing good language skills, communication is poor | Though limited in language skills, communication is often good |
| Pure linguistic deficits are not dominant | Pure linguistic deficits are dominant |

*Note: Right hemisphere damage in those few individuals whose right hemisphere is dominant for language results in aphasia, and for the same etiological factors.*

## Prognosis

- Variable, depending on the neuropathology and severity of deficits
- More severe initial symptoms suggest less favorable prognosis
- Smaller and unilateral lesions suggest more favorable prognosis

## Recommendations

- Treatment to improve communication and cognitive and perceptual functioning
- See the following cited sources and the companion volume, *Hegde's PocketGuide to Treatment in Speech-Language Pathology* (3rd ed.), for details

Blake, M. L., Duffy, J. R., Myers, P. S., & Tompkins, C. A. (2002). Prevalence and patterns of right hemisphere cognitive/communicative deficits: Retrospective data from an inpatient rehabilitation unit. *Aphasiology, 16*, 537–547.

Hegde, M. N. (2006). *A coursebook on aphasia and other neurogenic language disorders* (3rd ed.). Clifton Park, NY: Thomson Delmar Learning.

Myers, P. S. (1999). *Right hemisphere damage*. Clifton Park, NY: Thomson Delmar Learning.

Tompkins, C. A. (1995). *Right hemisphere communication disorders: Theory and management*. Clifton Park, NY: Thomson Delmar Learning.

S

**Sanfilippo Syndrome.** To assess this variety of mucopolysaccharidosis syndrome, see Syndromes Associated With Communication Disorders.

**Savant Syndrome.** Assess extraordinary skills in clients who otherwise have impaired intellectual and speech-language skills; case history is the most reliable indication of the need to assess such special skills in the context of significant limitations within the same individual; most likely an assessment concern in cases of autism; assessment of high level of writing, arithmetic, or musical skills may be necessary even though the client has a limited intellectual level and highly impaired oral communication skills.

**Scheie Syndrome.** To assess this variety of mucopolysaccharidosis syndrome, see Syndromes Associated With Communication Disorders.

**Semantic Aphasia.** To assess this type of aphasia, see Wernicke's Aphasia under Aphasia: Specific Types.

**Semantic Paraphasia.** To assess this characteristic problem of clients with aphasia, take note of any word substitutions that seem to be based on a relation between what is intended and what is actually produced; during interview and testing, take note of such semantic errors as saying *son* instead of *daughter*, *husband* instead of *wife*, *hammer* instead of *nail*, *fruits* instead of *vegetables*; see Aphasia for details on related assessment procedures.

**Semantic Relations.** Assessment of semantic relations is a part of evaluating child language disorders; impaired semantic relations may be an early sign of language disorders in preschool children; to assess semantic relations in young children:

- Record a conversational speech sample to analyze the specific kinds of language productions that suggest the mastery of abstract semantic relations
- Note that a typical conversational speech sample may not sample all the major semantic relations
- Select specific stimuli (e.g., objects of different size and color) to evoke the production of adjectives
- Manipulate objects to evoke responses related to events (e.g., show and hide under the table an object you hold to evoke productions that suggest the nonexistence of a semantic relation; put an object in a box to evoke locatives)
- Simulate an action like drinking or running or show pictures that show actions (to evoke such productions as agent + action)
- Generally, take note of the production of the following kinds of semantic relations that may be present in the child's speech:
    - Nomination: *this car; that doll*
    - Agent-Object: *daddy hammer* (daddy is hammering); *mommy cook* (mommy is cooking)
    - Agent-Action: *mommy run* (mommy is running)
    - Action-Object: *kick ball; hit nail*
    - Modifier-Head: *big ball; more juice*
    - X + Dative: *give Bobby* (give it to Bobby); *kiss mommy*
    - X + Locative: *ball box* (ball is in the box)

  - Nonexistence: *no truck; no baby*
  - Recurrence: *more juice; more jump*
  - Notice: *see this; hi Kermit*
  - Instrumental: *cut scissors* (cut it with scissors)
  - Attribution: *red car; big ball*
  - Rejection: *no milk* (I don't want milk)
  - Denial: *not hungry; not sleepy*
- Analyze the results and summarize the missing semantic relations the child is expected to have mastered
- Target missing semantic relations for treatment

**Sequential Motion Rate (SMR).** Assessment of rapid movement of articulators from one articulatory position to the other is important in ruling out neuromotor problems underlying speech disorders; sequential motion rate is routinely tested during speech and language evaluation and may be done in greater detail in clients with Dysarthria, Apraxia of Speech, Cerebral Palsy, and any other client in whom a neuromotor impairment is suspected; assessment procedures are the same as those for Diadochokinetic Rate; helps assess the structural and functional integrity of the lips, jaw, and tongue; related to alternating motion rates; SMRs usually follow AMRs; for procedures and analysis, see Alternating Motion Rates (AMRs).

**Single-Photon Emission Computed Tomography (SPECT).** A neurodiagnostic method that evaluates the amount of blood flowing through a structure; also known as regional cerebral blood flow (rCBF); in this procedure:
- The client inhales xenon 133
- The radioactive gas that immediately spreads throughout the cerebral hemispheres and enters the bloodstream
- A scanner detects radiation uptake in the cerebral blood
- A computer calculates the amount of blood flow in given regions and displays variations in blood flow in different colors
- Cerebral lesions associated with various neuropathologies causing communication disorders are diagnosed

**Sly Syndrome.** To assess this variety of mucopolysaccharidosis syndrome, see Syndromes Associated with Communication Disorders.

**Speech, Language, and Motor Development.** General guidelines on assessing speech, language, and motor development in infants, toddlers, and children; use them only as guidelines because individual differences in development are significant; guidelines are most useful in making broad judgments when the deviation is marked, less useful when subtle deviations need to be documented; many of the guidelines, especially at higher age levels, are vague and difficult to evaluate.

## Major Developmental Milestones

### 0–6 Months

#### Speech and Language Skills

- ❑ Repeats the same sounds
- ❑ Frequently coos, gurgles, and makes pleasure sounds
- ❑ Uses a different cry to express different needs
- ❑ Smiles when spoken to
- ❑ Recognizes voices
- ❑ Localizes sound by turning head
- ❑ Listens to speech
- ❑ Uses the phonemes /b/, /p/, and /m/ in babbling
- ❑ Uses sounds or gestures to indicate wants

#### Motor Skills

- ❑ Smiles
- ❑ Rolls over from front to back and back to front
- ❑ Raises head and shoulders from a face-down position
- ❑ Sits while using hands for support
- ❑ Reaches for objects with one hand but often misses
- ❑ Blows bubbles on lips
- ❑ Visually tracks people and objects
- ❑ Watches own hands

### 7–12 Months

#### Speech and Language Skills

- ❑ Understands *no* and *hot*
- ❑ Responds to simple requests
- ❑ Understands and responds to own name
- ❑ Listens to and imitates some sounds
- ❑ Recognizes words for common items (e.g., cup, shoe, juice)
- ❑ Babbles using long and short groups of sounds
- ❑ Uses a song-like intonation pattern when babbling
- ❑ Uses a large variety of sounds in babbling
- ❑ Imitates some adult speech sounds and intonation patterns
- ❑ Uses speech sounds rather than only crying to get attention
- ❑ Listens when spoken to
- ❑ Uses sound approximations
- ❑ Begins to change babbling to jargon
- ❑ Uses speech intentionally for the first time
- ❑ Uses nouns almost exclusively
- ❑ Has an expressive vocabulary of 1 to 3 words
- ❑ Understands simple commands

*(continues)*

*(continued)*

### Motor Skills

- ❑ Crawls on stomach
- ❑ Stands or walks with assistance
- ❑ Attempts to feed self with a spoon
- ❑ Rises to a sitting position
- ❑ Attempts to imitate gestures
- ❑ Uses smooth and continuous reaches to grasp objects
- ❑ Sits unsupported
- ❑ Drinks from a cup
- ❑ Pulls self up to stand by furniture
- ❑ Holds own bottle
- ❑ Plays ball with a partner
- ❑ Has poor aim and timing of release when throwing
- ❑ Enjoys games like peek-a-boo and pat-a-cake
- ❑ Uses a primitive grasp for writing, bangs crayon rather than writes
- ❑ Cooperates with dressing, puts foot out for shoe, and places arms through sleeves

## 13–18 Months

### Speech and Language Skills

- ❑ Uses adult-like intonation patterns
- ❑ Uses echolalia and jargon
- ❑ Uses jargon to fill gaps in fluency
- ❑ Omits some initial consonants and almost all final consonants
- ❑ Produces mostly unintelligible speech
- ❑ Follows simple commands
- ❑ Receptively identifies 1 to 3 body parts
- ❑ Has an expressive vocabulary of 3 to 20 or more words (mostly nouns)
- ❑ Combines gestures and vocalization
- ❑ Makes requests for more of desired items

### Motor Skills

- ❑ Points to recognized objects
- ❑ Runs but falls frequently
- ❑ Imitates gesture
- ❑ Removes some clothing items (e.g., socks, hat)
- ❑ Attempts to pull zippers up and down

## 19–24 Months

### Speech and Language Skills

- ❑ Uses words more frequently than jargon
- ❑ Has an expressive vocabulary of 50–100 or more words
- ❑ Has a receptive vocabulary of 300 or more words
- ❑ Starts to combine nouns and verbs

S

*(continues)*

*(continued)*

- ❑ Begins to use pronouns
- ❑ Maintains unstable voice control
- ❑ Uses appropriate intonation for questions
- ❑ Is approximately 25–50% intelligible to strangers
- ❑ Answers "what's that?" questions
- ❑ Enjoys listening to stories
- ❑ Knows 5 body parts
- ❑ Accurately names a few familiar objects

### Motor Skills

- ❑ Walks without assistance
- ❑ Walks sideways and backwards
- ❑ Uses pull toys
- ❑ Strings beads
- ❑ Enjoys playing with clay
- ❑ Picks up objects from the floor without falling
- ❑ Stands with heels together
- ❑ Walks up and down stairs with help
- ❑ Jumps down a distance of 12 inches
- ❑ Climbs and stands on chair
- ❑ Rotates head while walking
- ❑ Reaches automatically with primary concern on manipulation of object
- ❑ Inserts key into lock
- ❑ Stands on one foot with help
- ❑ Seats self in a child's chair
- ❑ Makes a tower 3 cubes high

## 2–3 Years

### Speech and Language Skills

- ❑ Speech is 50–75% intelligible
- ❑ Understands *one* and *all*
- ❑ Verbalizes toilet needs (before, during, or after act)
- ❑ Requests items by name
- ❑ Points to pictures in a book when named
- ❑ Identifies several body parts
- ❑ Follows simple commands and answers simple questions
- ❑ Enjoys listening to short stories, songs, and rhymes
- ❑ Asks 1- to 2-word questions
- ❑ Uses 3- to 4-word phrases
- ❑ Uses some prepositions, articles, present progressive verbs, regular plurals, contractions, and irregular past tense forms
- ❑ Uses words that are general in context
- ❑ Continues use of echolalia when difficulties in speech are encountered

*(continues)*

*(continued)*

- ❑ Has a receptive vocabulary of 500–900 or more words
- ❑ Has an expressive vocabulary of 50–250 or more words (rapid growth during this period)
- ❑ Exhibits multiple grammatical errors
- ❑ Understands most things said to him or her
- ❑ Frequently exhibits repetitions—especially starters, "I," and first syllables
- ❑ Speaks with a loud voice
- ❑ Increases range of pitch
- ❑ Uses vowels correctly
- ❑ Consistently uses initial consonants (although some are misarticulated)
- ❑ Frequently omits medial consonants
- ❑ Frequently omits or substitutes final consonants
- ❑ Uses approximately 27 phonemes
- ❑ Uses auxiliary "is" including the contracted form
- ❑ Uses some regular past tense verbs, possessive morphemes, pronouns, and imperatives

### Motor Skills

- ❑ Walks with characteristic toddling movements
- ❑ Begins developing rhythm
- ❑ Walks up and down stairs alone
- ❑ Jumps off floor with both feet
- ❑ Balances on one foot for one second
- ❑ Walks on tiptoes
- ❑ Turns pages one by one, or two to three at a time
- ❑ Folds paper roughly in half on imitation
- ❑ Builds a tower of 6 cubes
- ❑ Scribbles
- ❑ Uses a palmar grip with writing tools
- ❑ Paints with whole arm movements
- ❑ Steps and rotates body when throwing
- ❑ Drinks from a full glass with one hand
- ❑ Chews food
- ❑ Undresses self

## 3–4 Years

### Speech and Language Skills

- ❑ Understands object functions
- ❑ Understands differences in meanings (stop-go, in-on, big-little)
- ❑ Follows 2- and 3-part commands
- ❑ Asks and answers simple questions (who, what, where, why)
- ❑ Frequently asks questions and often demands detail in responses
- ❑ Produces simple verbal analogies

*(continues)*

*(continued)*

- ❑ Uses language to express emotion
- ❑ Uses 4 to 5 words in sentences
- ❑ Repeats 6- to 13-syllable sentences accurately
- ❑ Identifies objects by name
- ❑ Manipulates adults and peers
- ❑ May continue to use echolalia
- ❑ Uses nouns and verbs most frequently
- ❑ Is conscious of past and future
- ❑ Has a receptive vocabulary of 1200–2000 or more words
- ❑ Has an expressive vocabulary of 800–1500 or more words
- ❑ Uses up to 6 words in a sentence
- ❑ May repeat self often, exhibiting blocks, disturbed breathing, and facial grimaces during speech
- ❑ Increases speech rate
- ❑ Whispers
- ❑ Masters 50% of consonants and blends
- ❑ Speech is 80% intelligible
- ❑ Sentence grammar improves, although some errors still persist
- ❑ Appropriately uses *is, are,* and *am* in sentences
- ❑ Tells two events in chronological order
- ❑ Engages in long conversations
- ❑ Uses some contractions, irregular plurals, future tense verbs, and conjunctions
- ❑ Consistently uses regular plurals, possessives, and simple past tense verbs

### Motor Skills

- ❑ Kicks ball forward
- ❑ Turns pages one at a time
- ❑ Learns to use blunt scissors
- ❑ Runs and plays active games with abandonment
- ❑ Rises from squatting position
- ❑ Balances and walks on toes
- ❑ Unbuttons but cannot button
- ❑ Holds crayon with thumb and fingers, not fist
- ❑ Uses one hand consistently for most activities
- ❑ Traces a square, copies a circle, and imitates horizontal strokes
- ❑ Puts on own shoes, but not necessarily on the correct foot
- ❑ Rides a tricycle
- ❑ Builds a tower of 9 cubes
- ❑ Alternates feet while walking up and down stairs
- ❑ Jumps in place with both feet together
- ❑ Uses a spoon without spilling
- ❑ Opens doors by turning the handle

*(continues)*

*(continued)*

## 4–5 Years

### Speech and Language Skills

- ❑ Imitatively counts to 5
- ❑ Understands the concept of numbers up to 3
- ❑ Counts to 10 by rote
- ❑ Continues understanding of spatial concepts
- ❑ Recognizes 1 to 3 colors
- ❑ Listens to short, simple stories
- ❑ Answers questions about function
- ❑ Uses grammatically correct sentences
- ❑ Has a receptive vocabulary of 2800 or more words
- ❑ Has an expressive vocabulary of 900–2000 or more words
- ❑ Uses sentences of 4 to 8 words
- ❑ Answers complex 2-part questions
- ❑ Asks for word definitions
- ❑ Speaks at a rate of approximately 185 words per minute
- ❑ Reduces total number of repetitions
- ❑ Enjoys rhymes, rhythms, and nonsense syllables
- ❑ Produces consonants with 90% accuracy
- ❑ Significantly reduces number of persistent sound omissions and substitutions
- ❑ Frequently omits medial consonants
- ❑ Speech is usually intelligible to strangers
- ❑ Talks about experiences at school, at friends' homes, etc.
- ❑ Accurately relays a long story
- ❑ Pays attention to a story and answers simple questions about it
- ❑ Uses some irregular plurals, possessive pronouns, future tense, reflexive pronouns, and comparative morphemes in sentences

### Motor Skills

- ❑ Runs around obstacles
- ❑ Pushes, pulls, and steers wheeled toys
- ❑ Jumps over 6-inch-high object and lands on both feet together
- ❑ Throws ball with direction
- ❑ Balances on one foot for 5 seconds
- ❑ Pours from a pitcher
- ❑ Spreads substances with a knife
- ❑ Uses toilet independently
- ❑ Skips to music
- ❑ Hops on one foot
- ❑ Walks on a line
- ❑ Uses legs with good strength, ease, and facility
- ❑ Grasps with thumb and medial finger

S

*(continues)*

*(continued)*

- ❑ Releases objects with precision
- ❑ Holds paper with hand when writing
- ❑ Draws circles, crosses, and diamonds
- ❑ Descends stairs without assistance
- ❑ Carries a cup of water without spilling
- ❑ Enjoys cutting and pasting

## 5–6 Years

### Speech and Language Skills

- ❑ Names 6 basic colors and 3 basic shapes
- ❑ Follows instructions given to a group
- ❑ Follows 3-part commands
- ❑ Asks *how* questions
- ❑ Answers verbally to *hi* and *how are you?*
- ❑ Uses past tense and future tense appropriately
- ❑ Uses conjunctions
- ❑ Has a receptive vocabulary of approximately 13,000 words
- ❑ Continues to drastically increase vocabulary
- ❑ Names opposites
- ❑ Sequentially names the days of the week
- ❑ Counts to 30 by rote
- ❑ Reduces sentence length to 4 to 6 words
- ❑ Reverses sounds occasionally
- ❑ Exchanges information and asks questions
- ❑ Uses sentences with details
- ❑ Accurately relays a story
- ❑ Sings entire songs and recites nursery rhymes
- ❑ Communicates easily with adults and other children
- ❑ Uses appropriate grammar in most cases

### Motor Skills

- ❑ Walks backward heel-to-toe
- ❑ Does somersaults
- ❑ Cuts on a line with scissors
- ❑ Prints a few capital letters
- ❑ Cuts food with a knife
- ❑ Ties own shoes
- ❑ Builds complex structures with blocks
- ❑ Gracefully roller-skates, skips, jumps rope, and rides a bicycle
- ❑ Competently uses miniature tools
- ❑ Buttons clothes, washes face, and puts toys away
- ❑ Reaches and grasps in one continuous movement
- ❑ Catches a ball with hands
- ❑ Makes precise marks with crayon, confining marks to a small area

*(continues)*

*(continued)*

### 6–7 Years

**Speech and Language Skills**

- ❑ Names some letters, numbers, and currencies
- ❑ Sequences numbers
- ❑ Understands *left* and *right*
- ❑ Uses increasingly more complex descriptions
- ❑ Engages in conversations
- ❑ Has a receptive vocabulary of approximately 20,000 words
- ❑ Uses a sentence length of approximately 6 words
- ❑ Understands most concepts of time
- ❑ Recites the alphabet
- ❑ Counts to 100 by rote
- ❑ Uses most morphological markers appropriately
- ❑ Uses passive voice appropriately

**Motor Skills**

- ❑ Enjoys strenuous activities like running, jumping, racing, gymnastics, playing chase, and tag games
- ❑ Shows reduced interest in writing and drawing
- ❑ Draws a recognizable *man, tree,* and *house*
- ❑ Draws pictures that are not proportional
- ❑ Uses adult-like writing, but it is slow and labored
- ❑ Runs lightly on toes
- ❑ Walks on a balance beam
- ❑ Cuts out simple shapes
- ❑ Colors within lines
- ❑ Indicates well-established right- or left-handedness
- ❑ Dresses self completely
- ❑ Brushes teeth without assistance
- ❑ Follows advanced rhythms

From K. G. Shipley & J. G. McAfee, *Assessment in speech-language pathology: A resource manual* (pp. 32–40). San Diego, CA: Singular Publishing Group. Copyright © 1992 and used by permission.

**Sound Level Meter.** An instrument to assess vocal loudness; important components include the microphone and a voltmeter; magnifies and converts the acoustic signals into electrical signals and displays the sound pressure in decibels; the microphone is placed about 1 meter from the mouth; note that the loudness of voice measured on a sound level meter may not represent vocal loudness in natural settings.

S

**Spasmodic Dysphonia.** Assessment of this voice disorder requires a careful examination of voice quality and, if possible, an instrumental evaluation of laryngeal behavior during phonation; endoscopic examination may reveal hyperadduction of the vocal folds in most individuals and in a few cases, a sudden abduction of the folds may be evident.

- Assess spasmodic dysphonia of the adductor type
  - Assess strained or choked-off voice quality
  - Judge the presence of a severely hyperfunctional voice
  - Assess the periodic absence of phonation as the person tries to speak
  - Obtain endoscopic evidence of hyperadduction of the vocal folds, even adduction of the false vocal folds
  - Generally, judge the presence of extreme force in vocal fold adductions
- Assess spasmodic dysphonia of the abductor type
  - Assess the presence of periodic but sudden aphonia during conversational speech
  - Assess intermittent breathiness of voice
  - Relate sudden abduction to the production of unvoiced consonants
  - Obtain endoscopic evidence of the sudden abduction of folds that causes aphonia
- Recommend voice therapy, although the prognosis for sustained and long-standing treatment gains is doubtful
- See the following cited sources and the companion volume, *Hegde's PocketGuide to Treatment in Speech-Language Pathology* (3rd ed.), for details on treatment.

Boone, D. R., McFarlane, S. C., & Von Berg, S. L. (2005). *The voice and voice therapy* (7th ed.). Boston, MA: Allyn and Bacon.

Case, J. L. (2002). *Clinical management of voice disorders* (4th ed.). Austin, TX: Pro-Ed.

**Spastic Dysarthria.** To assess this type of motor speech disorder neurologically characterized by spasticity of the muscles, see Dysarthria for general procedures and Dysarthria: Speech Types for some additional assessment considerations.

**Specific Language Impairment (SLI).** Assessment of language disorders in children to determine that their language problems are not due to any other associated problems (e.g., intellectual impairments, sensory loss, emotional or behavioral disorders, or sensory loss) can be a challenging task; recent research suggests that language impairment in children who are thought to be otherwise normal may still have some subtle cognitive impairment; to make a thorough assessment of children with language difficulties who seem to be otherwise normal, use the procedures described under Language Disorders in Children; consider the following that especially apply to children with specific language impairment:

### *Assessment Objectives/General Guidelines*

- To assess the language skills with an emphasis on syntactic and morphological skills as compared with pragmatic skills
- To rule out the presence of any associated clinical condition that might explain the language disorder
- To help design a language treatment program that will integrate the child's academic goals and addresses the curricular needs

S

### *Case History/Interview Focus*

- Generally, the same as those described under Language Disorders in Children

- Ask the parents questions about early language delay
- Obtain information on potential intellectual deficits, early signs of hearing loss, or any behavioral or emotional disorders to rule out their contribution to the language problems

### *Ethnocultural Considerations*

- See Ethnocultural Considerations in Assessment
- At the very beginning, ascertain whether the child speaks a dialectal variety of English (e.g., African American English, Spanish-influenced English) or is bilingual with differential language skills in the two languages
- Assess family communication patterns, home literacy environment, resources, and supports the family may need
- Avoid the use of standardized tests that are inappropriate for an ethnoculturally different child; use alternative assessment procedures

### *Assessment*

- Record a representative speech and language sample from the child
- Assess semantic skills
- Assess morphological skills; assess these diagnostic markers in sufficient detail
- Assess syntactic skills; assess these diagnostic markers in sufficient detail
- Assess pragmatic skills
- Use the procedures described under Language Disorders in Children

### *Standardized Tests*

- Use selected standardized tests of language described under Language Disorders in Children

### *Related/Medical Assessment Data*

- Obtain psychological reports on cognitive functioning and behavioral deficits, including attentional problems
- Obtain any medical evaluation reports that are relevant to communication assessment

### *Educational Assessment Data*

- Obtain any educational assessment data that help evaluate the educational demands made on the child

### *Standard/Common Assessment Procedures*

- Complete the Standard/Common Assessment Procedures

### *Diagnostic Criteria*

- The main diagnostic criterion is the presence of significant language problems, especially syntactic and morphological problems, in the absence of sensory deficits, neurological impairment, and psychiatric disorders that could account for the problems



### *Differential Diagnosis*

- Compare the child's pragmatic language skills with syntactic and morphological skills; the two sets of skills may be differentially affected; the child's pragmatic language skills may be better than the syntactic and morphological skills

- Rule out the presence of such other factors as intellectual impairment, neurological deficits, sensory loss (e.g., hearing impairment), and behavioral or psychiatric disorders (e.g., autism spectrum disorders); obtain relevant assessment reports from other professionals to rule out these additional problems
- Diagnose specific language impairment only when no other serious problems seem to account for the predominantly syntactic and morphological problems

### *Prognosis*

- Prognosis for improved language skills with systematic treatment is good
- Most children improve with language treatment, although the possibility of persistent deficits exists

### *Recommendations*

- Language treatment to be initiated as early as possible
- Parent training in language stimulation at home, especially in the case of infants and toddlers
- Integration of language treatment with academic activities goals in school-age children
- Behavioral or psychological treatment in the case of children who have significant problems besides language problems
- See *PocketGuide to Treatment in Speech-Language Pathology* (3rd ed.) for details

**Standard/Common Assessment Procedures.** Assessment techniques used across disorders of communication; include case history, hearing screening, interview, orofacial examination, and speech and language sampling.

*Case History.* Detailed information on the client, communication disorder, family, health, education, occupation, and related matters that helps understand the client and his or her disorder; a common assessment procedure across disorders; relative emphasis on different aspects depends on the nature of the disorder and the age of the client; information collected through a printed case history form and interview of the client, family members, or both; obtain information on the following; select the relevant items depending on the age of the client:

- Identifying information: Obtain the client's name, date of birth, address, telephone number, and parents' names, ages, education, and occupations; name, address, and telephone number of the referring professional or person and client's physician; any other information the particular clinical or educational setting requires
- Whether on a printed form or during the interview, ask such questions as the following; note that some of the questions are alternative ways of getting the same information; modify the wording to suit the age and education of the client, parents, or both; skip questions that are not relevant for a particular client

S

- Client's or parents' description of the disorder
  - What do you think is your (your child's) communication problem?
  - How would you describe your (your child's) speech problem (voice problem, language problem)?
- Onset and development of the disorder
  - When did the problem (voice problem, stuttering, language difficulties) begin; or, when did you first notice the problem?
  - What were the early signs of the problem? Can you describe them? Can you imitate them?
  - What were the circumstances under which you first noticed the problem?
  - Were there any special circumstances surrounding the onset of the problem? Did anything special happen around the time the problem was first noticed? What do you think is the cause of the disorder?
  - How did the problem progress? Did the problem (stuttering, hoarseness, memory problems, language production) change over time? How did it change? Did it become progressively worse? Did it fluctuate? How did it fluctuate over time? Did you see any pattern in its change? What kind of pattern?
- Prior assessment and treatment of the disorder
  - Did you see any specialists? Who did you see? Could you supply the name and telephone number of the professional you saw? Could we contact the professional to get reports?
  - What did the professional recommend? Did you follow up on the recommendation?
  - Did you (the child) receive treatment? What kind of treatment? Can you describe what you did in a session? What were you asked to do? What were the results? Did the problem (stuttering, articulation problem, language difficulties, hoarseness) improve? How much did it improve? Did the improvement last? For how long? Why do you think the improvement did not last? Did the problem return suddenly or gradually?
- Family constellation and communication
  - How many brothers and sisters do you (does the child) have?
  - What language (or languages) do you speak at home? What is your (your child's) primary language? Second language? Do you (does the child) speak, read, and write the second language well? How well?
  - Is there any family history of communication problems? What kinds of problems? Who has them? For how long? Has it improved? Was it treated? If so, what were the results? What is the current status of the problem in the relative?
  - How does the child communicate with other members of the family? Words and phrases? Sentences? Gestures?
  - How does the child communicate with peers? How does the child play with others? How do they get along with each other?
  - Do the parents read stories to the child? Do they model reading and writing skills for the child?

  - Does the child have literacy resources at home? Does the child have a collection of books? Does the child have a separate area where he or she can read and write?
- Prenatal and birth history (mostly in the case of children)
  - What was the mother's health during pregnancy? Any major illnesses? Accidents? Medications? Any evidence of maternal substance abuse during pregnancy?
  - Full term or premature? Any birth complications? What type of delivery (head first, feet first, breech, cesarean)?
  - What was the birth weight of the child?
- Medical history
  - Did the child (did you) have any illnesses during the early childhood years? What kinds of illnesses?
  - What kinds of medical and/or surgical treatment did you (or your child) have?
  - Are you (is your child) on any medications? What kinds? Any negative side effects?
- Developmental history
  - When did the child crawl, sit, stand, walk, feed self, and dress self? Were there any feeding problems? How would you describe the child's physical development? If not normal, what were the problems?
  - Did you notice any signs of hearing loss? What kinds of problems or signs did you notice?
  - How would you describe your child's speech and language development? When did the child babble? Say first words? Use phrases? Produce sentences? Were you or were you not concerned about speech and language development? Why were you concerned?
- Educational history
  - What grade is the child in? How has the child done academically? Did the child receive special educational services? What kinds of services? How did the child do and benefit from the program? How did the child's communication problem affect his or her academic performance? What were the reactions of the teachers?
  - What level of education have you completed? How was your academic performance? How did your communication problem affect your academic performance?
- Occupational history
  - What is your current occupation? What do you do on your job? How does your communication problem affect your job performance?
  - What is your relationship with your colleagues? With your supervisors? How do they react to your communication problem? Are you concerned about their reactions?
  - Do you think you cannot get a job because of your communication problem? Why do you think so?
  - What is your occupational goal in seeking treatment now?

***Hearing Screening.*** A quick procedure to determine whether a person needs to be evaluated by an audiologist or can be assumed to have normal hearing.

- Screen hearing of all clients you assess
- Use a screening procedure adopted at your clinical site because the procedures vary
- Generally, screen hearing at 20 or 25 dB HL for 500, 1000, 2000, and 4000 Hz; for 500 Hz, screen at 25 dB HL
- Screen younger children at 15 dB HL for 500, 1000, 2000, 4000, and 8000 Hz
- Make sure the ambient noise in the screening situation is acceptable
- Refer the client who fails your screening test to an audiologist for a complete hearing evaluation

***Interview.*** A face-to-face contact with the client, parents, or both to obtain additional information, to get information given on the printed case history form clarified or expanded, to get familiarized with the client and family, and to make initial observations of the client and family.

- Note that the same questions as specified under **Case History** may be asked during the interview; however, information deemed satisfactory on the case history form may not be reexamined during the interview
- Before starting the interview, study the filled-out case history form; note areas that need to be addressed during the interview
- Take note of the client's ethnocultural background; if necessary, review information on the particular ethnocultural characteristics of interaction, language use, expected level of ease with which information can be gathered, special precautions to be taken, and so forth; see Ethnocultural Considerations in Assessment
- Go over the case history form and ask questions about unclear information or information that needs to be expanded
- Listen well, and offer comments to suggest that you understand and appreciate what the clients or family members say; do not give specific advice at this time; do not criticize or contradict; record their responses verbatim when appropriate (e.g., description of the disorder, prior treatment procedure, comments of colleagues or teachers, statements regarding causes and effects of the disorder)

***Orofacial Examination.*** An examination of the oral and facial structure to evaluate their structural and functional integrity from the standpoint of speech production; helps identify or rule out obvious structural abnormalities that may require medical attention; an important standard/common assessment procedure; use the following format from Peña-Brooks and Hegde (2007) to complete the assessment:

S

## Orofacial Examination Form

Name: ______________________ DOB: ____________ Age: _________________

Grade: ______ Teacher: ________________ Referred by: ___________________

Reason for Referral: ____________________ Date of Exam: _______________

(Items checked "YES" require closer examination and further evaluation by clinician or other specialist.)

### Structure and Function of the Facial Muscles

What to look for:
*General symmetry of the face at rest*

Questions to consider:

❑ Is there drooping at the corner of the mouth?
Yes_____ No_____

❑ Is an eyelid partially or completely closed?
Yes_____ No_____

❑ Is the mandible, or jaw, drooping on one side?
Yes_____ No_____

❑ Are there any abnormal movements (e.g., facial grimaces, spasms, twitching)?
Yes_____ No_____

❑ Are there any signs of mouth breathing or drooling?
Yes_____ No_____

What to look for:
*Symmetry of face while making specific movements*

Tasks and questions to consider:

❑ Ask the child to smile. Does the corner of the mouth deviate to one side?
Yes_____ No_____

❑ Ask the child to open the mouth wide. Does the jaw deviate to one side?
Yes_____ No_____

❑ Ask the child to raise both eyebrows. Do the eyebrows rise evenly?
Yes_____ No_____

❑ Ask the child to close the eyes tightly. Do both eyes close evenly?
Yes_____ No_____

*(continues)*

*(continued)*

**Structure and Function of the Lips**

What to look for:
*Structural integrity of the lips*

Questions to consider:

❑ Is there drooping at the corner of the mouth?

Yes_____ No_____

❑ Is there an adequate amount of tissue in the lips?

Yes_____ No_____

❑ Do the lips remain closed or apart while at rest?

Yes_____ No_____

❑ Are there any signs of mouth breathing or drooling?

Yes_____ No_____

❑ Does the lip tissue appear healthy?

Yes_____ No_____

❑ Is there any evidence of a repaired cleft lip or other scar tissue?

Yes_____ No_____

What to look for:
*Functional integrity of the lips*

Tasks and questions to consider:

❑ Ask the child to smile. Does the corner of the mouth deviate to one side?

Yes_____ No_____

❑ Ask the child to pucker. Does the amount of lip puckering favor one side?

Yes_____ No_____

❑ Ask the child to alternate between a pucker and a smile. Does the range of motion appear adequate for speech?

Yes_____ No_____

❑ Ask the child to puff the cheeks and hold air. Can the child maintain the air in the mouth to at least the count of 5?

Yes_____ No_____

❑ Is any nasal emission perceived or evident when a mirror is placed under the nares?

Yes_____ No_____

*(continues)*

*(continued)*

- ❑ Ask the child to say "ooo-eee-ooo-eee" in alternating fashion. Does the range of motion and strength of the lips seem appropriate?
  Yes_____ No_____

**Structure and Function of the Tongue**

What to look for:
*Structural integrity of the tongue*

Questions to consider:

- ❑ Does the coloration of the tongue appear normal?

  Yes_____ No_____

- ❑ Does the size of the tongue appear appropriate in relation to the child's oral cavity?

  Yes_____ No_____

- ❑ Are there any signs of atrophy (muscle loss)?

  Yes_____ No_____

- ❑ Are there any abnormal movements (e.g., spasms, fasciculations, writhing, twitches)?

  Yes_____ No_____

What to look for:
*Functional integrity of the tongue*

Tasks and questions to consider:

- ❑ Ask the child to protrude the tongue as far as possible.

  Can the child do this without effort?

  Yes_____ No_____

  Does the speed and range of motion appear appropriate?

  Yes_____ No_____

  Does the tongue deviate to one side on protrusion?

  Yes_____ No_____

- ❑ Ask the child to maintain the tongue in the protruded position to at least the count of 5.

  Can the child do this without resting the tongue on the lower lip?

  Yes_____ No_____

S

*(continues)*

*(continued)*

Does the tongue rest or hang over the lower lip?

Yes_____ No_____

❑ While the tongue is protruded, ask the child to move the tongue tip up and down, to the right and then to the left, and finally from side to side as quickly as possible.

Is the range of motion and excursion appropriate?

Yes_____ No_____

Are there any signs of groping, uncoordinated movement, or weakness?

Yes_____ No_____

❑ Ask the child to retract the tongue. Do the speed and range of motion appear adequate?

Yes_____ No_____

❑ Ask the child to open the mouth and lift the tongue so that the lingual frenulum is observed. Is there any sign of ankyloglossia (tongue-tie)?

Yes_____ No_____

❑ Ask the child to repeat "**la-la-la-la**." Does the range of motion, strength, and excursion of the tongue seem appropriate?

Yes_____ No_____

❑ Ask the child to repeat "**ka-ka-ka-ka**." Does the range of motion, strength, and excursion of the tongue seem appropriate?

Yes_____ No_____

❑ Ask the child to repeat "**ka-ka-ka-ka**." Does the range of motion, strength, and excursion of the tongue seem appropriate?

Yes_____ No_____

### Structure of the Hard Palate

What to look for:
*Structural integrity of the hard palate*

Questions to consider:

❑ Does the coloration of the hard palate appear normal along its midline?

Yes_____ No_____

❑ Does the height and width of the hard palate vault appear within normal range for speech production?

Yes_____ No_____

S

*(continues)*

*(continued)*

- ❑ Are there any signs of repaired or unrepaired clefts, fistulas, or fissures?

  Yes_____ No_____

- ❑ Are there any signs of surgical removal of any portion of the hard palate?

  Yes_____ No_____

- ❑ Are there any prostheses (e.g., dentures, obturators, palatal lifts)?

  Yes_____ No_____

### Soft Palate Structure and Function

What to look for:
*Structural integrity of the soft palate*

Questions to consider:

- ❑ Does coloration of the soft palate appear normal along its midline (normal coloration is white and pink)?

  Yes_____ No_____

- ❑ Is the uvula normal or bifid?

  Yes_____ No_____

- ❑ Are there any signs of repaired or unrepaired clefts, fistulas, or fissures?

  Yes_____ No_____

- ❑ Are there any signs of surgical removal of a portion of the soft palate?

  Yes_____ No_____

- ❑ Are there any prostheses (e.g., dentures, obturators, palatal lifts)?

  Yes_____ No_____

- ❑ Does the velum appear symmetrical?

  Yes_____ No_____

- ❑ Does the length of the velum appear sufficient for adequate posterior movement in velopharyngeal closure?

  Yes_____ No_____

What to look for:
*Functional integrity of the soft palate*

Tasks and questions to consider:

- ❑ Engage the child in conversation.

  Does the child's speech sound hypernasal or hyponasal?

  Yes_____ No_____

*(continues)*

*(continued)*

Are the pressure consonants produced correctly?

Yes_____ No_____

Are there any unusual substitutions such as pharyngeal fricatives and glottal stops for pressure consonants?

Yes_____ No_____

- ❑ Ask the child to produce a prolonged "ah." Does the velum move up and back to meet the pharyngeal wall?

  Yes_____ No_____

- ❑ Ask the child to make repeated productions of "ah." Does the velum move up and back to meet the pharyngeal wall?

  Yes_____ No_____

- ❑ Ask the child to produce isolated sounds, syllables, or words loaded with nonnasal sounds, while placing a small mirror under the child's nostrils. Is there any clouding or fogging of the mirror? (It is important to instruct the child not to exhale because the sounds or words are made to rule out normal exhalation as the cause of the mirror fogging.)

  Yes_____ No_____

### Teeth and Other Related Structures

What to look for:
*Integrity of the teeth and dental arches*

Tasks and questions to consider:

- ❑ Ask the child to open the mouth.

  Are there any missing teeth?

  Yes_____ No_____

  Are the teeth jumbled, tilted, or malpositioned?

  Yes_____ No_____

  Are there full or partial dentures in place?

  Yes_____ No_____

  Are there dental appliances such as braces in place?

  Yes_____ No_____

*(continues)*

*(continued)*

❑ Ask the child to bite down gently and separate the lips so that the teeth can be observed.

What is the molar occlusal relationship?

Normal occlusion ______

Neutrocclusion ______

Distocclusion ______

Mesiocclusion ______

What is the occlusal relationship of the teeth?

Open bite ______

Overjet ______

Closebite ______

Crossbite ______

What is the general condition of the teeth? (e.g., hygiene, cavities, breaks) ______________________

Diadochokinetic Syllable Rates (see Diadachokinetic Rate for norms)

[pʌ-pə-pə] # of repetitions__________ # of seconds__________

[tʌ-tə-tə] # of repetitions__________ # of seconds__________

[kʌ-kə-kə] # of repetitions__________ # of seconds__________

[fʌ-fə-fə] # of repetitions__________ # of seconds__________

[lʌ-lə-lə] # of repetitions__________ # of seconds__________

[pʌ–tə-kə] # of repetitions__________ # of seconds__________

Other Observations:______________________________________________

________________________________________________________________

Speech-Language Pathologist ______________________________________

**Key:**

*Normal occlusion:* Lower first molar is approximately half a tooth ahead of the upper molar. Very few individuals have a normal occlusion.

*Neutrocclusion:* Upper and lower dental arches are in normal occlusion; however, individual teeth are misaligned, rotated, or jumbled.

*Distocclusion:* Lower dental arch is too far back in relation to the upper dental arch. This can often be observed when the mouth is closed; the person has a receding chin (commonly referred to as *overbite*).

*(continues)*

*(continued)*

*Mesiocclusion:* Lower dental arch is too far forward in relation to the upper dental arch. This is also often observed when the mouth is closed; person has a protruding chin (commonly referred to as *underbite*).

*Open bite:* Lack of contact between upper and lower front teeth despite normal occlusion of the first molars. A central space is created.

*Overjet:* Excessive horizontal distance between the surfaces of the incisors. A normal distance of 1–3 mm of the upper central incisors in relation to the lower central incisors can be expected.

*Closebite:* Excessive vertical overlapping of the upper front teeth over the lower front teeth. The upper front teeth cover more than the usual half to one-third of the lower teeth. Occlusion of the molars is normal.

*Crossbite:* Lateral overlapping of the upper and lower dental arches. The lower jaw is either to the right or to the left of a normal, central position in relation to the upper jaw.

Peña-Brooks, A., & Hegde, M. N. (2007). *Articulation and phonological disorders: Assessment and treatment resource manual.* Austin, TX: Pro-Ed.

**Speech and Language Sample.** A primary means of assessing speech, language, voice, and fluency in children and adults, speech and language sampling is a standard aspect of evaluation; it is an audio-recorded sample of speech and language from a child or an adult; it is more naturalistic than the results of standardized tests; the clinician may contrive or manipulate to varying extents to evoke specific constructions; ideally, a conversational speech between a client and his or her caregiver on the one hand and the client and the clinician on the other gives the best possible means to achieve communication skills; recording a speech and language sample often involves selecting specific stimuli designed to evoke conversational speech; when the concern is speech production, the sample may be described as a speech sample and when the concern is language, it may be described as a language sample; in either case, the goal is to obtain a representative sample of a person's speech and language skills; because connected speech is important for phonological analysis, a language sample may be just as important for assessing articulation and phonological disorders; many basic procedures of evoking speech and language are the same; however, the primary concern is on language structures in the case of clients with language disorders and speech sound production in single words and connected speech in the case of clients with articulation and phonological disorders; see Language Disorders in Children for procedures that focus on language structures and Articulation and Phonological Disorders for procedures that focus on connected speech production; physical stimuli, questions, and topics of conversation need to be modified to suit the age and ethnocultural background of the client.

## Standard/Common Assessment Procedures

- Tape-record the entire speech and language sample
- Record in stereo for a more dynamic range
- Obtain 50 to 100 utterances; expect to spend about 30 minutes
- Observe carefully and take notes on the context of utterances that may not be clear from the audio-taped sample
- Use a quiet room and avoid noisy stimulus materials
- Carefully select stimuli that are appropriate for the client's age, education, occupation, and ethnocultural background
- In the case of adults, use pictures and objects only when necessary; in most cases, engage them in conversation
  - Use pictures and objects in the case of adults with neurogenic communication disorders
  - Use natural conversation in the case of adults with stuttering and voice disorders
  - Judge the necessity of physical stimulus materials in the case of adult clients who are mentally retarded; select stimuli carefully to match the adult client's level of functioning
- In the case of children, use a variety of stimulus materials to evoke and sustain conversation
  - Have the parents bring a few of the child's favorite toys
  - In the case of younger children, use toys, objects, pictures, pretend situations, role playing, storytelling and story retelling, and such other devices to evoke speech and language structure
  - Engage the older child in conversational speech; use appropriate stimulus materials as found necessary
  - In the case of most children, first have the mother, father, or any accompanying family member and the child interact with each other; let them interact in their usual manner; supply soft toys and toys that can be assembled and disassembled; supply picture books the child prefers; consider the child's interests and ethnocultural background in selecting stimulus materials; observe from the one-way mirror and take notes
  - Next, engage the child in communicative interaction using the same stimulus materials that the family member used; if necessary, add new stimulus materials
  - Use a bag or box that conceals materials to induce curiosity and questioning; pull something out of the container to surprise the child and thus to sustain the child's interest in talking
- Do not talk all the time, but do talk enough to make it a natural conversation between you and the client
- Listen carefully
- Do not make it a session of interrogation
- Let the client initiate conversation; tolerate some periods of silence to encourage speech initiation
- Repeat what you think the child just said when the child's speech is not clear
- Let the client initiate new topics; give hints of new topics (e.g., *What about this?* or *You want to talk about___?*); if hints do not work, suggest specific

topics (e.g., *Do you want to talk about your birthday party? Do you want to tell me about your trip to Disney Land? Can you tell me about your favorite cartoon show?*)

- Let the client continue to talk on a topic; do not interrupt the client
- Do not ask yes/no questions; ask open-ended questions
- Ask questions that evoke single-word responses when it is important (e.g., *What is this?* or *What color is this?*); ask questions that evoke phrases and sentences when this is needed (e.g., *What did you do last weekend?* or *Tell me about your friends*)
- Use both simple and complex sentences to see the effects on the client's speech, especially in the case of children
- Encourage conversation after picture description because the former tends to evoke more complex language from children
- Evoke single word productions for assessing vocabulary and speech sound productions
- Evoke conversation with a variety of strategies: picture descriptions, descriptions of games and toys, play activities that promote verbal interactions; conversations about siblings and grandparents, vacations, school and teachers; friends in the neighborhood; briefly mentioning your own vacations or hobbies that prompt the child to talk about his or her own similar experiences, and so forth
- Evoke specific language structures of interest by designing task-specific procedures; see Language Disorders in Children
- Have the child tell a story by looking at picture cards; see Articulation and Phonological Disorders for procedures
- Ask the child to narrate a story
- Tell a story and ask the child to retell it
- Role play activities (e.g., cooking, shopping, planning a picnic)
- See Language Disorders in Children and Articulation and Phonological Disorders for all procedural details
- Obtain a home sample; ask the parents to observe your interaction with the child and have them repeat it at home
- Repeat language sampling before beginning treatment
- Supplement language sampling with standardized tests if preferred
- Supplement language sampling with baserates established before treatment
- Transcribe the entire sample for analysis; identify the speakers involved (e.g., C for the clinician, M for the mother, CL for the client)
- Mark utterance endings with a slash (/)
- Number all utterances and obtain their total count
- Make further analysis as dictated by the purpose of speech and language sampling; see Language Disorders in Children and Articulation and Phonological Disorders for all procedural details
- Use a computerized method of transcript analysis if preferred



**Stopping.** To assess this phonological process or a pattern of misarticulations, see Articulation and Phonological Disorders and Phonological Processes.

**Stridency.** To assess this type of voice disorder characterized by an unpleasant, shrill, and metallic-sounding voice caused by excessive pharyngeal constriction and an elevated larynx, see Voice Disorders.

**Stroboscopy.** An instrumental method of assessing structures in motion; it may be used to assess vibratory patterns of vocal folds; used in combination with an endoscope or laryngeal mirror; in this method:

- A flashing light at varying frequency is directed into the laryngeal area
- The light flash rates are adjusted to match the frequency of vocal fold vibration
- The vibrating folds are then observed as static structures, due to an optic illusion
- The light flash rate is varied so it is different from the fold vibratory cycles
- The motion then is observed to have slowed down
- Various structural and functional aspects of vocal folds including fundamental frequency, the health of the folds, different phases of vibration, the degree of contact between the two folds, and symmetry of movement of the two folds may be assessed

**Stuttering.** Assessment of stuttering, a speech problem with impaired fluency, is done on the basis of excessive amounts of dysfluencies often produced with a fast tempo and with muscular tension; assessment of other associated features, including associated motor behaviors, negative emotional reactions, and avoidance behaviors is also important; needs to be distinguished from such other fluency disorders as cluttering and neurogenic stuttering; see Stuttering under Fluency Disorders for details on assessment procedures and differential diagnosis.

**Subcortical Aphasia.** To assess this variety of aphasia due to damage to the subcortical regions of the brain, see Aphasia and Aphasia: Specific Types.

**Substitution Processes.** To assess this phonological process or an error pattern in speech sound production, see Articulation and Phonological Disorders and Phonological Processes.

**Suffixes.** To assess these bound grammatical morphemes that are added at the end of words (e.g., the plural /s/ added at the end of the words), see Grammatical Morphemes and Language Disorders in Children.

**Syndromes Associated With Communication Disorders.** Assessment of communication disorders associated with inherited or congenital syndromes requires a thorough knowledge of the phenotype of each syndrome; in some cases, a diagnosis of a syndrome may have been made by other professionals, mostly medical professionals, before a speech-language pathologist evaluates the child or an adult for communication disorders; in many cases, an assessment of communication disorders may be part of the initial interdisciplinary assessment with a view to diagnose the syndrome, often in a child; detailed case history and interview; examination of the individual to establish the physical and behavioral features of the client; medical, dental, and neurological examinations; psychological evaluation; assessment of intellectual, sensory, educational, and communication functions; and various kinds of laboratory tests are all essential to diagnose genetic or congenital syndromes.

## Assessment of Syndromes: General Guidelines

- Use the Common/Standard Assessment Procedures; pay special attention to the orofacial examination, hearing screening, and audiological assessment
- **Case History** and the **Interview** are important initial steps in diagnosing a syndrome
- Obtain reports from other professionals before conducting an interview; parents themselves and the records may provide an initial diagnosis that may provide a framework for assessment; relevant interview questions can then be framed before the appointment
- Obtain detailed information on familial incidence of various clinical conditions; to facilitate this investigation, the clinician, at the time of scheduling an appointment, may ask the adult client or family members of a child client to find out whether any of their blood relatives have a similar clinical condition or have conditions that may be related to the problem to be assessed
- Concentrate on the following during the interview/history taking
  - Seek a clear and detailed description of the problems in the client's or parents' own language
  - Investigate the family background, including the family's ethnic, socioeconomic, educational, and occupational background
  - Investigate the family history of inheritable disorders; information should be obtained not only on the familial incidence of the specific clinical condition the client presents, but also on various related conditions that might be associated with genetic syndromes; for example, familial prevalence of cleft palate and other craniofacial anomalies, intellectual disabilities, hearing loss, congenital or acquired vision loss due to degenerative diseases, musculoskeletal problems, various neurological diseases, autism and other pervasive developmental disorders, cardiovascular diseases, kidney diseases, twinning and multiple births, high rate of infantile mortality, and so forth
  - Get detailed prenatal history; a detailed history of pregnancy is essential to understand the influence of teratogenic influences (e.g., drug abuse, alcoholism, excessive smoking, ingestion of harmful substances); mechanical forces that affect the fetal growth (accidental injury of the unborn); maternal infections, illnesses, vitamin deficiencies, and anemia; number of previous pregnancies, especially any history of spontaneous abortions, stillbirths, or infantile mortality; duration of pregnancy; medical and radiological treatment during pregnancy; and so forth
  - Get detailed information on perinatal history; information on the birth process is useful to evaluate any injury or distress that may play a role in creating the total clinical picture of the client; it is essential to know the duration of labor to assess prematurity; whether it was a cesarean, vaginal, or natural birth; use of local or general anesthesia; any complications and how they were handled, and so forth
  - Get detailed immediate postnatal history; information on the weight of the newborn; any need for special support; hospitalization of the baby; need to admit the baby to the newborn intensive care unit; when the baby was taken home; whether the baby had any feeding or sucking problems; and whether there was an initial failure to thrive, and so forth

  - Get a detailed developmental history; trace the child's development in all areas of concern, including physical, intellectual, and communication development; diseases and disabilities and their treatment or rehabilitation; seek information on the specific ages and stages of development and general health not only of the child to be assessed, but also of the siblings
- Work with a geneticist or genetic counselor who may construct a pedigree, which shows the pattern of inheritance in the family; this becomes a part of the client's medical records; if not involved in its development, consult the pedigree to understand the potential pattern of inheritance
- Examine the results of the client's karyotype—the result of a chromosomal analysis from a geneticist or cytogeneticist that shows a client's chromosomes and their abnormalities; karyotypes help identify specific chromosomal abnormalities that cause various genetic syndromes
- To assess communication disorders, use the assessment procedures described under Language Disorders in Children and Articulation and Phonological Disorders; administer selected tests described under these entries
- Use other procedures as found necessary (e.g., procedures described under Fluency Disorders: Stuttering, Voice Disorders, Cleft Palate, Hearing Impairment, Intellectual Disabilities, Cerebral Palsy, and Dysarthria)
- Obtain assessment reports from other professionals and work with the team serving the child
- Integrate your findings with those of the other specialists
- Make periodic assessments to document positive or negative changes

***Aicardi Syndrome.*** To assess this genetic syndrome with craniofacial anomalies including cleft lip and palate and central nervous system disorders:

### Review the Case History and Medical Records

- Establish from the case history and medical records a pattern of X-linked dominant inheritance
- Establish brain and corpus callosum abnormalities from the medical records
- Obtain evidence of intellectual disabilities from the case history and interview of family members

### Observe and Assess Physical and Behavioral Characteristics

- Assess cleft lip and palate that are a common feature of Aicardi syndrome
- Observe abnormalities of the choroid coating of the eye and the retina (chorioretinal lacunae) and rib and other skeletal abnormalities
- Assess signs of intellectual disabilities and the associated behavioral deficits

S

### Assess Speech, Language, and Hearing

- Rule out a possible conductive hearing loss due to middle ear infections associated with cleft palate
- Obtain an intellectual assessment report, which may document a severe disability

- Assess speech and language skills, which may be minimal or negligible, depending on the degree of intellectual disabilities; in most cases, the retardation is severe enough to prevent speech and language development
- Assess speech errors that may be comparable to those found in children with Cleft Palate and Intellectual Disabilities

***Alport Syndrome.*** A genetic syndrome that affects kidney functions and causes hearing loss and speech and language problems; also known as *hereditary nephritis*; the disease is more severe in males with a more rapidly progressing course.

#### Review the Case History and Medical Records

- Look for evidence of an autosomal dominant inheritance in most cases and X-linked inheritance in some cases
- Ascertain whether nephritis had begun in early childhood and whether kidney failure or need for transplant has been a concern
- Find out whether a bilateral sensorineural progressive hearing loss started around age 10

#### Observe and Assess Physical and Behavioral Characteristics

- Take note of current kidney problems
- Observe such ocular abnormalities as cataract and myopia that are present in some cases

#### Assess Speech, Language, and Hearing

- Assess articulation disorders; make periodic reassessments to document a progressive deterioration in articulatory skills, especially in males
- Screen hearing and recommend a complete audiological assessment to diagnose or rule out (the commonly found) bilateral, sensorineural, progressive hearing loss

***Angelman Syndrome.*** A genetic syndrome that affects more males than females, characterized by intellectual disabilities, unique facial features, and muscular disorders; genetic abnormality is similar to that found in Prader-Willi Syndrome; craniofacial and central nervous system abnormalities are common.

#### Review the Case History and Medical Records

- Ascertain whether a DNA analysis has been made to establish a deletion of DNA material on the long arm of chromosome 15 (15q11-q13)
- Obtain information on early feeding disorders and any evidence of impaired sleep patterns
- Ask the parents about their observation of congenital cranial abnormalities



#### Observe and Assess Physical and Behavioral Characteristics

- Assess feeding disorders in the case of infants
- Assess such physical characteristics as open-mouth posture with a protruded tongue, cranial abnormalities, including microcephaly, brachycephaly (*brachy* means short), and large mouth and chin

- Take note of any neurological disorders including seizures, progressive ataxia, hyperactive reflexes, and hypotonia during infancy
- Observe and record such behavioral deviations including uncontrolled outbursts of laughter, arm flapping, and severe intellectual disabilities with limited attention and social interaction

### Assess Speech, Language, and Hearing

- Obtain information on early speech and language development, which may be severely impaired
- Assess speech and language production and comprehension
- Note that there may be no significant hearing loss that explains the severe communication deficits (including comprehension deficits)
- Assess the voice, which may be limited to a few random vocalizations

*Apert Syndrome.* A genetic syndrome whose dysmorphology includes cranial Synostosis, Syndactyly of hands and feet, midfacial Hypoplasia, Strabismus, hearing loss, and speech problems; affects growth, nervous system, and craniofacial structures; also known as *acrocephalosyndactyly*.

### Review the Case History and Medical Records

- Ascertain any evidence for spontaneous autosomal dominant mutations and abnormalities on the long arm of chromosome 10
- Interview the parents about any congenital physical abnormalities associated with the syndrome
- Ask the parents about the early signs of intellectual disabilities

### Observe and Assess Physical and Behavioral Characteristics

- Assess such physical features as syndactyly (fusing of fingers, toes, or both, typically, second, third, and fourth digits may be fused); cranial synostosis resulting in a smaller anterior-posterior skull diameter, flat frontal and occipital bones, and high forehead; hydrocephalus; midfacial hypoplasia (incomplete development) with a small nose; low set and posteriorly rotated ears
- Assess oral structural abnormalities including a forward carriage of the tongue, an arched and grooved hard palate, thickened alveolar process, long or thickened soft palate, and cleft of the hard palate
- Assess malocclusion and dental abnormalities (a Class III malocclusion and irregularly placed teeth are common)
- Assess intellectual disabilities and attending behavioral deficits, including communication deficits

### Assess Speech, Language, and Hearing

- Assess feeding disorders
- Assess such resonance disorders as hyponasality and hypernasality associated with clefts and related oral-pharyngeal structural anomalies
- Assess such articulation, especially of alveolar or anteriorly produced consonants (e.g., /s/ and /z/) and labial dental sounds (e.g., /f/ and /v/)
- Assess language skills, which may be minimal in cases of severe intellectual disabilities

- Screen hearing and make a referral to an audiologist for an evaluation because of a high incidence of conductive hearing loss

***Ataxia-telangiectasia Syndrome.*** A neurodegenerative, autosomal recessive syndrome that results in death in the early 20s, although some survive into their early 40s; also known as *Louis-Bar syndrome*.

### Review the Case History and Medical Records

- Note that there may be no family history of the syndrome in many cases
- Establish from the detailed case history that there was a period of normal development of the child followed by significant degeneration in behavior and skills
- Review the medical records for a possible deficient immune system, leukemia, and Hodgkin's and non-Hodgkin's lymphoma that are present in many clients
- Ask questions about frequent infections of the upper and lower respiratory systems

### Observe and Assess Physical and Behavioral Characteristics

- Assess the physical features: a thin, drawn, and mask-like face with little expressiveness; any progressive cerebellar ataxia and dystonia; focal red lesions on the skin or on mucous membranes (telangiectasia), which begin to appear after the onset of ataxia
- Assess feeding disorders, often found in clients who have ataxia; assess especially disorders of mastication, drooling, and impaired oral-motor control

### Assess Speech, Language, and Hearing

- Assess arrested language development (which may be normal until age 3 years) and perhaps normal language comprehension; take note of normal hearing and normal intellectual development until infancy and early childhood years
- Assess dysarthric speech associated with cerebellar ataxia and dystonia; rate the speech intelligibility problem, which tends to increasingly worsen
- Assess such voice disorders as progressively worsening tremulous and weak voice
- Assess hypernasality, the main resonance disorder

***Beckwith-Wiedemann Syndrome.*** A syndrome that includes multiple anomalies and overgrowth (*gigantism syndrome*); speech and language impairments, craniofacial, gastrointestinal/abdominal, and central nervous system abnormalities characterize this syndrome.



### Review the Case History and Medical Records

- Look for evidence of an autosomal dominant pattern of inheritance
- Ascertain whether a gene defect on chromosome 11 (11p15) has been mapped
- Ask the parents about any early signs of hypotonia due to hypoglycemia

- Ascertain whether the child's development improves as hypoglycemia is treated
- Question the parents about overgrowth
- Ascertain from the interview and medical records about potential; ask the parents about gastrointestinal and abdominal abnormalities, umbilical hernia and enlarged liver, and tumors of the kidneys
- Ascertain the presence of chronic ear infections

### Observe and Assess Physical and Behavioral Characteristics

- Assess overgrowth of the body, which may have slowed down after puberty
- Assess orofacial structures and take note of a large mouth, large mandible (mandibular prognathism), unusually big tongue, and cleft palate or submucous cleft

### Assess Speech, Language, and Hearing

- Assess feeding difficulties due to the large tongue (macroglossia) and hypotonia
- Screen hearing and refer the child to an audiologist to rule out conductive hearing loss, commonly found in children with cleft palate
- Assess speech disorders including the frequent distortions of speech sounds; assess such compensatory articulation as the production of glottal stop substitutions, pharyngeal fricatives, and pharyngeal stops associated with cleft palate; take note of any fronting errors due to the large and protruding tongue
- Assess language disorders and delayed language development in cases of intellectual deficiency associated with the syndrome
- Evaluate voice disorders including hoarseness, hypernasality, and hyponasality

***Binder Syndrome.*** A genetic syndrome characterized by midfacial retrusion (backward positioning or movement of the mandible) and speech disorders; also known as *maxillonasal dysplasia.*

### Review the Case History and Medical Records

- Establish early signs of speech delay and disorders
- May not be possible to establish a pattern of inheritance for this syndrome
- Ask the parents about lack of maxillary growth after the childhood years

### Observe and Assess Physical and Behhavioral Characteristics

- Observe and record such craniofacial features as a flat facial profile (midface deficiency), lack of growth in the maxilla from the childhood years on, mandibular prognathism, short nose, and short anterior cranial base
- Assess possibly impaired chewing activity

### Assess Speech, Language, and Hearing

- Assess speech disorders, especially distortion of anteriorly produced speech sounds, especially lingua-alveolar and lingua-dental sounds
- Assess possible compensatory bilabial sound productions (contact between the upper teeth and lower lip)

- Note that language disorders, hearing disorders, or voice disorders may not be significant
- Assess possible hyponasality

***Bronchio-Oto-Renal Syndrome.*** A genetic syndrome characterized by malformations of the auricle, bronchial fistulas or cysts, and abnormalities of the kidneys; also known as *Melnick-Fraser syndrome*; a relatively common syndrome of multiple anomalies, hearing loss, and resulting speech-language problems.

#### Review the Case History and Medical Records

- Review medical and laboratory test evidence of autosomal dominant inheritance, abnormalities on the long arm of chromosome 8 (8q13.3), and highly varied expression in different individuals
- Check medical records for bronchial fistulas or cysts and kidney problems

#### Observe and Assess Physical and Behavioral Characteristics

- Observe and record auditory anomalies, including such outer ear anomalies as easily visible preauricular pits, narrow or malformed external auditory canal, displaced or malformed auditory ossicles, fused or unconnected stapes, and hypoplastic apex of the cochlea
- Assess craniofacial anomalies including cleft palate (submucous variety) and varieties of malocclusion

#### Assess Speech, Language, and Hearing

- Screen hearing and refer the client for audiological evaluation to diagnose a possible conductive, sensorineural, or mixed hearing loss
- Assess articulation disorders, mainly distortions and substitutions, typically associated with hearing loss, cleft palate (when present), and severe forms of malocclusions of the dental arches
- Assess language disorders of the kind associated with hearing loss
- Assess resonance disorders associated with hearing loss and submucous cleft palate

***Cat Eye Syndrome.*** Also known as *chromosome 22 partial tetrasomy* and *Schmid-Fraccaro syndrome,* the cat eye syndrome is so named because of the iris coloboma (any defect of the eye or iris) that is a dominant feature of this syndrome; speech, language, and hearing disorders are parts of this syndrome.

#### Review the Case History and Medical Records

- Review medical records for any evidence of genetic abnormality on chromosome 22 (q11) in the form of extra chromosome material
- Ask the parents about the iris coloboma and when they noticed it
- Ascertain whether the infant had early feeding disorders
- Ascertain whether a medical diagnosis of cardiac abnormalities or kidney diseases has been made

#### Observe and Assess Physical and Behavioral Characteristics

- Observe and take note of iris coloboma, the most distinguishing feature
- Observe other physical features, including small protuberant ears with preauricular tags or pits

### Assess Speech, Language, and Hearing

- Assess feeding disorders, a consequence of hypotonia
- Assess speech development and speech sound production; assess compensatory articulation associated with cleft palate, found in a quarter of the children
- Screen hearing loss and refer to an audiologist for a possible mild conductive hearing loss, probably due to middle ear infections in children with cleft palate and ear anomalies
- Assess language disorders that may be the kind associated with potential intellectual impairment
- Assess such resonance disorders as hypernasality

***CHARGE Association.*** A syndrome of multiple anomalies, CHARGE is an acronym for **C**oloboma, **H**eart anomalies, **A**tresia choanae, **R**etarded growth, **G**enital hypoplasia, and **E**ar anomalies; a consistent pattern of expression across individuals has not been identified; speech, language, and hearing may all be affected.

### Review the Case History and Medical Records

- Ascertain whether an autosomal dominant pattern can be established, although in most cases, the occurrence may be sporadic
- Ask the parents about early feeding disorders, congenital heart problems, and retarded physical growth

### Observe and Assess Physical and Behavioral Characteristics

- Assess feeding disorders and a failure to thrive
- Observe and record choanal atresia (abnormal opening of the nasal cavity into the nasopharynx on either side, causing feeding disorders)
- Ascertain evidence of intellectual dysfunctions or obtain intelligence test reports
- Observe and record craniofacial and ocular anomalies, including facial paresis, microcephaly, and low-set, posteriorly rotated ears; protuberant eyes; cleft palate; cleft lip in a few cases, and micrognathia, abnormalities of the iris, choroid, retina, and optic nerve coloboma
- Take note of any retarded physical growth, resulting in a short stature
- Assess behavioral characteristics associated with intellectual impairment

### Assess Speech, Language, and Hearing

- Assess feeding disorders
- Assess articulation disorders; take note of errors commonly associated with hearing loss and other craniofacial abnormalities
- Assess language disorders; take note of extremely limited language in many cases
- Assess hoarseness as the dominant voice disorder
- Have the child's hearing assessed because all kinds of hearing impairments, including conductive, sensorineural, and mixed types, may be evident in most cases



***Cornelia de Lange Syndrome.*** A congenital syndrome characterized by microcephaly, intellectual disabilities, and severe speech and language problems; also known as *de Lange syndrome* and *Brachman-de Lange syndrome*.

### Review the Case History and Medical Records

- Interview the parents about the retarded physical growth of the child
- Ask the parents about excessive hair growth on the forehead and neck
- Take note of any unclear or varied genetic basis of the syndrome
- Obtain details on the early signs of intellectual disabilities and speech and language delay
- Chromosomal abnormalities may be observed in a few cases

### Observe and Assess Physical and Behavioral Characteristics

- Take note of any retarded physical growth
- Observe and record other physical characteristics including brachycephaly (shortness of the head); such auricle anomalies as low-set ears; bushy eyebrows; coarse, shaggy, and excessive hair growth on the forehead and neck; webbed neck; small nose; upward-tilted nares; down-turned upper lip; and flat hands with short and tapering fingers
- Observe and record behavioral characteristics of severe intellectual disabilities

### Assess Speech, Language, and Hearing

- Screen hearing and refer the child to an audiologist to diagnose a potential sensorineural hearing loss
- Assess articulation disorders, which may be severe
- Assess language disorders associated with intellectual disabilities and behavioral deficits; language disorder may be severe in many cases
- Assess voice disorders, especially hoarseness

***Cri du Chat Syndrome.*** An autosomal chromosome disorder that tends to be associated with intellectual disabilities, cleft palate, hearing impairment, communication deficits, and a distinctive cry that resembles that of a cat (hence the name); the characteristic cry, however, is not heard in all children with this syndrome.

### Review the Case History and Medical Records

- Ascertain whether an absence of a part of the short arm of chromosome 5 (5p15.2) or its complete deletion has been established
- Ask the parents about any early feeding problems and failure to thrive (more likely in cases of clefts)
- Obtain information on early signs of such neurological disorders as hypotonia or hypertonia and hyperflexia

### Observe and Assess Physical and Behavioral Characteristics

- Assess hypotonia, hypertonia, and hyperreflexia
- Observe and record such physical characteristics as microcephaly, cerebral asymmetry, retrognathia, cleft palate, cleft lip, low set, posteriorly rotated ears, narrow oral cavity, and small hands and feet
- Take note of any laryngeal hypoplasia
- Assess the behavioral characteristics of intellectual deficiencies

### Assess Speech, Language, and Hearing

- Assess a high-pitched cry if it still persists
- Assess severe articulation disorders, compounded by the frequent presence of cleft palate and cleft lip
- Assess language development, which tends to be severely limited; may be absent in cases of severe intellectual deficiencies

***Crouzon Syndrome.*** A genetic syndrome characterized by cranial and midface abnormalities, ocular hypertelorism, strabismus, hearing loss, and speech and language problems.

### Review the Case History and Medical Records

- Ascertain whether an autosomal dominant pattern of inheritance or abnormality of a gene (FGFR2, fibroblast growth factor receptor 2) located on the long arm of chromosome 10 has been documented
- Take note that the phenotype of the syndrome is highly varied
- Ask the parents about any early signs of intellectual deficiencies

### Observe and Assess Physical and Behavioral Characteristics

- Observe and record such craniofacial abnormalities due to craniosynostosis (fusion of the cranial suture, especially that of the coronal sutures); hypoplasia of the midface, maxilla, or both; ocular hypertelorism (bulging eyes that are set far apart); small maxillary structure (maxillary hypoplasia); facial asymmetry; malocclusion Class II; highly arched palate; shallow oropharynx; long and thick soft palate; short front-to-back cranial diameter (brachycephaly), and "parrot-like" nose
- Assess such neurological symptoms as headaches and ataxia, possibly due to increased intracranial pressure
- Assess cognitive or intellectual deficiencies

### Assess Speech, Language, and Hearing

- Screen hearing and have the child assessed for hearing impairment, especially a common conductive hearing loss
- Assess articulation disorders associated with hearing loss palatal abnormalities
- Assess such resonance disorders as hyponasality
- Assess language disorders that may be a function of hearing loss and cognitive deficits

***Down Syndrome.*** A common genetic syndrome associated with varying degrees of intellectual disabilities; also known as *trisomy 21*; speech and language disorders consistent with the degree of intellectual deficits and the severity of hearing loss that is commonly associated with the syndrome.



### Review the Case History and Medical Records

- Ascertain whether an extra whole number chromosome 21, resulting in 47, rather than the normal 46, chromosomes has been established
- Ascertain the maternal age at which the child was delivered; the risk of trisomy 21 increases with advanced maternal age
- Be aware that people with Down syndrome are predisposed to Alzheimer's Disease

- Take detailed information on early motor and speech and language development and signs of intellectual deficits
- Look for possible diagnosis of cardiac malformations

### Observe and Assess Physical and Behavioral Characteristics

- Observe and record such craniofacial abnormalities as Brachycephaly (short front-to-back cephalic dimension), microcephaly, maxillary hypoplasia, midface Dysplasia, flat facial profile, small ears, small nose, small chin, malocclusion, epicanthal folds, short neck with excess skin on the back of it, obesity, small stature, short fingers and toes (*brachydactyly*), and permanently deflected fingers (*clinodactyly*)
- Assess abnormalities of the oral and pharyngeal structures that may include shortened oral and pharyngeal cavities, narrow and high arched palate, relatively large and fissured tongue that tends to protrude, and dental anomalies
- Assess early feeding difficulties
- Assess behavioral signs of intellectual disabilities
- Assess cleft palate found in some children

### Assess Speech, Language, and Hearing

- Screen hearing and get an audiological evaluation of the child to rule out conductive hearing loss, sensorineural hearing loss, or mixed hearing loss
- Assess the numerous articulation disorders, especially distortions, a general slurring of speech, and an increased speech rate; judge the speech unintelligibility
- Assess language disorders and compare their better vocabulary with severely impaired morphological and syntactic skills
- Assess fluency disorders, especially stuttering, which is often associated with Down syndrome
- Assess hypernasality, nasal emission, hoarseness, breathier voice, and lower pitch

***Dysautonomia.*** Also known as *Riley-Day syndrome*, a genetic syndrome characterized by an impaired autonomic nervous system; its incidence is limited to Ashkenazi Jews from Eastern Europe.

### Review the Case History and Medical Records

- Establish the ethnocultural background of the child with this syndrome (Ashkenazi Jews from Eastern Europe)
- Ascertain whether the specific gene defect located on chromosome 9 (9q31-q33) has been mapped
- Take a careful family history
- Ask the parents about any early feeding problems, aspiration, and vomiting; check the records or the parents for aspiration pneumonia

S

### Observe and Assess Physical and Behavioral Characteristics

- Assess the early feeding problems and associated difficulties
- Assess or ascertain from medical reports such neurological disorders as hypotonia, hypothermia (low body temperature), syncopy (fainting episodes), absence of reflexes, ataxia, and low blood pressure

### Assess Speech, Language, and Hearing

- Assess articulation disorders, including symptoms of dysarthria and hypernasality
- Screen hearing, although hearing loss is not a significant part of the syndrome
- Assess voice and prosodic disorders; listen especially for a monotone vocal quality
- Assess language disorders that are likely to appear along with neurological disorders; take note of normal early language development

***Ectrodactyly-Ectodermal Dysplasia-Clefting Syndrome (EEC Syndrome).*** A genetic syndrome of multiple anomalies that affects the development of ectodermal and mesodermal tissue; associated with clefts of the lip and palate with infrequent occurrence of intellectual disabilities.

### Review the Case History and Medical Records

- Establish an autosomal dominant inheritance pattern with variable and sometimes incomplete expression
- Check the medical records to see whether abnormalities on chromosome 7 (7q11.2-q21.3) have been diagnosed
- Check the medical records for evidence of absent sweat glands that predispose the individual to heat strokes

### Observe and Assess Physical and Behavioral Characteristics

- Observe and record the congenital absence of fingers and toes (Ectrodactyly), and Ectodermal Dysplasia (sparse and brittle hair and scanty eyebrows, absence of eyelashes, and dystrophied nails)
- Assess cleft lip and palate (more common than cleft lip alone); check the hands and feet for clefts
- Take note of such craniofacial anomalies as microcephaly, maxillary hypoplasia, choanal atresia, missing or malformed teeth, or other craniofacial features
- Assess behavioral and language signs of intellectual disabilities, which may be observed but only in a few cases

### Assess Speech, Language, and Hearing

- Assess feeding problems
- Screen hearing and refer the child to an audiologist for a diagnosis of moderate conductive hearing loss in some cases
- Assess articulation disorders, especially distortions and lingual protrusions; assess compensatory articulatory strategies associated with cleft palate
- Assess hoarseness of voice and hypernasality
- Assess delayed language acquisition and disorders and relate them to the degree of hearing loss and intellectual disabilities, if present

S

***Fetal Alcohol Syndrome (FAS).*** A congenital syndrome (not genetically inherited) in which the prenatal and postnatal growth is affected by the toxic effects maternal alcoholism during pregnancy had on the embryo; associated with physical abnormalities, intellectual disabilities, and speech and language problems.

### Review the Case History and Medical Records

- Establish maternal alcoholism during pregnancy
- Seek information on the frequency and duration of drinking, and the embryonic stage at which the abuse was intensive
- Ask the parents about the low birth weight and early feeding problems—the two initial signs of the syndrome
- Check medical records about heart anomalies and kidney disorders

### Observe and Assess Physical and Behavioral Characteristics

- Assess feeding disorders, mainly due to hypotonia and micrognathia
- Assess or take note of craniofacial anomalies including Microcephaly, Maxillary Hypoplasia, posterior rotation of the ears, prominent forehead and mandible, short palpebral (eyelid) fissures, thin upper lip, epicanthal folds, small eyes, small teeth with faulty enamel, and cleft palate, cleft lip, or both
- Take note of severe growth retardation, especially nail growth problems and small hands and feet
- Assess the behavioral and speech and language characteristics of the intellectual deficiencies
- Get reports on the child's potential learning disabilities

### Assess Speech, Language, and Hearing

- Screen hearing for a potential conductive hearing loss
- Assess articulation disorders; assess aggravated speech and resonance problems and compensatory articulation if clefts are or have been repaired
- Assess language disorders including deficits in the syntactic, semantic, and pragmatic aspects of language
- Assess limited fluency, partly because of their limited language skills
- Assess voice problems, especially hoarseness and hypernasality

***Fragile X Syndrome.*** An X-linked genetic syndrome caused by a chromosomal abnormality; also known as *X-linked mental retardation* and *Martin-Bell syndrome*; associated with intellectual disabilities.

### Review the Case History and Medical Records

- Ascertain whether an X-linked inheritance pattern and the defective gene's location (Xq27.3) have been mapped

### Observe and Assess Physical and Behavioral Characteristics

- Observe and record the physical features, which include a large, long, and poorly formed pinna; and a big jaw, high forehead, mandibular prognathism, thick lips, macrocephaly, dental abnormalities, and submucous cleft in some cases
- Assess behavioral and speech and language characteristics associated with intellectual deficiencies

#### Assess Speech, Language, and Hearing

- Screen hearing, although hearing loss is not a characteristic of the syndrome
- Assess language production (resembling the language characteristics of children with autism), which may be filled with jargon, perseveration, echolalia, telegraphic utterances, inappropriate and irrelevant language, and self-talking in a low monotonous voice; note their predominance in male rather than female children
- Take note of lack of verbal expression in some; in such cases, assess their nonverbal communication skills; note that the lack of nonverbal means of communication that normally accompany speech is a characteristic of the syndrome
- Assess voice problems, including an occasional hoarseness or a high-pitched voice
- Assess articulation disorders and relate them to the various craniofacial anomalies; assess compensatory articulation that may be associated with cleft palate
- Assess fluency disorders and take note that features similar to those found in Cluttering may be found in persons with fragile X syndrome
- Assess motor speech disorders (Apraxia of Speech and Dysarthria)

***Goldenhar Syndrome.*** A genetic syndrome characterized by oculo-auriculo-vertebral dysplasia; rarely associated with intellectual disabilities.

#### Review the Case History and Medical Records

- Note that a family history of the disorder may be missing because it is of sporadic occurrence, although when a parent is affected, autosomal dominant inheritance is suspected
- Ask the parents about any early feeding problems; check the medical records for diagnosed congenital heart and kidney diseases

#### Observe and Assess Physical and Behavioral Characteristics

- Observe and record such craniofacial anomalies as an underdeveloped mandible; hypoplastic or dysfunctional facial, masticatory, and palatal muscles; cleft-like lateral extension of the mouth; high-arched palate, cleft palate, cleft lip, and unilateral hypoplasia of the pharynx or palate; Microtia and Preauricular Tags; clefts of the eyelids or orbits, microphthalmia, strabismus, and clefts of the eyelids or orbits
- Assess feeding disorders
- Observe and record cervical spine anomalies, spina bifida, club foot, and other limb anomalies
- Assess cognitive impairments and resulting behavioral deficiencies that may be present in a few children



#### Assess Speech, Language, and Hearing

- Screen hearing loss and refer the child for audiological assessment because a conductive hearing loss (more common) or sensorineural loss (in a few children) may need to be diagnosed
- Assess delayed speech onset and disorders of articulation, especially distortions and substitutions; relate them to noted craniofacial abnormalities, including the clefts of the palate

- Assess resonance problems typically associated with palatal clefts; assess hypernasality
- Assess voice disorders, including hoarse or breathy voice, partly due to the unilateral vocal fold paresis
- Assess any associated language problems

***Laurence-Moon Syndrome.*** A genetic syndrome characterized by retinitis pigmentosa, hypogonadism, obesity, and intellectual disabilities; previously also known as *Laurence-Moon-Biedl syndrome, Bardet-Biedl syndrome*, and *Laurence-Moon-Bardet-Biedl syndrome*; however, four subtypes of Bardet-Biedl syndromes have been recognized and are now considered separate from Laurence-Moon syndrome; polydactyly, a feature of Bardet-Biedl syndromes, is absent in Laurence-Moon syndrome; the latter is associated with spastic paraplegia, which is absent in the former four types.

### Review the History and Medical Records

- Note that a specific gene abnormality or definite pattern of inheritance has been established
- Ask the parents about early neurological symptoms (spastic paraplegia and hypotonia)

### Observe and Assess Physical and Behavioral Characteristics

- Observe, assess, and record spastic paraplegia, hypotonia, and obesity due to endocrine disorders
- Ascertain vision problems due to retinitis pigmentosa and initial difficulty in night vision
- Ascertain information on retarded sexual development (hypogonadism)
- Assess intellectual deficits and associated behavioral limitations
- Assess motor control problems due to neurological involvement

### Assess Speech, Language, and Hearing

- Screen for hearing loss and refer to an audiologist when warranted
- Assess speech onset and articulation disorders that are significant; relate the speech production problems to hypotonia and intellectual deficits
- Assess language disorders that are typical of children with intellectual deficits
- Assess potential hypernasality and breathy voice

***Moebius Syndrome.*** Also spelled as *Möbius* syndrome, a genetic syndrome characterized by congenital bilateral facial palsy; mild intellectual disabilities in 10% to 15% of the affected individuals, occasional hearing loss, articulation disorders, and some language problems; it is a rare genetic disorder.



### Review the Case History and Medical Records

- Note that no specific gene abnormality has been identified
- Note that the main neuropathology is Agenesis or Aplasia of the motor nuclei of the cranial nerves
- Ascertain early neurological signs of the syndrome and early feeding disorders

### Observe and Assess Physical and Behavioral Characteristics

- Observe and record paralysis of the facial and eye muscles and tongue weakness
- Assess feeding problems, aspiration, choking, and drooling
- Conduct a thorough orofacial examination to document bilabial paresis and weak tongue control for lateralization, elevation, depression, and protrusion; take note of a short or deformed tongue; assess the strength, range, and speed of articulatory movements
- Observe and record such ocular problems as unilateral or bilateral paralysis of the abductors of the eyes, eyelids that may not fully close, lack of blinking and lateral eye movements, strabismus that may be surgically corrected, and eye sensitivity to light (due to lack of blinking)
- Assess difficulty expressing emotions through such facial expressions as smiling and frowning; take note of the child's mask-like face
- Assess a high palate, submucous cleft palate, and abnormal dentition
- Assess behavioral limitations associated with intellectual deficiencies

### Assess Speech, Language, and Hearing

- Screen hearing, although hearing loss is not a characteristic of the syndrome
- Assess dysarthria; pay special attention to bilabial, linguadental, and lingua alveolar sound productions
- Assess delayed language and language disorders; pay special attention to language development in children with frequent hospitalization and intellectual deficiencies

***Mohr Syndrome.*** A genetic syndrome characterized by cranial, facial, lingual, palatal, and digital anomalies; a subtype of a large group of syndromes called *oral-facial-digital syndromes* with differing etiologies; Mohr syndrome is classified as *oral-facial-digital syndrome type II*; the syndrome affects craniofacial structures and limbs along with the central nervous system.

### Review the Case History and Medical Records

- See whether you can establish an autosomal recessive pattern of inheritance through the case history
- Interview the parents about any congenital craniofacial anomalies

### Observe and Assess Physical and Behavioral Characteristics

- Observe and record abnormalities of the extremities including shortness of fingers and toes (brachydactyly); deflected fingers (clinodactyly); supernumerary toes or fingers (polydactyly), often a bilateral reduplication of the big toe (hallux); and fused fingers or toes (syndactyly)
- Observe and record cranial and orofacial abnormalities including midline partial tongue cleft, lobate tongue with nodules, midline cleft lip, cleft palate, broad or bifid nasal tip, mandibular hypoplasia, and external auditory canal atresia
- Assess the behavioral deficits associated with intellectual disabilities (if evident)

S

### Assess Speech, Language, and Hearing

- Screen hearing and refer to an audiologist for a complete evaluation

- Assess delayed speech and articulation disorders that may be a result of a combination of intellectual disabilities, hearing loss, lingual anomalies, and cleft lip and palate
- Assess language delay and disorders

***Mucopolysaccharidoses (MPS) Syndromes.*** A group of syndromes characterized by a metabolic disorder; excessive storage of complex carbohydrates in the body, due to a lack of enzymes that break down mucopolysaccharides (sugar molecules), leads to their excessive accumulation in the systems; causes progressive intellectual disabilities, clouding of the corneas, skeletal dysplasia, thick coarse hair and bushy eyebrows, hearing loss, large tongue, anomalies of the hand, flat nasal bridge, and Hypertelorism; varieties include Hunter syndrome, Hurler syndrome, Maroteau-Lamy syndrome, Morquio syndrome, Sanfilippo syndrome, and Scheie syndrome; the syndrome is known for its extremely variable clinical expression.

### Review the Case History and Medical Records

- Check whether autosomal recessive inheritance patterns can be established for all varieties of MPS syndromes except for Hunter syndrome
- Check whether an X-linked recessive inheritance pattern can be established for Hunter syndrome

### Assess Physical, Behavioral, and Communication Problems

- ***Hunter Syndrome:*** Assess symptoms that are less severe than those found in children with Hurler syndrome; generally:
  - Assess and record corneal clouding; slower progression of symptoms
  - Screen hearing loss and refer the child to an audiologist
  - Assess feeding and swallowing problems that become evident in later childhood
  - Assess speech disorders associated with oral and cranial abnormalities
  - Establish an initially normal language development and language disorders in later childhood when the progression is stopped
  - Assess such voice characteristics as chronic wet hoarseness and hyponasality
- ***Hurler Syndrome:*** The most severe of the MPS syndromes; also called *MPS Type I*; generally:
  - Assess or observe and record coarse facial features, clouded corneas, skeletal dysplasia, thick coarse hair, enlargement of viscera, and bushy eyebrows; anomalies of the middle ear; thick lips, large tongue, thickened palate and alveolar ridge, and depressed nasal bridge; short fingers and short broad hands; short neck and trunk; thickened and stiff joints; severe and progressive intellectual deterioration
  - Screen hearing and refer the child to an audiologist for a complete assessment of a potential conductive hearing loss
  - Review medical records for heart anomalies, enlarged liver, and the spleen
  - Assess speech development, which may be severely limited; assess severe articulation disorders associated with the syndrome
  - Assess language skills, which may be extremely limited
  - Assess such voice disorders as hoarseness and hyponasality

- ***Maroteaux-Lamy Syndrome:*** This syndrome is similar to Hurler syndrome except for normal or near-normal intelligence; generally:
    - Note that the mild forms are similar to Scheie syndrome
    - Take note of chronic otitis media and conductive or sensorineural hearing impairment
    - Assess articulation disorders that may be due to tongue enlargement and alveolar ridge abnormalities
    - Screen language skills that may be normal or nearly so; assess when warranted
    - Assess hyponasality and hoarseness
- ***Morquio Syndrome:*** Also called *MPS Type IV*; abnormalities are found on chromosome 16; the most distinguishing feature of this syndrome is dwarfism due to bone dysplasia; generally:
    - Observe and record hip dysplasia, short neck and trunk; dwarfism; extremely mild corneal clouding
    - Review medical records for evidence of liver and heart anomalies
    - Screen hearing and refer the child to an audiologist for diagnosing a progressive and mixed or sensorineural hearing loss
    - Screen speech and language skills that may be within normal limits; assess when warranted
    - Assess high-pitched hoarse voice and hyponasality
- ***Sanfilippo Syndrome:*** Also called *MPS Type III*; this syndrome is similar to Hurler syndrome, though with milder somatic symptoms; generally:
    - Observe and record an enlarged head, somewhat aggressive behavior, and rapid mental deterioration resulting in dementia
    - Screen hearing impairment and refer the child to an audiologist when warranted
    - Assess speech and language skills that may be initially normal but follow the same rapid course of deterioration as the intellectual skills
- ***Scheie Syndrome:*** A milder form of Hurler syndrome; hence, difficult to diagnose before age six; generally:
    - Take note of near normal intellectual skills because significant intellectual disabilities are not found in this syndrome
    - Take note of normal physical stature and life expectancy
    - Screen hearing because hearing impairment may be found in 20% of the cases
    - Assess as you would the children with Hurler syndrome.

**Noonan Syndrome.** Also known as *pterygium coli syndrome*, characterized by neck webbing; a genetic syndrome with congenital heart disease, facial and skeletal anomalies, cryptorchidism, and intellectual disabilities in 50% to 60% of the cases; physically, children with Noonan syndrome resemble those with Turner syndrome, although etiologically the two are different; Turner syndrome is found only in females and is due to chromosome X abnormalities; Noonan syndrome is not related to sex chromosome abnormalities and occurs in both males and females.

### Review the History and Medical Records

- See whether an Autosomal Dominant inheritance pattern can be established
- Ask parents about congenital heart problems and examine the medical records for their diagnosis
- Question the parents about early feeding problems

### Observe and Assess Physical and Behavioral Characteristics

- Observe and record such craniofacial abnormalities as the webbing of the neck (pterygium), a triangular facial shape, a deeply furrowed philtrum, generally narrow growth of the face, malocclusion, constricted maxillary arch, low-set and posteriorly rotated ears, down-slanting eyes, epicanthal folds, open-bite, short stature, shield-shaped chest, and an occasional cleft palate
- Examine medical records that may have documented genitourinary deficiencies including Hypertelorsim, Ptosis of the eyelids, cryptorchidism, and male infertility
- Assess intellectual and behavioral deficiencies including perceptual problems and learning disabilities; note that some individuals with Noonan syndrome may be normal or above normal in intelligence

### Assess Speech, Language, and Hearing

- Screen hearing and refer the child to an audiologist for a possible diagnosis of conductive or sensorineural hearing loss, though they are not characteristic of the syndrome
- Assess articulation problems that are typically associated with maxillary abnormalities
- Assess whether a submucous cleft exists, and, if it does, assess any compensatory articulation of speech sounds
- Assess delayed language development and limited expressive language skills associated with limited intelligence
- Compare spoken language skills with language comprehension; the latter may be better
- Assess an occasional high-pitched voice and hypernasality associated with a submucous cleft

***Oral-Facial-Digital (OFD) Syndromes.*** Eight varieties of genetic disorders with different etiological factors are grouped under this common name; all share certain common characteristics, although different varieties have somewhat different involvement; the syndrome is characterized by cranial, facial, lingual, palatal, and digital anomalies; also called *Mohr syndrome*.

### Review the Case History and Medical Records

- Take note of varied etiological factors; see the sources cited at the end of this main entry and the companion volume, *Hegde's PocketGuide to Communication Disorders* for details
- See whether known patterns of inheritance may be established for each variety of this syndrome

- Ask the parents about any early feeding problems
- Check medical records for a diagnosis of any kidney diseases

### Observe and Assess Physical and Behavioral Characteristics

- Assess feeding disorders in children with all subtypes of OFD
- Observe and take note of any limb abnormalities, especially polydactyly in all OFD variations
- Take note of corpus callosum and cognitive impairments in all subtypes except for OFD5
- Assess midline cleft of the upper lip or just a notch in children with OFD1, OFD5, and OFD7
- Assess cleft palate with or without cleft lip in children with OFD4, OFD6, and OFD7
- Assess midline partial tongue cleft and lobate tongue with nodules in most subtypes

### Assess Speech, Language, and Hearing

- Screen hearing loss and refer the child to an audiologist for an assessment of conductive hearing loss associated with OFD1 and OFD4
- Assess speech onset and speech sound acquisition, which may be delayed in all subtypes of OFD
- Assess dysarthria in OFD1
- Screen for language disorders and assess a possible language disorder especially when intellectual deficiencies are present; note that the disorders may be severe in all subtypes except for OFD5; some children may never develop functional communication skills.
- Assess hypernasality if cleft palate is part of the symptom complex; more likely to occur in OFD1, OFD4, and OFD6.

***Otopalatodigital Syndromes.*** A genetic syndrome characterized by otological, palatal, and digital anomalies; associated with cleft palate, hearing loss, and mild intellectual disabilities; two types of otopalatodigital syndromes have been identified, although the symptoms associated with the two types are quite different; both are summarized in this single entry.

### Review the Case History and Medical Records

- Ascertain whether an X-linked recessive inheritance pattern can be established for both types of this syndrome
- Ascertain from the parents any early feeding disorders and signs of intellectual deficits

### Observe and Assess Physical and Behavioral Characteristics

- To assess otopalatodigital syndrome Type I:
  - Observe and record cleft palate, micrognathia, malocclusion, hypertelorism, broad nasal root, widely spaced toes, short fingers, short and broad fingertips, short fingernails, small stature, hypodontia, and congenital malformations of the ossicular chain
  - Assess feeding disorders
  - Assess mental intellectual deficits and associated behavioral deficits

- To assess otopalatodigital syndrome Type II:
  - Observe and record extremely small oral and pharyngeal cavities, cleft palate, maxillary and mandibular hypoplasia, hypertelorism, broad and high forehead, syndactyly, clinodactyly, bowed limbs, and narrow chest
  - Assess feeding disorders
  - Take note of hydrocephalus and intellectual disabilities in some cases

### Assess Speech, Language, and Hearing

- Assess speech, language, and hearing characteristics of children with otopalatodigital syndrome Type I:
  - Screen hearing and have the child evaluated for a bilateral conductive hearing loss, possibly due to otitis media
  - Assess delayed speech onset and articulation disorders
  - Assess compensatory articulation and hypernasality due to cleft palate
  - Assess delayed language and language disorders associated with intellectual deficits
- Assess speech, language, and hearing characteristics of children with otopalatodigital syndrome Type II:
  - Screen hearing and have the child evaluated for potential conductive hearing loss
  - Assess articulation disorders that are often more severe than those found in Type I; note that because of the extremely small oral and pharyngeal cavities, the place of articulation for most sounds may be shifted to the posterior parts of the mouth
  - Assess hypernasality and muffled resonance
  - Assess language disorders and in greater detail if intellectual deficits are evident

***Pendred Syndrome.*** A genetic syndrome characterized by congenital, bilateral, and sensorineural hearing loss and Goiter in middle childhood; intellectual disabilities in some cases; due to thyroid gland abnormality and a major cause of congenital deafness.

### Review the Case History and Medical Records

- Review the case history to possibly establish a pattern of autosomal recessive inheritance
- Ascertain whether goiter has been diagnosed
- Question the parents about any hearing loss

### Observe and Assess Physical and Behavioral Characteristics

- Through the case history and medical records, document enlarged thyroid (goiter) and possibly hypothyroidism in early years
- Take note of the delayed skeletal maturation as the child grows older



### Assess Speech, Language, and Hearing

- Screen hearing and get a complete audiological assessment to diagnose bilateral, mild to profound sensorineural hearing loss; schedule periodic hearing assessments because the loss may be progressive

- Assess language learning and disorders; take note of the often severe delay in language acquisition; relate the severity of language disorders to the severity of the hearing loss
- Assess errors of articulation, which may be significant; relate the articulation errors to the hearing impairment in the child

***Pierre-Robin Syndrome.*** A controversial genetic syndrome characterized by Mandibular Hypoplasia, Glossoptosis, and cleft of the soft palate; some do not consider it a separate syndrome; instead, they describe it as the Robin sequence; features of this syndrome (technically, the Robin sequence) may be found in several other syndromes, including Stickler Syndrome, Treacher Collins Syndrome, and Velo-Cardio-Facial Syndrome; there is much variability in its diagnosis.

### Review the Case History and Conduct an Interview

- Ascertain from the case history and medical records whether a pattern of Autosomal Recessive inheritance can be established
- Evaluate the possibility of Autosomal Dominant inheritance if the features are a part of Stickler Syndrome
- Take note of the possibility of sporadic occurrence
- Check history for maternal drug use or mechanical disruption of the embryonic growth

### Observe and Assess Physical and Behavioral Characteristics

- Observe and record such craniofacial anomalies as Mandibular Hypoplasia, Glossoptosis (downward displacement of the tongue), cleft of the soft palate in most cases (typically without cleft lip), velopharyngeal incompetence due to the soft palate cleft, dental abnormalities, deformed pinna, low-set ears, and temporal bone and ossicular chain deformities
- Assess early feeding difficulties and failure to thrive because of the tongue placement that may create breathing difficulties, apnea, and dysphagia; check for vomiting
- Assess behavioral and communicative impairments that might suggest intellectual impairment

### Assess Speech, Language, and Hearing

- Screen hearing and obtain a complete audiological evaluation to diagnose a possible unilateral or bilateral conductive hearing loss associated with otitis media and cleft palate
- Assess delayed language and language disorders and relate them to the hearing loss and possibly to intellectual impairment
- Assess voice and resonance characteristics to rule out hypernasality and nasal emission due to the velopharyngeal incompetence associated with the cleft of the soft palate
- Assess articulation disorders and compensatory articulation as likely consequences of the cleft



***Prader-Willi Syndrome.*** A genetic syndrome characterized by Hypotonia, slow motor development, small hands and feet, underdeveloped genitals, almond-shaped eyes, obesity due to insatiable appetite, and intellectual deficiencies in most but not all cases; genetically, but not phenotypically, somewhat related to Angelman Syndrome.

### Review the Case History and Medical Records

- Check the medical records for evidence of deletion in the region of the long arm of paternal chromosome 15 (15q11.2-15q12) or maternal uniparental disomy of chromosome 15

### Observe and Assess Physical and Behavioral Characteristics

- Assess such neurological symptoms as low muscle tone, hypotonia, and seek information on possible high threshold for pain
- Assess feeding difficulties during early infancy and take note of a failure to thrive initially
- Observe and record such craniofacial abnormalities as a thin upper lip and upslanting almond-shaped eyes, strabismus, and myopia
- Observe and record such physical anomalies as small hands and feet, scoliosis, and osteopenia
- Assess the behavioral and communication characteristics of intellectual deficiencies
- Observe and record such behavioral problems as excessive and compulsive eating that causes obesity, sleep disturbances, and self-destructive behavior

### Assess Speech, Language, and Hearing

- Screen hearing; hearing loss is not a typical characteristic of Prader-Willi syndrome
- Assess articulation disorders and rate speech intelligibility
  Assess the effects of hypotonia and velopharyngeal insufficiency on articulation errors; take note of the typical omissions, distortions, and weak consonant productions
- Assess a likely delay in initial language development; take note that most children tend to catch up with their normally developing peers; relate language deficits to the degree of intellectual deficits
- Assess hypernasality and nasal air emission possibly due to hypotonia

***Refsum Syndrome.*** A genetic syndrome characterized by progressive sensorineural hearing loss, neurological deterioration and cerebellar ataxia, chronic Polyneuritis, and Retinitis Pigmentosa

### Review the History and Medical Records

- Ascertain whether a pattern of Autosomal Recessive inheritance can be established
- Review medical records for evidence of biochemical imbalance involving excessive storage of Phytanic Acid in tissue or plasma, chronic inflammation of the peripheral nerves (Polyneuritis), and heart diseases

### Observe and Assess Physical and Behavioral Characteristics

- Observe and record disturbed balance (cerebellar ataxia)
- Take note of eye and vision problems including pigmentary degeneration of the retina and night blindness
- Observe and record such skeletal abnormalities as Spondylitis and Kyphoscoliosis

### Assess Speech, Language, and Hearing

- Screen hearing and obtain an audiological evaluation to diagnose a slowly progressive sensorineural hearing loss that begins during the second or third decade of life in 50% of the cases; schedule periodic audiological assessments to document the deterioration in hearing
- Assess articulation disorders in the context of the acquired hearing loss
- Assess dysarthria especially if the facial muscles are involved
- Assess such voice disorders as harsh voice and variable pitch and loudness
- Assess hypernasality and nasal emission
- Assess such prosodic problems as altered rate of speech and stress patterns typically associated with dysarthria

***Stickler Syndrome.*** A genetic syndrome characterized by facial deformities, ophthalmological problems, musculoskeletal deficiencies, Pierre-Robin sequence including cleft palate or submucous cleft, and hearing impairment; intelligence is generally within normal limits.

### Review the Case History and Medical Records

- Ascertain whether a pattern of Autosomal Recessive inheritance can be established
- Check the medical records for ophthalmological problems including cataracts, retinal detachments, and severe myopia
- Review evidence for upper airway obstructions

### Observe and Assess Physical and Behavioral Characteristics

- Observe and record such musculoskeletal problems as joint diseases, juvenile rheumatoid arthritis; prominent ankle, knee, and wrist bones; and long and thin legs and hands
- Observe and record such craniofacial deviations as micrognathia, midface Hypoplasia, Cleft Palate, submucous cleft or bifid uvula, round face, depressed nasal root, and epicanthal folds
- Observe and record any auricular malformations

### Assess Speech, Language, and Hearing

- Assess early feeding, sucking, and swallowing problems, complicated by upper airway obstructions
- Screen hearing and have an audiological assessment done to diagnose a more frequently found bilateral conductive hearing loss or less frequently found sensorineural loss
- Assess language problems associated with hearing loss and Cleft Palate
- Assess hypernasality and nasal emission associated with clefts; also take note of hyponasality, which may be observed in some children
- Assess articulation disorders associated with cleft palate along with those associated with micrognathia

***Tourette's Syndrome.*** A genetic syndrome characterized by patterned, stereotypic, and compulsively performed movements called tics; individual may suppress them but only for a short duration; may be associated with such psychiatric symptoms as obsessive-compulsive behavior, phobia, and hyperactivity.

### Review the Case History and Conduct an Interview

- Check the medical records and case history for possible evidence of autosomal dominant inheritance
- Rule out other neurological diseases or drug effects

### Observe and Assess Physical and Behavioral Characteristics

- Observe and assess multiple motor tics (eye blinks, facial twitches, shoulder shrugging, grimaces)
- Take note of various behavioral deviations, including depression, inattention, impulsivity, anxiety, sexual disorders, and aggressive behaviors

### Assess Speech, Language, and Hearing

- Assess vocal tics that may start as grunting and evolve into such other forms as throat clearing, humming, yelling, screaming, spitting, and making barking noises
- Assess coprolalia (compulsive swearing or utterance of obscenities)
- Assess palilalia (repetition of one's own utterances) and echolalia (repetition of what is heard)
- Assess stuttering because it is frequently associated with Tourette's Syndrome
- Assess dysarthric speech, especially hyperkinetic dysarthria
- Observe a tendency to talk to oneself and carry on a conversation by assuming different roles

***Treacher Collins Syndrome.*** A somewhat rare genetic syndrome characterized by mandibulofacial Dysostosis, hearing impairment, cleft or velopharyngeal incompetence, dental problems, and external ear malformations; intellectual disabilities are not a typical characteristic.

### Review the Case History and Medical Records

- Examine the case history and medical records for possible evidence of autosomal dominant inheritance
- Ask the parents about any early sucking and feeding problems

### Observe and Assess Physical and Behavioral Characteristics

- Observe and record the dominant craniofacial anomalies including a long face, beaklike nose, underdeveloped facial bones (small chin and underdeveloped cheeks), dental malocclusion, downwardly slanted palpebral fissures, Coloboma of the lower eyelid, high hard palate, short or immobile soft palate, cleft palate in about 30% of the cases, submucous cleft in some cases, cleft lip and palate in a few cases, pharyngeal hypoplasia (small pharynx), hair growth on the cheeks, absence of lower eyelashes, and strabismus
- Observe and record such auditory abnormalities as stenosis or Atresia of the external auditory canal, malformations of the pinna, preauricular ear tags, and middle and inner ear malformations including a fixation of the footplate of the stapes
- Assess sucking or swallowing problems and potential airway obstruction if warranted

### Assess Speech, Language, and Hearing

- Screen hearing and have an audiological assessment done to diagnose a potential congenital, bilateral, or conductive hearing loss in most cases and sensorineural loss in some
- Assess speech disorders, especially anteriorly produced speech sounds because of micrognathia which may force the tongue toward the back of the mouth; assess compensatory articulation associated with cleft palate
- Assess language skills, especially syntactic and morphological skills, and relate evident problems to hearing impairment
- Assess resonance disorders in the context of cleft palate (hypernasality, hyponasality, and nasal emission)

***Turner Syndrome.*** A genetic syndrome characterized by defective gonadal differentiation; congenital edema of neck, hands, or feet; webbing of the neck; low posterior hair line; intellectual disabilities in only 10% of the cases; occurs only in the female because the cause is a missing X chromosome; a similar syndrome that occurs in both males and females is called *Noonan syndrome.*

### Review the Case History and Medical Records

- Review the medical records for possible evidence of a missing X chromosome, missing secondary sex characteristics, and cardiac defects
- Interview clients about hearing loss, which may be noticed around age 10

### Observe and Assess Physical and Behavioral Characteristics

- Observe and record congenital swelling of the foot, neck, and hands; and webbing of the neck (excess skin over the neck)
- Observe and record such abnormalities as broad chest with widely spaced nipples, hip dislocation, skeletal dysplasia, dysplastic nails, low posterior hairline, and pigmented skin lesions
- Observe and record such craniofacial anomalies as Micrognathia (abnormally small lower jaw); maxillary Hypoplasia (underdeveloped or very small maxilla); high arched and narrow palate; and cleft palate in some cases
- Observe and record such anomalies of the auricle as low-set, elongated, and cup-shaped ears and thick earlobes
- Assess features of right hemisphere dysfunction present in some cases
- Obtain educational assessment reports because some children may experience learning disabilities, even though intellectual impairments are uncommon

### Assess Speech, Language, and Hearing

- Screen hearing and obtain an audiological assessment to diagnose a likely sensorineural loss in many cases and conductive or mixed loss in some cases
- Assess speech and language skills which may show deviations that are consistent with hearing impairment
- Assess auditory processing skills and visual, spatial, and attentional problems as warranted

S

***Usher Syndrome.*** A genetic syndrome characterized by Retinitis Pigmentosa (night blindness) and nonprogressive congenital hearing loss; disturbed gait in many cases; intellectual disabilities in some cases; 50% of individuals who are deaf and blind may have this syndrome; there are four types of Usher syndrome: Usher Type I, Usher Type II, Usher Type III, and Usher Type IV.

### Take a Case History and Conduct an Interview

- Review the family history and medical records for possible evidence of Autosomal Recessive inheritance for Usher syndromes Types I, II, and III and for X-linked recessive trait in the case of Usher syndrome Type IV
- Obtain detailed information on progressive blindness

### Observe and Assess Physical and Behavioral Characteristics

- To assess Usher syndrome Type I, take note of the onset of night blindness before the age of 10 years, and limited and progressively worsening peripheral vision, terminating in total blindness; have an audiological assessment done to diagnose congenital sensorineural deafness
- To assess Usher syndrome Type II, take note of any visual field problems that vary in severity, and have an audiological assessment done to diagnose congenital sensorineural deafness
- To assess Usher syndrome Type III, take note of normal development until puberty because this is not a congenital disorder, and have an audiological assessment done to diagnose a progressive hearing loss
- To assess Usher syndrome Type IV, take note of any vision impairment, and have an audiological assessment done to diagnose hearing loss

### Assess Speech, Language, and Hearing

- Assess speech acquisition, which is typically delayed (may even be absent or extremely limited) because of both visual and auditory impairments Assess acquisition of sign language, although even this may be affected because of blindness
- Assess articulation disorders and relate them the hearing impairment; assess speech intelligibility, which may be severely impaired
- Assess language disorders and relate them to the hearing impairment
- Assess hypernasality and nasal emission as warranted

***van der Woude Syndrome.*** A genetic syndrome characterized by lower lip pits and cleft lip with or without cleft palate; a relatively common syndrome involving clefts; mixing of the cleft types among relatives (incidence of cleft palate only, cleft lip only, and cleft lip and cleft palate) is a characteristic of this syndrome.

### Review the Case History and Medical Records

- Review the family history and medical records for possible evidence of Autosomal Dominant inheritance
- Interview the parents about such congenital abnormalities as cleft palate and subsequent middle ear infections
- Ask the parents about any early feeding difficulties

### Observe and Assess Physical and Behavioral Characteristics

- Assess such craniofacial anomalies as pits or cysts of the lower lip in all cases; cleft lip and cleft palate in many cases; ankyloglossia; and missing premolars

### Assess Speech, Language, and Hearing

- Screen hearing and obtain an audiological assessment to diagnose a likely conductive loss associated with cleft palate
- Assess early feeding problems, mostly because of the cleft palate
- Assess articulation disorders that may be consistent with hearing loss and cleft palate; take note that early speech development may be normal; assess compensatory articulation associated with palatal clefts and velopharyngeal insufficiency
- Assess language skills, which may be normal for the most part; errors found are likely to be consistent with hearing loss (e.g., missing morphological features)
- Assess hypernasality and nasal emission associated with cleft palate and velopharyngeal insufficiency

***Velo-Cardio-Facial Syndrome (VCFS).*** A common genetic syndrome of multiple anomalies, with over 180 clinical features; associated with congenital heart disease, psychiatric problems, and communication disorders.

### Take a Case History and Conduct an Interview

- Review the family history and medical records for possible evidence of Autosomal Dominant inheritance
- Review the medical records for evidence of cardiovascular abnormalities, including ventral and atrial septal defects, right-sided aorta, interrupted aorta, aortic valve anomalies, defective subclavian arteries, abnormal origin of the carotid artery, and structural abnormalities of the internal carotid and vertebral arteries
- Review the medical records for evidence of such neurological disorders as seizures, hypotonia, cerebellar growth abnormalities, spina bifida, and enlarged sylvian fissure
- Review the medical records for evidence of digestive, respiratory, renal, endocrine, and genitourinary disorders

### Observe and Assess Physical and Behavioral Characteristics

- Assess and record such craniofacial, oral, and laryngeal anomalies as a flat skull base, microcephaly, a long and asymmetrical face, small or missing teeth characterized by deficient enamel, occasional cleft lip, prominent nasal bride, narrow nostrils, upper airway obstruction, laryngeal web, deficient adenoids, arytenoid hyperplasia, thin pharyngeal muscle, and unilateral vocal cord paresis
- Observe and record such auditory anomalies as overfolded helix; small, protruded, asymmetrical, and cup-shaped ears; and narrow external ear canal
- Observe and record such optic anomalies as small eyes, strabismus, narrow palpebral fissure, iris nodules, and puffy eyelids
- Observe and record such skeletal abnormalities as small hands and feet, short fingers, polydactyly, and syndactyly
- Take note of such behavioral (psychiatric) problems as bipolar affective disorders, schizophrenia, obsessive-compulsive disorders, anxiety, and phobia

### Assess Speech, Language, and Hearing

- Assess airway obstruction and any early feeding and swallowing problems
- Screen hearing and obtain an audiological assessment to diagnose a likely conductive hearing loss (more common) or a sensorineural hearing loss (less common)
- Assess articulation disorders and related error patterns with severe velopharyngeal insufficiency associated with VCFS
- Assess early language acquisition which may be delayed; take note of a tendency to catch up with their normally developing peers, unless severe hearing loss impedes language learning
- Assess voice disorders and take note of high-pitched, hoarse, and breathy voice that characterizes children with VCFS
- Assess hypernasality associated with velopharyngeal insufficiency

***Waardenburg Syndrome, Type I and Type II.*** A genetic syndrome subclassified into two types; Type I is characterized by a wide bridge of the nose caused by lateral displacement of inner (nasal) canthi, pigmentary disturbances, and hearing impairment in about 25% of the cases; Type II is characterized by cranial and facial anomalies, brachydactyly, cleft palate, cardiac defects, and hearing impairment in about 50% of the cases.

### Take a Case History and Conduct an Interview

- Review the family history and medical records for possible evidence of Autosomal Dominant inheritance Type I Waardenburg syndrome and Autosomal Recessive inheritance in Type II
- Interview the parents about any early feeding and swallowing problems and cardiac anomalies

### Assess or Observe Physical Characteristics, Type I

- Assess or observe and record the physical features of Type I, which include a lateral displacement of the inner (nasal) Canthi (causing a wide bridge of the nose), medial flare of the eyebrows, and white eyelashes; take note of any pigmentary anomalies including white forelock and Heterochromia irides; check the medical and audiological records for evidence of cochlear anomalies

### Assess or Observe Physical Characteristics, Type II

- Assess or observe and record the physical features of Type II, which include a high-domed skull called Acrocephaly, orbital and facial deformities, cleft palate, shortness of fingers (Brachydactyly), fusion (Syndactyly) of soft tissue, and a variety of glaucoma (Hydrophthalmos)

### Assess Speech, Language, and Hearing

- Assess early feeding and swallowing problems consistent with cleft palate
- Screen hearing and obtain an audiological assessment to diagnose a likely congenital unilateral or bilateral sensorineural loss which is more common in Type II than in Type I
- Assess language disorders, especially syntactic and morphological deficiencies that are consistent with congenital hearing impairment

- Assess hypernasality and nasal emission, especially when cleft palate is evident
- Assess articulation disorders consistent with hearing impairment and compensatory articulatory gestures consistent with cleft palate

Baraitser, M., & Winter, R. M. (1996). *Color atlas of congenital malformation syndromes*. London: Mosby-Wolfe.

*Dorland's Illustrated Medical Dictionary* (1994, 28th ed.). Philadelphia, PA: W. B. Saunders.

Jones, K. L. (2005). *Smith's recognizable patterns of human malformations* (6th ed.). Philadelphia, PA: W. B. Saunders.

Jung, J. H. (1989). *Genetic syndromes in communication disorders*. Austin, TX: Pro-Ed.

Kahn, A. (2000). *Craniofacial anomalies*. San Diego, CA: Singular Publishing Group.

Shprintzen, J. R. (2000). *Syndrome identification for speech-language pathology*. San Diego, CA: Singular.

Shprintzen, J. R. (1997). *Genetics, syndromes, and communication disorders*. San Diego, CA: Singular.

Wiedemann, H. R., & Kunze, J. (1997). *Clinical syndromes* (3rd ed.). London: Mosby-Wolfe.

**Syntactic Aphasia.** To assess this type of aphasia, also known as *Wernicke's aphasia*, see Aphasia and Wernicke's Aphasia under Aphasia: Specific Types.

S

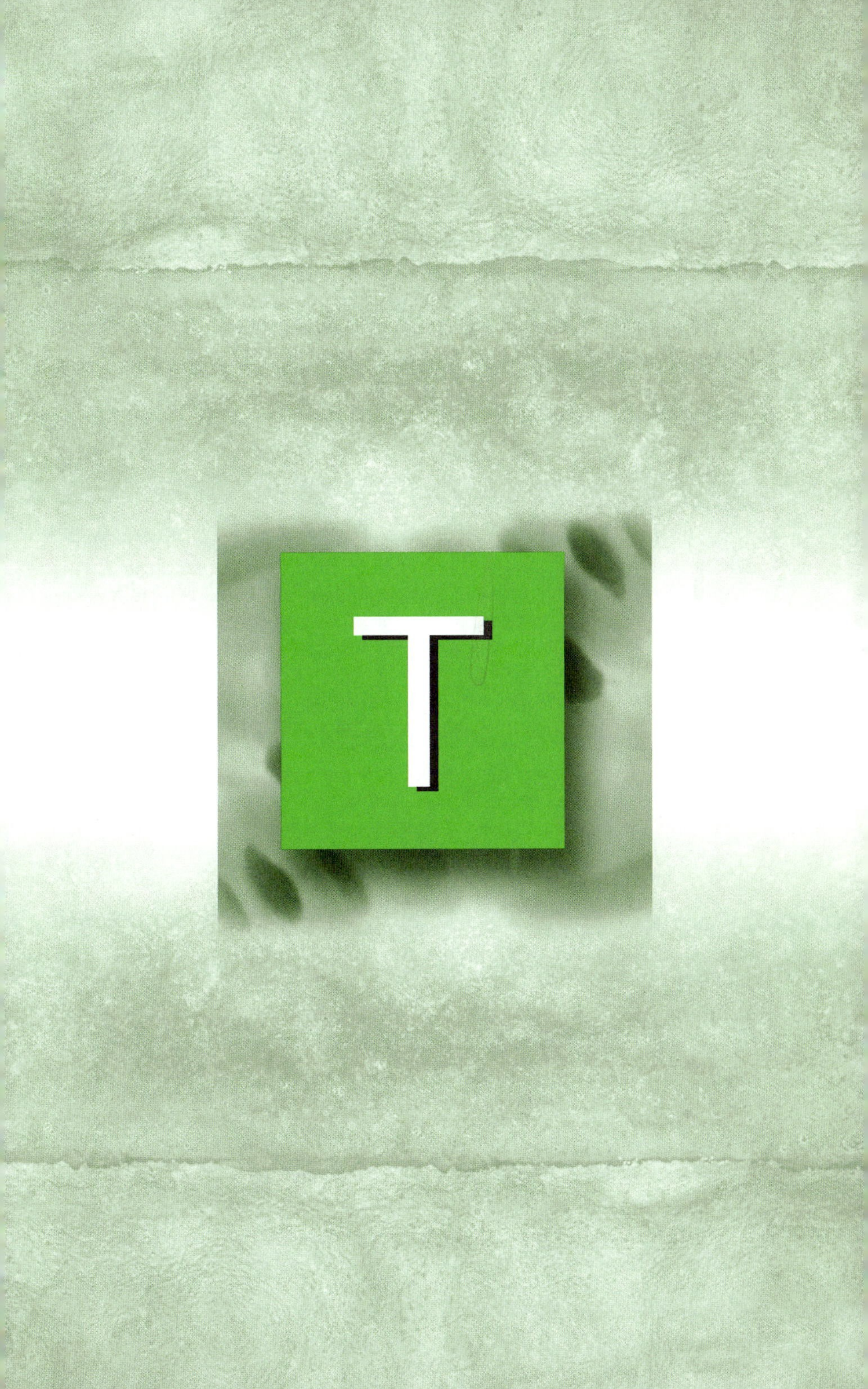
T

**Tactile Agnosia.** To assess this neurological impairment that causes difficulty recognizing objects that are touched and felt, but are not seen, see Agnosia.

**Taybi Syndrome.** To assess this syndrome, also called *oto-palatal-digital syndrome*, see Syndromes Associated With Communication Disorders.

**Telegraphic Speech.** To assess speech that is devoid of many grammatical morphemes that render speech telegraphic, take a speech sample and analyze the missing grammatical morphemes and limited syntactic structures; see Language Disorders in Children for assessment details.

**Third Alexia.** To assess reading problems associated with brain pathology, also known as frontal alexia, see Alexia.

**Tomography.** A computerized radiographic method of taking pictures of different planes of body structures; a method of scanning brain structures; useful in neurodiagnostics; see Computerized Axial Tomography.

**Tongue Thrust.** Assessment of tongue thrust, also known as deviant swallow, may be important in assessing its potential effects on speech articulation, although the relationship between deviant swallow and articulation disorders is not well established; in assessing tongue thrust, consider the following:

- Note that tongue thrust does not really mean that the tongue is thrusting against the front teeth; it means a forward tongue gesture during swallowing; take note of this tongue posture during assessment
- Observe whether the tongue tip is in contact with the lower lip; it is in most cases
- Observe whether the mandible is slightly open
- Assess the fronting of the tongue during speech production
- From the case history, judge whether the tongue thrust is habitual
- Assess whether such structural problems as enlarged adenoids or tonsils partially block the posterior airway passage; such a blockage may force the tongue into a more forward position in the oral cavity
- Check whether there is any evidence of malocclusion
- Assess articulation if there is evidence of an articulation disorder
- Pay special attention to a lisp (distortions of /z/ and /l/) because this may be found in some children

**Topic Initiation.** To assess this pragmatic or conversational language skill in children and adults with communication disorders, hold a conversation with the client and:

- Note the number of times the client introduced a new topic of conversation
- Judge whether the client introduced topics abruptly, interrupting your speech
- Assess whether the client introduced topics when opportunities were available
- See Language Disorders in Children for procedural details

T

**Topic Maintenance.** To assess the conversational skill of talking on the same topic for an extended and socially acceptable duration, hold a conversational speech with the client and:

- Note the duration for which the client continued to speak on the same topic of conversation that either the client or you introduced

- Judge the duration for multiple topics, three being the minimum
- Make clinical judgments on whether the client spoke for an acceptable duration on each topic, offered sufficient details, and gave substantive information on the topic
- Note the number of times the client abruptly switched to another topic
- See Language Disorders in Children for procedural details

**Tourette's Syndrome.** To assess tics and communication disorders that characterize this syndrome, see Syndromes Associated With Communication Disorders.

**Transcortical Motor Aphasia.** To assess this nonfluent variety of aphasia, take a conversational speech sample and assess the fluency of speech production, along with other language difficulties; see Aphasia and Aphasia: Specific Types for procedural details.

**Transcortical Sensory Aphasia.** To assess this type of fluent aphasia, take a conversational speech sample and take note of fluent but highly paraphasic speech with impaired meaning; see Aphasia and Aphasia: Specific Types for procedural details.

**Traumatic Brain Injury (TBI).** Assessment of neurological, behavioral, and communication deficits associated with traumatic brain injury is a complex task that requires the participation of multiple professionals, including general physicians and neurologists, medical and nonmedical rehabilitation specialists, psychologists, speech-language pathologists, physical and occupational therapists, and other specialists; the main symptoms that need to be assessed include restlessness, irritation, disorientation to time and place, disorganized and inconsistent responses; impaired memory, attention, reasoning, drawing, naming, repetition, and pragmatic communication deficits.

### *Assessment Objectives/General Guidelines*

- To assess the communication deficits associated with TBI
- To evaluate the strengths and limitations that might help in planning treatment
- To evaluate communicative deficits in relation to cognitive, sensory, and physical deficits
- To evaluate the need for augmentative and alternative modes of communication
- Make an initial, brief assessment at the bedside; make a detailed assessment as soon as the client's condition permits it
- Give frequent breaks from assessment tasks because the client with TBI is likely to get tired soon; complete the assessment in more than one session if necessary
- Repeat selected portions of the assessment as the client's condition improves
- Integrate communication assessment data with assessment results obtained by other professionals
- Continue to assess the client during treatment

### Case History/Interview Focus

- See **Case History** and **Interview** under Standard/Common Assessment Procedures
- Interview the family members or other informants about the premorbid language skills, literacy, and employment history to gauge negative changes due to TBI
- During the interview, ask the informants about the client's interests, hobbies, and any special skills that may be useful in treatment sessions
- If possible, interview those who were present at the time of TBI to understand the conditions associated with TBI (e.g., those who were in the car that had an accident)

### Ethnocultural Considerations

- See Ethnocultural Considerations in Assessment
- Find out whether the client is bilingual or monolingual; if bilingual, find out the dominant language; if necessary, make arrangements for a bilingual assessment or assessment with the help of an interpreter
- Evaluate the family communication patterns and the resources and supports the family may need because TBI rehabilitation may be expensive and prolonged

### Assessment of Clients with TBI

- Screen the client
  - Use the *Mini-Mental Status Examination* (M. Folstein, S. Folstein, & P. McHugh) or the *Brief Test of Head Injury* (N. Helm-Estabrooks & G. Hotz)
  - Make a brief and initial bedside evaluation of consciousness and cognition with client-specific questions
- Make an initial assessment of verbal skills
  - Assess simple responses to verbal commands; for example, ask the client to:
    - "Open your eyes"
    - "Move your feet"
    - "Wiggle your toes"
    - "Nod your head"
    - "Raise your hand"
    - "Move your fingers"
  - Assess the presence or absence of verbal responses; note the speed, relevance, and appropriateness of all responses given; note whether the client:
    - Can say "Hi"
    - Gives only single word responses; and if so, the kinds of words produced
    - Uses sentences; and if so, note the types of sentences
    - Responds spontaneously; and if so, note the types and length of utterances spontaneously produced
    - Responds only to questions and commands
    - Responds only nonverbally, but appropriately
    - Tries to respond nonverbally, but not successfully
    - Cannot show signs of a response of any kind

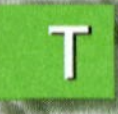

- Assess simple memory skills and basic orientation; note whether the stimuli have to be repeated; ask the client such questions as:
  - "How old are you?"
  - "What is your name?"
  - "What is your [wife's, husband's, mother's, father's] name?"
  - "Where do you live?"
  - "What do you do?"
  - "Where are you now?"
  - "What time is it?"
  - "What day is it?"
  - "What year is it?"
  - "What month is it?"
  - "Can you count to ten?"
  - "Can you recite the days of the week?"
- Assess cognitive deficits
  - Wait until the client's initial symptoms subside to assess cognitive deficits in detail
  - Assess memory deficits
    - Question the client about events prior to brain injury to assess pretraumatic amnesia
    - Ask such questions as "Where were you when the accident happened?," "What were you doing when the accident happened?," and "Where were you going when the accident happened?"
    - Question the client about events subsequent to the brain injury to assess posttraumatic amnesia
    - Ask such questions as "How long have you been in the hospital?," "What did you eat for breakfast this morning?," "Who visited you this afternoon?," and "What did you do after lunch today?"
    - Have the client read a list of words and ask him or her to recall as many words as possible
    - Have the client read the list repeatedly and by requesting interspersed recall, assess the number of trials needed to learn the list in meeting such a performance criterion as 90% accuracy
    - Assess recognition by presenting a list of words that contains previously shown words and new words that were not shown and ask the client to point to the ones previously presented
    - Read a paragraph aloud to the client and immediately ask questions about the content
    - Read a paragraph aloud to the client and ask questions about the content after a delay of about 20 to 30 minutes
    - Ask the client to read a short paragraph repeatedly and assess repeatedly to find out the number of readings necessary to meet a criterion such as 90% recall
    - Administer a standardized test such as the *Wechsler Memory Scale-Revised*
    - Obtain neuropsychological reports for more a detailed assessment of memory functions

        - Take note of any errors and analyze the client's strategies (e.g., repeating only the last few words of a list or a read paragraph, repeating the same words, intrusion of novel or nontarget words)
    - Assess attention span and distractibility
        - Observe the client during the assessment and interview to judge attention and distractibility as the assessment tasks are presented or questions are asked about the client's history or current status
        - Take note of lack of attention as evidenced by the need to repeat instructions, represent test items, or repeatedly give alerting stimuli (e.g., *look at me*, *look at this picture*)
        - Ask the client to repeat clusters of two, three, four, five, six, and seven digits to assess memory span for digits
        - Ask the client to repeat sentences of varying length to assess the attention span for words
        - Take note of response to extraneous stimuli such as people passing by and noise to assess distractibility
        - Take note of fatigue during assessment and how fast it sets in
    - Assess reaction time
        - Take note of the speed of response to questions
        - Take note of the speed of response when spontaneous speech is offered
        - Make a judgment about the reaction time
- Assess visual and perceptual deficits
    - Assess visuospatial, drawing, and constructional deficits
        - Ask the client to copy selected, simple line drawings that you present
        - Ask the client to copy geometric figures
        - Ask the client to draw a face, a cup, a pencil, and such other common items from memory
        - Ask the client to copy a block design
        - Ask the client to copy a stick figure
- Assess communication problems
    - Assess dysarthria; if necessary, determine its type
        - Initially, observe speech sound production as the client talks; take note of any articulatory problems
        - When feasible, record a conversational speech sample
        - Analyze the sample for the kinds of speech sound problems; take note especially of imprecise consonant productions
        - Administer selected tests described under Dysarthrias
        - Use the additional assessment procedures described under Dysarthrias
        - If a particular type of dysarthria seems a likely diagnosis, use the assessment procedures described under the specific types of dysarthrias
        - Rate the severity of dysarthria following the guidelines given under Dysarthrias
    - Assess the rate of speech
        - Measure the speech rate in segments of multiple speech samples
        - Calculate the number of words or syllables spoken per minute
        - Take note of slower speech rate or variability in the rate in segments of speech

- Assess apraxia of speech
  - Use the recorded conversational speech sample to assess apraxia of speech
  - Assess the imitative and spontaneous production of syllables, words, phrases, and sentences that are described under Apraxia of Speech
  - Make a detailed orofacial examination to assess nonverbal oral apraxia
  - Determine the presence of oral apraxia; use the procedures described under Apraxia of Speech
- Assess confused, bizarre, inappropriate, and incoherent language
  - Assess the relevance, appropriateness, and meaningfulness of answers to questions
  - Evaluate any extended language productions for their appropriateness and social acceptability
  - Look for signs of any confabulation and irrational and illogical statements
  - Consider the general state of the client (confusion and disorientation) in evaluating speech productions
- Assess mutism or aphonia
  - Assess the reasons for any lack of responses
  - Rule out motor problems that prevent expression
  - Take note of any attempts on the part of the client to communicate in any manner possible; such attempts negate mutism
- Assess problems in auditory comprehension of spoken language and gestures
  - Take note of any problems in auditory comprehension during the interview and speech samples as evidenced by wrong responses or requests for repetitions
  - Assess any problems in understanding the meaning of facial gestures, hand gestures, and such other nonverbal means of communication
- Assess persistent word finding problems
  - Ask the client to name selected common objects or pictures of objects
  - Ask the client to name family members and friends
  - Ask the client to point to the correct stimuli among several as you name them
  - Observe signs of word finding difficulty in conversational speech (e.g., undue pauses, word repetitions, interjections, gestures, word substitutions, circumlocution, and the use of vague or general words instead of specific terms)
- Assess the production of syntactic and morphologic features
  - Record a conversational speech (discourse) sample note that may be adequate in most clients; if warranted, make a detailed analysis
  - Analyze the length of typical sentences
  - Assess the grammatical complexity of any sentences that lack syntactic and morphological features
  - Take note of the transformational variety of sentences, which may be limited
  - Judge the word order and their appropriateness within sentences

    - Assess the production of such grammatical morphemes as the plural, the possessive, the present progressive, prepositions, pronouns, auxiliary verbs, and copula
  - Assess conversational skills (pragmatic features of language)
    - Make judgment as you interview the client and while recording a conversational speech sample
    - Judge the appropriateness of conversational turn taking; take note of the frequency of interruptions, silence when it is the client's turn to talk, and yielding to your speech attempts
    - Judge the frequency with which the client initiates conversation or a topic of conversation; judge the adequacy of such initiations
    - Evaluate the rough duration for which the client sustains conversation on given topics; judge the adequacy of topic maintenance, topic expansion, and topic shifting
    - Judge the adequacy of eye contact, use of gestures, facial expressions, and so forth
    - Judge the appropriateness of emotional expressions that accompany verbal expressions
  - Assess any prosodic impairments including difficulty in monitoring rate, pitch, and vocal loudness
    - Measure the speech rate and judge its appropriateness
    - Judge the appropriateness of vocal loudness
    - Judge the appropriateness of the client's vocal pitch
    - Evaluate the client's intonational patterns
    - Assess the client's linguistic stress patterns
- Assess reading and writing problems
  - Obtain a sample of the client's premorbid writing
  - Have the client read a printed passage silently, and ask questions to test the comprehension of what is read
  - Have the client read a printed passage orally, and assess the kinds of reading problems exhibited
  - Ask the client to write a brief essay and analyze for spelling errors, syntactic structures, overall organization of writing, details of information supplied, and so forth
  - Ask the client to copy a printed paragraph and analyze the type of errors
  - Analyze the client's writing errors in relation to the premorbid writing skills
- Assess related problems
  - Assess dysphagia; use the procedures described under Dysphagia
  - During assessment sessions, observe and take note of persistent physical and sensory disabilities
    - Screen hearing and, if warranted, refer the client to an audiologist
    - Refer the client to a vision specialist

### *Assessment of Children with TBI*

- Generally, the assessment goals and targets are the same as those for adults with TBI

- Essentially, the assessment procedures are also the same as those for adults with TBI
- Consider the child's special needs in assessing the effects of TBI
  - Interview the parents in detail to assess the family's concerns and expectations from rehabilitation and treatment programs
  - Assess the family's resources and needs and support systems that are essential to promote home training and management
  - Assess the child's academic needs and demands
  - Talk to the teachers and find out what kinds of demands are placed on the child
  - Assess reading, writing, and literacy skills more thoroughly than you would in the case of adults with TBI; obtain a reading passage that is appropriate for the child's grade level to assess oral reading and comprehension of read material
  - If evaluated by a reading specialist, obtain the report
  - If the child is in a special educational program, assess the communication demands placed on the child within the program
  - Obtain psychological reports from the school psychologist to better understand the intellectual and behavioral status of the child
  - Concentrate on evaluating the communication deficits as described previously
  - Integrate your findings with those of the special educators, teachers, and psychologists to obtain a more complete picture of the child's strengths and limitations
  - Suggest a treatment plan that facilitates the child's re-entry to the classroom as soon as possible and promotes academic achievement

### *Standardized Tests*

- Note that although some tests of aphasia may seem appropriate to assess clients with TBI, generally it is not advisable to use them because very few clients with TBI are aphasic
- Tests of aphasia tend to underestimate the communicative deficits of people with TBI because such tests do not assess the special kinds of impairments TBI produces
- To conduct an initial bedside screening for awareness, responsiveness, and memory, administer the *Mini-Mental Status Examination* (M. Folstein, S. Folstein, & P. McHugh) or the *Brief Test of Head Injury* (N. Helm-Estabrooks & G. Hotz)
- To assess memory, orientation, cognitive and behavioral deficits, and communication impairments, administer the latest edition of one or more of the following tests:

T

| Test | Purpose |
|---|---|
| *Comprehensive Level of Consciousness Scale* (D. E. Stanczak & associates) | To assess behavior in several dimensions and to assess communicative effort |

*(continues)*

*(continued)*

| Test | Purpose |
|---|---|
| *Disability Rating Scale* (M. Rappoport & associates) | To assess the current level of functioning and employability |
| *Galveston Orientation and Amnesia Test* (H. S. Levin, V. M. O'Donnel, & R. G. Grossman) | To make a bedside screening of memory and orientation |
| *Glasgow Coma Scale* (G. Teasdale & B. Jennett) | To make a bedside screening of general awareness and responsiveness |
| *Glasgow Outcome Scale* (B. Jennett & G. Teasdale) | To assess outcome for, or course of recovery from, TBI |
| *Ranchos Los Amigos Scale of Cognitive Levels* (C. Hagen & D. Malkamus) | To assess the cognitive and behavioral level and recovery |
| *Ross Information Processing Assessment* (D. G. Ross) | To assess memory, orientation, problem solving, reasoning, and other intellectual skills |
| *Scales of Cognitive Ability for Traumatic Brain Injury* (B. B. Adamovich & J. Henderson) | To assess perception and discrimination, orientation, organization, recall, and reasoning skills |
| *Wechsler Memory Scale—Revised* (E. W. Russell) | To assess memory skills |

- A few additional tests, even if they are not standardized on people with brain injury, may be appropriate to administer because they target specific skills that may be impaired in individuals for different reasons:
    - *The Peabody Picture Vocabulary Test* (L. M. Dunn & L. M. Dunn) may be helpful in assessing receptive vocabulary skills
    - *The Word Fluency Measure* (J. G. Borkowski, A. L. Benton, & O. Spreen) may be useful in assessing how well the client can generate semantically related words within a specified time duration
    - *The Gates-MacGinitie Reading Test* (A. Gates & W. MacGinitie) may be useful in assessing basic reading and reading comprehension skills
    - *The Test of Adult/Adolescent Word Finding* (D. J. German) may be administered to assess impairment in word finding
    - *The Boston Naming Test* (E. Kaplan, H. Goodglass, & S. Weintraub), typically used to assess naming problems of clients with aphasia, may be appropriate to assess this specific aspect of communication in clients with TBI
    - *The Test for Auditory Comprehension of Language* (E. Carrow-Woodfolk) may be useful in assessing the comprehension of grammatical and syntactic aspects of language
    - Various subtests of intelligence that help assess such specific skills as reasoning and judgment, verbal absurdities, and logical relationships may

be useful in assessing these specific skills in clients with TBI; the *Wechsler* (D. Wechsler) and *Stanford-Binet* (L. M. Terman & M. A. Merrill) scales have such subtests
  - Abstract thinking and categorization tests with low verbal demand may be assessed with such tests as the *Standard Progressive Matrices* (J. C. Raven) and *Wisconsin Card Sorting Test* (D. A. Grant & E. A. Berg) because these skills may be impaired in clients with TBI

### Related/Medical and Neuropsychological Assessment Data

- Review the client's medical diagnosis that may specify the type and extent of brain injury
- Understand the current medication and their side effects that may have an effect on speech-language treatment (e.g., client who is drowsy because of medication may not perform well during treatment)
- Review the medical records for current and future medical treatment plans for the client
- Check the medical records for additional problems such as sleep disorders, fatigue, and depression associated with TBI
- Check the medical prognosis for the client
- Review radiological and brain imaging data that might be integrated or correlated with the speech diagnosis
- Understand the physical rehabilitation plans that might affect communication treatment
- Obtain audiological reports and integrate the hearing assessment results with the communication assessment
- Obtain reports from the neuropsychologist on cognitive impairment, intellectual functioning, and emotional and behavioral disorders or deficits; relate these to the communication deficits of the client

### Standard/Common Assessment Procedures

- Complete the Standard/Common Assessment Procedures

### Analysis of Assessment Data

- Analyze and summarize the assessment data relative to any physiological and neuromotor problems
- Integrate the findings with the medical-neurological and neuropsychological assessment data to obtain a comprehensive profile of the client's physiological, neurological, neuropsychological, and behavioral (including communication) performance
- Rate the severity of the disturbances noted
- Summarize the communication problems in relation to any cognitive deficits

T

### Diagnostic Criteria

- History and medical evidence of TBI is essential to diagnose TBI and any communication deficits associated with it
- Dominant neurophysiological consequences of TBI need to be documented
- Communicative disorders in the context of attentional, memory, and other cognitive deficits need to be documented to justify TBI

- Relatively intact language functions, but ineffective communication and a dominance of pragmatic language problems are essential to relate communication deficits to TBI
- Presence of dysarthria offers additional supportive evidence to diagnose TBI

### *Differential Diagnosis*

- Distinguish TBI from dementia; characteristics of dementia that contrast with those of TBI include gradual onset (vs. sudden onset of TBI), progressive course (vs. improving course of TBI), and symptoms and medical evidence of a degenerative neurological disease (vs. head trauma in the case of TBI)
- Distinguish TBI from schizophrenia; characteristics of schizophrenia that contrast with those of TBI include gradual onset (vs. sudden onset of TBI), such serious thought disorders as delusions (vs. attentional and perceptual problems of TBI), no evidence of head trauma (vs. evidence of head trauma in TBI), and persistent or deteriorating mental and behavioral symptoms (vs. improving course of TBI)
- Distinguish TBI from right hemisphere syndrome; characteristics of right hemisphere syndrome that contrast with those of TBI include left sided neglect (which is absent in TBI), denial of illness (not a significant symptom of TBI), and medical evidence of right hemisphere injury (vs. variable, diffuse injury in TBI)
- Distinguish TBI from aphasia with which it is most likely to be confused; use the following grid in making a differential diagnosis:

### Traumatic Brain Injury or Aphasia?

| Traumatic Brain Injury | Aphasia |
|---|---|
| Pure linguistic problems are not dominant | Pure linguistic problems are dominant |
| Grammatical errors not significant | Significant grammatical errors |
| Dysarthria part of the syndrome | Dysarthria not part of the syndrome |
| Initially, confused language | Language not confused |
| Faster improvement in language | Slower improvement in language |
| More serious pragmatic problems | Less serious pragmatic problems |
| Social interaction seriously impaired | Social interaction not as seriously impaired |
| Initially disorganized and confused | Not disorganized or confused |
| Initially disoriented to time and space | Not disoriented to time and space |
| Responses may be inconsistent or irrelevant | Responses not inconsistent or irrelevant |
| Serious attentional problems including distractibility, impulsivity, poor social judgment, and lack of insight | Attentional problems not as serious |

### Prognosis

- Prognosis is variable depending on the nature and extent of brain injury; prognostic guidelines are only suggestive and in need of stronger empirical support
- Prognosis for improvement with treatment is generally good
- Persistent mutism after initial recovery may suggest relatively poor prognosis for more complete recovery of verbal skills
- Possibly, the longer the duration of posttraumatic amnesia, the poorer the prognosis for more complete recovery

### Recommendations

- Communication treatment with an emphasis on improving dysarthria and pragmatic language disorders in the context of cognitive rehabilitation is recommended for almost all clients with traumatic brain injury
- See the following cited sources and *Hegde's PocketGuide to Treatment in Speech-Language Pathology* (3rd ed.) for details

Beukelman, D. R., & Yorkston, K. M. (1991). *Communication disorders following traumatic brain injury: Management of cognitive, language, and motor impairments*. Austin, TX: Pro-Ed.

Bigler, E. D. (Ed.). (1990). *Traumatic brain injury*. Austin, TX: Pro-Ed.

Cooper, P. R., & Golfinos, J. G. (2000). *Head injury* (4th ed.). New York: McGraw-Hill.

Gillis, R. J. (1996). *Traumatic brain injury: Rehabilitation for speech-language pathologists*. Boston, MA: Butterworth-Heinemann.

Hegde, M. N. (2006). *A coursebook on aphasia and other neurogenic language disorders* (3rd ed.). Clifton Park, NY: Thomson Delmar Learning.

High, W. M., Sander, A. M., Struchen, M. A., & Hart, K. A. (2006). *Rehabilitation for traumatic brain injury*. New York: Oxford University Press.

Murdoch, B. E., & Theodoros, D. G. (2000). *Traumatic brain injury: Associated speech, language, and swallowing disorders*. Clifton Park, NY: Thomson Delmar Learning.

Silver, J. M., McAllister, T. W., & Yudofsky, S. C. (Eds.) (2005). *Textbook of traumatic brain injury*. Arlington, VA: American Psychiatric Publishing Inc.

**Turn Taking.** To assess this conversational skill (pragmatic language skill) that may be impaired in adults and children with language disorders:

- Hold a conversation with the client and record it for later analysis
- Analyze the number of times the client appropriately took turns to talk and let you talk
- See Language Disorders in Children for procedural details

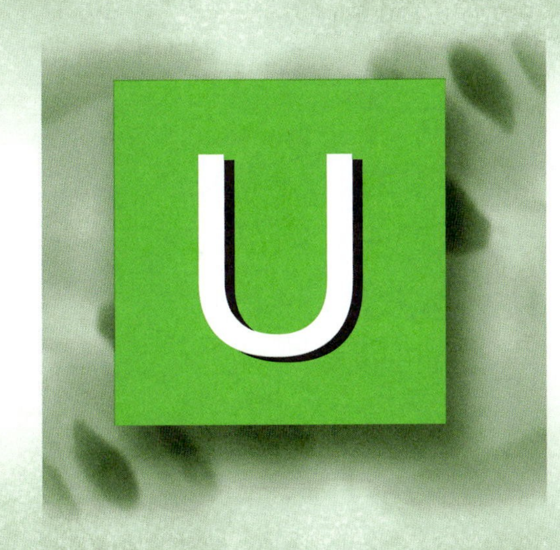
U

**Unilateral Upper Motor Neuron Dysarthria.** To assess this type of dysarthria, see Dysarthria and Dysarthria: Specific Types.

**Underextensions.** To assess this otherwise normal language phenomenon seen in young children, but may be an indication of a language disorder when it persists beyond age 3 or so:

- Hold a conversation with the child or show various stimulus items and have the child talk about them
- Take note of any overly restricted production of words
- Check to see whether the words are not generalized appropriately; for instance, take note whether the child:
  - Says "doll" only to a particular doll, but not to other dolls
  - Says "car" only to a car of certain color or shape, but not other cars
  - Says "cat" or "doggie" to pictures of only a specific cat or dog respectively, but not when pictures of other cats or dogs are presented
  - Says "house" only when a house of certain shape or color is presented, but not when pictures of houses of different shape and color are presented
- Present such additional stimuli to assess whether the child's concepts are restricted to certain specific stimuli, preventing generalized responses within classes of stimuli

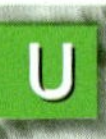

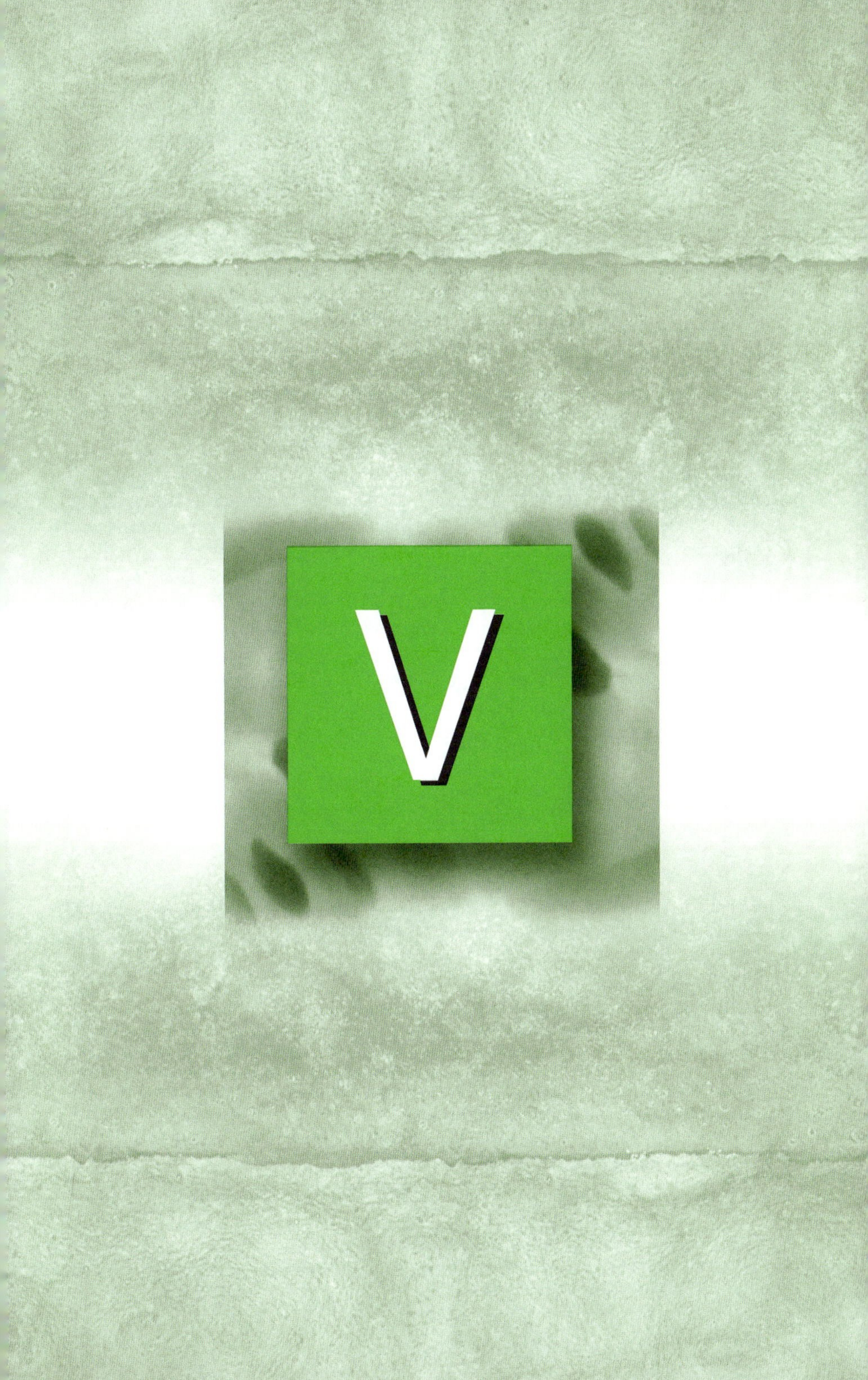
V

**Validity.** The degree to which a measuring instrument measures what it purports to measure; a criterion for test selection; clinicians should select only those tests that are known to be valid for the purpose of assessing a particular skill; may be demonstrated in many ways, resulting in different kinds of validity; validity measures of standardized tests include the following:

- Concurrent validity: The degree to which a new test correlates with an established test of known validity; too high a correlation suggests that the new test may be as valid as the old one and that the two tests are too similar, questioning the need for the new test; considered a form of criterion-related validity.
- Construct validity: The degree to which test scores are consistent with theoretical constructs or concepts; a language test, for example, that shows higher scores for older children compared to younger children is consistent with the theoretical construct that language changes (improves) with age.
- Content validity: A measure of validity of a test based on a thorough examination of all test items to determine whether the items are relevant to measuring what the test purports to measure and whether the items adequately sample the full range of the skill being measured; a test of articulation, for example, should include all speech sounds in all word positions and in phrases and sentences; omissions of sounds or inclusion of items not relevant to measuring articulation would reduce the validity of a test; often based on expert evaluation of test items and agreement among experts that the items are appropriate for assessing a given behavior.
- Predictive validity. The accuracy with which a test predicts the future performance of a related task; for example, a test of language competence may be shown to predict academic performance; also known as criterion-related validity; future performance is the criterion used to evaluate the validity.

**Vascular Dementia.** Assessment of vascular dementia follows the same general principles and procedures described under Dementia; the clinician needs to assess three common types of vascular dementia: multi-infarct dementia, lacunar state, and Binswanger disease.

***Multi-infarct Dementia.*** To assess this type of dementia, also known *multiple bilateral cortical infarcts* (that lead to dementia):

#### Take a Case History and Review Medical Records

- Take note of the following distinguishing features of multi-infarct dementia as revealed by the case history and medical records:
  - Document repeated strokes associated with a history of hypertension and arteriosclerosis
  - Review medical records to establish the occurrence of repeated strokes in the past
  - Note abrupt onset and step-wise deterioration
  - Note the relatively younger age of onset compared to dementia of the Alzheimer type

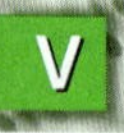

### Assess Neurological and Behavioral Symptoms

- Assess the following distinguishing features of multi-infarct dementia:
  - Cognitive impairments, including confusion, which may be the early symptoms
  - Inconsistent memory impairments that may range from total difficulty to recall an event and sudden recall of the same event
  - Focal versus the more typical diffuse neurological impairments
  - Somewhat better preserved personality and behavior patterns than those with other forms of dementia

***Lacunar State.*** To assess dementia due to lacunar states:

### Take a Case History and Review Medical Records

- Take note of the following distinguishing features of lacunar state-related dementia as revealed by the case history and medical records:
  - Through a detailed case history, establish a prolonged hypertension
  - Review the medical records to document any occlusion of small-end arteries deep in the brain, causing ischemia
  - Review the neurodiagnostic evidence for any multiple, small, ischemic strokes in the basal ganglia, thalamus, midbrain, and brainstem

### Assess Neurological and Behavioral Symptoms

- Assess the following distinguishing features of dementia associated with the lacunar state:
  - Assess any symptoms of stroke, including hemiplegia from which the client may recover or may have recovered by the time of the examination
  - Observe any muscular rigidity, plasticity, pseudobulbar palsy, and limb weakness
  - Assess Dysarthria
  - Assess Dysphagia which may be present in most clients
  - Assess any symptoms of dementia, which may remain nonspecific until the late stage of the disease
  - Take note that language problems appear only in the late stage
  - Observe such psychiatric symptoms as apathy, disinhibition (inappropriate social behavior), and frequent mood swings

***Binswanger's Disease.*** To assess dementia associated with this disease, also known as *subcortical arteriosclerotic encephalopathy:*

### Take a Case History and Review Medical Records

- Assess the following distinguishing features of Binswanger's disease as revealed by the case history and medical records:
  - Establish a long-standing history of hypertension and other factors that lead to vascular diseases
  - Take note of any multiple infarcts in the past
  - Review the medical records for evidence of leukoareosis (atrophy of the subcortical white matter) and lacunar states in the basal ganglia and thalamus

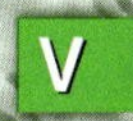

### Assess Neurological and Behavioral Symptoms

- Assess the following features of dementia associated with Binswanger's disease:
  - Symptoms that are similar to those found in clients with lacunar states
  - Take note of any acute strokes and a slow accumulation of focal neurological symptoms
  - Observe such motor symptoms as those associated with pseudobulbar palsy
  - Note that intellectual deterioration and eventual dementia are the final consequences of the disease

American Psychiatric Association (1994). *Diagnostic and statistical manual of mental disorders* (4th ed.) Washington, DC: Author.

Clark, C. M., & Trojanowski, J. Q. (2001). *Neurodegenerative dementias.* New York: McGraw-Hill.

Hegde, M. N. (2006). *A coursebook on aphasia and other neurogenic language disorders* (3rd ed.). Clifton Park, NY: Thomson Delmar Learning.

Jagust, W. (2001). *Understanding vascular dementia. Lancet, 358,* 2097–2098.

**Velopharyngeal Dysfunction.** Assessment of velopharyngeal dysfunction is important in understanding resonance disorders and in distinguishing resonance disorders that may be confused with articulation disorders in some clients, especially those with cleft palates; impaired velopharyngeal function needs to be assessed in children with clefts, those with dysarthria, and many clients who present voice and resonance disorders; because velopharyngeal dysfunction has multiple causes, it is important to differentiate *velopharyngeal inadequacy, velopharyngeal incompetence, velopharyngeal insufficiency,* and *velopharyngeal mislearning;* resonance disorders that need to be assessed include hypernasality, hyponasality, denasality, cul-de-sac nasality, nasal air emission, weak consonant productions, and compensatory articulation errors; see the sources cited at the end of this main entry and the companion volume, *Hegde's PocketGuide to Communication Disorders*, for etiological and symptomatic details; the following specific clinical conditions should be differentially diagnosed:

***Velopharyngeal Inadequacy.*** A general term that suggests that regardless of etiological factors, there is a problem in achieving an adequate closure of the velopharyngeal mechanism; this condition needs to be diagnosed in children with clefts of the palate (even with repaired clefts) and clients with dysarthria; generally, any client who exhibits hypernasality is a candidate for assessment of the velopharyngeal mechanism; to diagnose velopharyngeal inadequacy, assess and document the presence of:

- Hypernasal speech production; use phrases and sentences without nasal sounds in them to make a clinical judgment; see also Cleft Palate and Voice Disorders for details on assessment procedures
- Nasal air emission; to assess audible or inaudible air emission during speech, see Cleft Palate and Voice Disorders
- Weak consonant production; to assess this problem, see Cleft Palate and Voice Disorders; also see Dysarthria

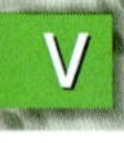

- Compensatory errors of articulation; to assess them, see Cleft Palate
- Hyperfunctional voice disorder; to assess, see Voice Disorders
- Reduced utterance length due to loss of air through an inadequate velopharyngeal closure; to assess, see Dysarthria

***Velopharyngeal Incompetence.*** Distinguish velopharyngeal incompetence from insufficiency and mislearning by:

- Inadequate movement of the velopharyngeal mechanism, not insufficiency of the tissue mass in the velum
- History of cleft palate repair in the client that might suggest a neuromuscular problem
- Wrong insertion of the levator veli palatini in cases of submucous clefts that extend into the velum
- Inadequate lateral pharyngeal wall movements
- Weakness of the oral and pharyngeal muscles that results in poor movement of the velopharyngeal mechanism; observe and record symptoms of Dysarthria
- Evidence of cranial nerve defects that cause the movement problems

***Velopharyngeal Insufficiency.*** Distinguish velopharyngeal insufficiency from incompetence and mislearning by:

- Insufficient tissue mass surrounding the velopharyngeal port
- Relatively short velum, as viewed in relation to the posterior pharyngeal wall; in essence, a short velum and a deep pharynx
- History of adenoidectomy; examine whether the child has a deeper nasopharynx because of adenoidectomy
- History of normal velopharyngeal function until the onset of puberty when inadequate closure causes hypernasality and related problems; the differential diagnosis in such cases might be the shrunken adenoids that reduce the overall tissue mass
- Other features that help diagnose velopharyngeal insufficiency include a history of surgery of the maxilla and the mandible, irregular adenoids, and hypertrophic tonsils

***Velopharyngeal Mislearning.*** Distinguish velopharyngeal mislearning from insufficiency and incompetence by:

- Lack of evidence of reduced tissue mass; observe and document normal tissue mass
- A history of surgical repair of the clefts of the hard and soft palates, resulting in adequate tissue mass, but continued speech production problems; this suggests mislearning or continuation of presurgical, inappropriate, and habitual speech production patterns
- A history of hearing loss; if suspected, get an audiological evaluation to assess whether hearing loss is the cause of velopharyngeal mislearning

Kummer, A. W. (2001). *Cleft palate and craniofacial anomalies.* Clifton Park, NY: Thomson Delmar Learning.

Peterson-Falzone, S. J., Hardin-Jones, M. A., & Karnell, M. P. (2001). *Cleft palate speech* (3rd ed.). St. Louis, MO: Mosby.

**Ventricular Dysphonia.** To diagnose this voice disorder resulting from the use of the ventricular (false) vocal folds for phonation:

- Take note of the characteristic low pitch, monotone, decreased loudness, harshness, and arrhythmic voicing
- Make an assessment through endoscopy, X-ray, or stroboscopy to observe the behavior of the vocal folds and that of the ventricular folds

**Verbal Aphasia.** To make an assessment of this type of aphasia, better known as Broca's aphasia, see Aphasia: Specific Types.

**Verbal Apraxia.** To assess this type of motor speech disorder, see Apraxia of Speech.

**Videofluoroscopy.** A radiological method of examining the movement of internal structures and video recording the movement patterns for assessment and diagnosis; useful in assessing the functions of the velopharyngeal mechanism, vocal folds, swallowing, and respiratory movement; preferred because it needs less radiation than cineradiography; in this procedure:

- X-rays are transmitted through the tissue under observation
- The soft tissue is coated with barium with the help of a nasal spray, or in the diagnosis of swallowing disorders, the client is asked to swallow barium-coated boluses of foods of various consistencies or drink liquid barium
- Multiple views of the structures (e.g., frontal, lateral, base, and oblique views of the velopharyngeal mechanism) and their movements are observed
- The images are shown on a fluorescent screen
- The images are recorded on videotape for later examination and diagnosis

**Videofluorographic Worksheet.** A detailed protocol for systematically observing and recording relevant structures, functions, symptoms, and disorders related to swallowing during videofluoroscopic studies; developed by J. A. Logemann and:

- Contains two sections: One for recording the results of liquid swallow tests and the other for recording the results of semi-solid and solid food swallow tests
- Provides space for recording additional observations
- Makes a clear distinction between various swallowing disorders and their symptoms
- Useful in recording detailed and systematic observations during videofluoroscopic examination of clients with swallowing disorders.

Logemann, J. A. (1998). *Evaluation and treatment of swallowing disorders* (2nd ed.). Austin, TX: Pro-Ed.

**Vocal Fold Paralysis.** Assessment of vocal fold paralysis is essential to understand certain kinds of aphonias, dysphonias, or dysarthrias; complete neurological examination to document neural pathology that affects the functioning of vocal folds and endoscopic examination of the paralyzed fold or folds are essential to make a reliable diagnosis; see Voice Disorders for details.

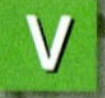


**Vocal Fundamental Frequency in Males and Females.** Typical vocal pitch levels of the male and female voice; various data sources suggest either the following ranges for the two genders or averages when no information on range is available; use them in evaluating the appropriateness of assessed pitch for clients with voice disorders:

| Age | Male | Female |
|---|---|---|
| 1–2 | 340–470 | 340–470 |
| 3 | 255–360 | 255–360 |
| 4–8 | 340–210 | 340–215 |
| 9–12 | 285–195 | 290–200 |
| 13 | 275–140 | 280–195 |
| 14–18 | 215–105 | 270–175 |
| 20–29 | 119 | 192–275 |
| 30–40 | 112 | 171–222 |
| 40–50 | 107 | 168–208 |
| 50–60 | 118 | 176–241 |
| 60–70 | 112 | 143–235 |
| 80–90 | 146 | 170–249 |

**Vocal Hyperfunction.** To assess this vocally abusive behavior, which involves excessive muscular effort and force in speaking, see Voice Disorders.

**Vocal Nodules.** Assessment of the presence or absence of vocal nodules is essential to differentially diagnose voice disorders; to diagnose vocal nodules:

- Obtain a report from a laryngologist who may have diagnosed vocal nodules
- Conduct an endoscopic examination to observe nodules at the junction of the anterior one-third and posterior two-thirds of the true vocal folds
- Make an analysis of voice quality to establish hoarseness, harshness, periodic aphonia, frequent throat clearing, hard glottal attacks, tension, and a dry vocal tract that result from nodules; see Voice Disorders for details.

**Voice Disorders.** Assessment of voice disorders requires a perceptual and instrumental examination of abnormal or inappropriate loudness, pitch, quality, and resonance of speech; assessment needs to consider the underlying pathology, behavioral patterns, or a combination of the two that produces voice disorders; general voice assessment procedures follow; see the sources cited at the end of this main entry and the companion volume, *Hegde's PocketGuide to Communication Disorders*, for the epidemiology, etiology, and symptomatology of voice disorders.

### *Assessment Objectives/General Guidelines*

- To assess all aspects of voice and its effects on communication
- To assess whether the voice helps meet the social and occupational demands of communication that a client faces
- To assess voice qualities in the context of what is expected of his or her vocal behavior based on age, culture, or gender

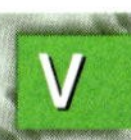

- To work closely with the physician of the client; in most cases, be a member of a multidisciplinary team
- To be a coordinator of different services if necessary
- To assist the medical professionals when a diagnosis of voice disorders is of medical significance (such as the diagnosis of vocal pathology, including cancer or central nervous system lesion)
- To make periodic assessments of voice in clients under medical treatment
- To integrate the voice assessment with medical, psychological, educational, and occupational information of relevance to the voice disorder and its management
- Note that careful observation of the client and listening to his or her speech and voice production is indispensable
- Note that it is necessary to combine clinical judgment (perceptual analysis) with instrumental measures; some instrumental measures may not directly correspond to clinical judgments; some insurance companies may require instrumental measures to reimburse for clinical services
- Note that information from family members should supplement the observations of voice parameters especially when some voice problems may not be consistently observed in the clinic (e.g., in some cases, loudness problem, especially excessive loudness, may be more often noticed in natural settings than in the clinic)

### *Case History/Interview Focus*

- See **Case History** and **Interview** under Standard/Common Assessment Procedures
- Take a detailed case history to assess the presence of vocal abuse; concentrate on such vocally abusive behaviors as excessive talking, habitually loud talking, frequent yelling and screaming, hard glottal attacks, habitual and forceful throat clearing, drug abuse including excessive intake of alcohol, smoking, and so forth
- In cases of laryngeal trauma, seek information on the accident or other traumatic conditions (e.g., burning) that injured the larynx
- Take note of any neurological signs or symptoms; request the client's neurologist for his or her report that may specify certain neuropathologies (e.g., amyotrophic lateral sclerosis, multiple sclerosis, cerebellar lesions, or upper motor neuron lesions)
- Obtain reports from the client's otolaryngologist if a consultation has been made
- Obtain information on any previous medical or surgical treatment for laryngeal pathologies, voice disorders, or both

### *Ethnocultural Considerations*

- See Ethnocultural Considerations in Assessment
- Note that vocal characteristics including vocal intensity and acceptable levels of nasal resonance may be culturally determined
- Note that various laryngeal pathologies that are associated with voice disorders are differentially distributed in different ethnocultural segments of society; see the companion volume, *Hegde's PocketGuide to Communication Disorders*,

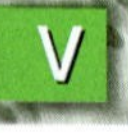

for details on incidence of voice disorders as they relate to ethnocultural variables

## Assessment

- Interview the client and record a speech and language sample for a complete communication analysis (speech, language, fluency, and voice); see Standard/Common Assessment Procedures
- Keep audiotaped samples of speech and voice to assess changes due to treatment or other factors
- Observe general behaviors
  - General bodily tension; tensed postures; tension in the neck, jaw, and chest; tics
  - Signs of neurological involvement including lack of facial emotional expression (mask-like); tremor, rigidity, flaccidity; paresis, and paralysis
  - Extent of mouth opening
  - Loud or excessive talking
  - Soft or inaudible speech
- Observe general phonatory behaviors
  - Frequency of throat clearing and coughing
  - Sound initiations: Soft and gentle or forceful and with hard glottal attacks
  - Emotional expression in speech
  - Prosodic features
  - Signs of allergy or cold (sneezing, sniffing, nose blowing)
  - Flow of speech: Smooth, effortless, and fluent; or jerky, effortful, and dysfluent
- Assess vocally abusive behaviors
  - Note that unless the laryngeal pathology is physically based (e.g., cancer), many cases of voice disorders, including some that have laryngeal pathology (e.g., vocal nodules or polyps), have a behavioral origin; vocally abusive behaviors are the main causes of these disorders
  - Assess vocally abusive behaviors through a detailed case history and interview; ask questions about the following vocally abusive behaviors:
    - Excessive talking
    - Excessively loud voice
    - Talking in inappropriate pitch
    - Argumentative behavior patterns
    - Habitually hard and abusive laughing
    - Excessive talking during menstruation
    - Excessive talking during allergy and upper respiratory diseases
    - Frequent shouting, screaming, cheering, throat clearing
    - Occupational use of voice (e.g., teaching, preaching, sports coaching, singing, aerobic instruction, pep club activities)
    - Working and talking in noisy conditions (e.g., bars and sports arenas, construction sites)
    - Smoking
    - Working in smoke-filled rooms (e.g., bars and other places with no regulation on smoking); general exposure to second-hand smoke

- Excessive alcohol intake
- Persistent, excessive laryngeal tension
- Inadequate breath support
- Constant and excessive grunting during exercising and weight lifting
- Habitual name shouting (calling) from a distance
- Not drinking enough water
- Play activity with much vocal activity (e.g., children who make loud mechanical and animal noises as they play)

- Ask the client or a family member to document the occurrence of vocally abusive behaviors in natural settings
  - Ask the client or a parent to keep a diary of vocally abusive behaviors for a week
  - Have the person record the frequency of vocally abusive behaviors
  - Have the person record the amount of talking on a daily basis

- Assess functional aphonia
  - Obtain first a medical evaluation that clears the client of any organic pathology leading to lack of voice (e.g., bilateral paralysis of the vocal folds due to neurological diseases)
  - Identify possible stress factors in life through a careful and detailed interview
  - During the interview, make some jokes to assess phonation accompanying laughter
  - Take note of phonation during throat clearing; ask the client to demonstrate his or her throat clearing
  - Take note of phonation during coughing; ask the client to demonstrate his or her coughing
- Assess disorders of loudness (intensity)
  - Probe the client and family members about the client's vocal intensity in natural settings
  - Observe and make clinical judgments about the vocal intensity; note whether the loudness of the voice is adequate (normal loudness), inadequate (too soft), or inappropriate (too loud)
  - Take note of variations in loudness; note whether a normal loudness level is maintained during conversation, whether variations in loudness are acceptable, and whether loudness varies unpredictably and inappropriately
  - Ask the client to vary the loudness to assess the range of intensity the client can exhibit; ask the client to whisper, speak softly, and to speak as loudly as possible; ask the client to shout; ask the client to count from 1 to 20, gradually increasing the intensity as counting is continued
  - Use the **Clinical Voice Evaluation Form** described later to make clinical judgments about the client's vocal intensity
  - Use the Sound Level Meter to obtain instrumental measures of loudness and evaluate them versus the normal range of vocal intensity levels in most social situations
    - Typical speech intensity level: 60 dB SPL at about 1 meter
    - Maximum speech intensity level: 100 to 110 dB SPL at about 1 meter
    - Minimum speech (not whispered) intensity level: 40 dB SPL

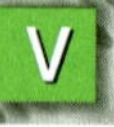

- Compare clinical judgments with instrumental measures; make an evaluation

- Assess disorders of pitch (frequency)
  - Use voice models to assess the client's pitch levels
    - Have recorded models of a male and female adult, and male and female children's voice samples; record the production of prolonged (about 3 sec) vowels; play back an appropriate sample and ask the client to match the pitch
    - Tape-record a sample of speech; later, play back the tape; at random intervals, match the client's pitch with a piano or a pitch pipe
    - Ask the client to vary the pitch, producing the lowest, intermediate, and highest pitch levels while prolonging vowels
    - Ask the client to say "mmmhhumm" in response to a question that is answered *yes* and "hhmm-mmm" in response to a question answered *no*; the pitch of the "mmm" may indicate the client's most desirable (habitual) pitch
    - Identify the best pitch (pitch that is produced with little effort and good sound)
  - Use one of the Instruments for Voice and Speech Analysis to measure the frequency range, best pitch, and habitual pitch of the client (e.g., the Visi-Pitch, Phonatory Functional Analyzer, or Fundamental Frequency Indicator)
  - Note that normal pitch for an individual is closer to the lowest pitch produced by that person
  - Compare the client's habitual pitch with the normative data; see Vocal Fundamental Frequency in Males and Females
- Assess disorders of voice quality
  - Listen carefully and take note of:
    - Vocal hyperfunction (tensed production of voice with pressed approximation of vocal folds)
    - Vocal hypofunction (too lax or inadequate approximation of vocal folds)
    - Breathiness of voice
    - Vocal spasticity and periodic voice cessation indicating possible neurological involvement
    - Hoarseness of voice with or without voice breaks and diplophonia
    - Colds and allergic reactions that may cause temporary hoarseness
    - Nodules and other laryngeal pathologies that may cause more permanent hoarseness
    - Jitter and shimmer
    - Diplophonia
    - Glottal fry
- Assess disorders of resonance
  - Judge hyponasality and hypernasality as you listen to the client's speech; be aware that clinical judgment of nasality may not always be reliable; therefore, in addition to making judgments, tape-record the client's production of:
    - Prolonged vowels with low pressure oral consonants (e.g., /a/ with *Ollie* or /u/ with *Lulu*)

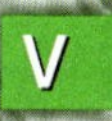

        - Sentences that are devoid of nasal sounds (e.g., *he wore a bow tie and cowboy boots; the dishwasher washes the dishes; Bob took Steve to the store*)
        - Sentences that are loaded with nasal sounds (e.g., *Nanny makes marshmallows; Jenny and Nancy joined the navy*)
        - Make judgments of nasality by listening to the taped productions
    - Have the client produce phrases or sentences devoid of nasal sounds while holding and releasing the nose; reduced nasality while holding the nose suggests hypernasality and velopharyngeal incompetence
    - Have the client produce phrases that are loaded with nasal sounds while holding and releasing the nose; if nose holding and releasing make no difference, conclude that the problem is denasality
    - Have the client produce "maybe baby, maybe baby"; the problem is hypernasality if both words sound like *maybe,* hyponasality if both sound like *baby*
    - Test stimulability for oral sounds; provide models of oral sounds, phrases, and sentences and ask the client to imitate; successful imitation suggests adequate velopharyngeal closure
    - Use measures of articulation to assess nasal resonance; administer the *Iowa Pressure Articulation Test*; nasal emission during the production of plosives and fricatives suggests velopharyngeal incompetence
    - Make an oral examination; take note of a short palate and obvious problems; note that subtle problems of velopharyngeal closure cannot be determined by visual inspection
    - Use Instruments for Resonance Assessment to evaluate nasal resonance (e.g., the Nasometer from the Kay Elemetrics Corporation)
    - Make an endoscopic examination or obtain the results of the examination from a physician; see Endoscopy
    - Make a videofluoroscopic examination of the velopharyngeal closure; see Videofluoroscopy
    - Assess assimilated nasality by having the client produce:
        - Words that contain a nasal sound in the initial or final positions (e.g., *nice* and *mice*; *Ben* and *him*) with enough mouth opening
        - Judge assimilated nasality by the presence of nasal resonance on the adjacent oral sounds
    - Assess cul-de-sac resonance by noting muffled or hollow oral resonance
- Assess maximum phonation duration
    - To assess general phonatory efficiency and the use of air flow:
        - Ask the client to phonate /s/ and /z/ as long as possible; measure the duration in seconds
        - Obtain measures on at least three trials
        - Compare the durations against norms (about 15 to 20 seconds for adults and 10 seconds for children); note that the durations may be highly variable and may increase with additional trials
        - Calculate the /s/ and /z/ durations by dividing z durations into /s/ durations
        - Judge the appropriateness of the ratio (about .90 being normal); /z/ durations are slightly longer than /s/ durations; note that laryngeal pathology shortens the /z/ durations, resulting in s/z ratios over 1.4

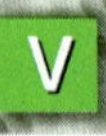

- Make an aerodynamic evaluation
  - Measure the phonatory air flow rate
    - Use an instrument described under Instruments for Aerodynamic Measures of Phonatory Functions (e.g., a pneumotachometer, Phonatory Function Analyzer, or Aerophone II)
    - Note that the normal flow rate is between 100–150 cc per second
    - Flow rates in excess of 300 cc/second suggest such laryngeal pathology as vocal cord paralysis
    - Markedly reduced flow rates may suggest spasmodic dysphonia
  - Measure subglottal air pressure and resistance
    - Place the open end of a small tube in the oral cavity and attach the other end to a pressure transducer
    - Ask the client to produce /**pi**/ at the rate of 1.5 syllables a second with normal pitch and loudness; evoke at least 10 productions
    - Note that the peak intraoral pressure obtained through this procedure is assumed to equal the subglottic pressure (normal average pressures: 5 to 10 cm $H_2O$)
- Evaluate the voice parameters; use one of the published voice rating scales (see the sources cited at the end of this main entry or the following **Clinical Voice Evaluation Form**)

*Make an evaluation of each voice parameter; then, if preferred, assign an overall numerical rating to the parameter; use a 5- or 7-point rating scale to assign a number to suggest the severity beyond the categorical, clinical evaluation (for example, after having evaluated hard glottal attacks as excessive, you also may assign a 5 or a 7 as the highest numerical rating).*

## Clinical Voice Evaluation Form

| Voice Parameter | Clinical Evaluation | | | Numerical Rating |
|---|---|---|---|---|
| Hard glottal attacks | ❑ none | ❑ some | ❑ excessive | |
| Comments: | | | | |
| Hyperfunctional voice (tensed) | ❑ none | ❑ occasional | ❑ frequent | |
| Comments: | | | | |
| Hypofunctional voice (lax, weak) | ❑ none | ❑ occasional | ❑ frequent | |
| Comments: | | | | |
| Voice breaks | ❑ none | ❑ occasional | ❑ frequent | |
| Comments: | | | | |

V

*(continues)*

*(continued)*

| Voice Parameter | Clinical Evaluation | | | Numerical Rating |
|---|---|---|---|---|
| Vocal tremors | ❑ none | ❑ some | ❑ excessive | |
| Comments: | | | | |
| Breath support | ❑ adequate | ❑ somewhat inadequate | ❑ inadequate | |
| Comments: | | | | |
| Loudness | ❑ too soft | ❑ normal | ❑ too loud | |
| Loudness variations | ❑ too few | ❑ normal | ❑ excessive | |
| Comments: | | | | |
| Pitch | ❑ too low | ❑ normal | ❑ too high | |
| Diplophonia | ❑ none | ❑ occasional | ❑ frequent | |
| Pitch breaks | ❑ none | ❑ occasional | ❑ frequent | |
| Pitch inflections | ❑ monopitch | ❑ normal | ❑ uncontrolled | |
| Comments: | | | | |
| Quality | | | | |
| Breathiness | ❑ none | ❑ occasional | ❑ excessive | |
| Harshness | ❑ none | ❑ occasional | ❑ excessive | |
| Hoarseness | ❑ none | ❑ occasional | ❑ excessive | |
| Comments: | | | | |
| Strained/strangled voice | ❑ none | ❑ occasional | ❑ excessive | |
| Comments: | | | | |

*(continues)*

*(continued)*

| Voice Parameter | Clinical Evaluation | | | Numerical Rating |
|---|---|---|---|---|
| Resonance | | | | |
| Oral | ❑ limited | ❑ normal | | |
| Nasal | ❑ hyponasal | ❑ normal | ❑ hypernasal | |
| Comments: | | | | |
| Muscle tension (face, neck, and shoulders) | ❑ lax | ❑ normal | ❑ excessive | |
| Comments: | | | | |
| Body posture during speech | ❑ appropriate | | ❑ inappropriate | |
| Comments: | | | | |

### *Instrumental Assessment*

- Consider supplementing clinical assessment and judgment of voice parameters with instrumental assessment; the following instruments, measures, or procedures are briefly described under their main alphabetical entries:
  - Electroglottography
  - Endoscopy
  - Instruments for Aerodynamic Measures of Phonatory Functions
  - Instruments for Resonance Assessment
  - Instruments for Voice and Speech Analysis
  - Sound Level Meter
  - Stroboscopy

### *Related/Medical Assessment Data*

- Obtain medical reports, including those from the client's general physician, otorhinolaryngologist, and neurologist
- Integrate voice assessment with medical assessment data
- Obtain psychological and behavioral assessment data if available and relevant to the case
- Obtain educational information from teachers in the case of children
- Obtain occupational information of relevance from adult clients

### *Standard/Common Assessment Procedures*

- Complete the Standard/Common Assessment Procedures
- If the client fails the hearing screening, get a complete audiological assessment because hearing loss is a source of voice disorders

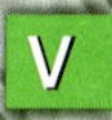

### Analysis of Results

- Integrate information from different sources
- Evaluate your assessment data in light of information from the case history, other professional sources, and any instrumental assessment
- Complete a voice profile by summarizing the findings

### Diagnostic Criteria/Guidelines

- Clear evidence of deviant voice as indicated by the assessment; depending on the client and potential diagnosis, one or more of the following:
    - Abnormal loudness
    - Abnormal pitch, pitch breaks, and pitch deviations
    - Deviant voice quality including breathiness, hoarseness, and harshness
    - Deviant resonance including hypernasality, hyponasality, assimilated nasality, and cul-de-sac nasality
    - Other characteristics including muscle tension, hard glottal attacks, and abnormal aerodynamic measures
    - Evidence of vocal abuse or misuse
    - Evidence of organic pathology from medical, radiological, and other examinations

### Differential Diagnosis

- Distinguish various voice disorders (e.g., loudness disorders, pitch disorders, quality disorders, and resonance disorders)
- Distinguish between laryngeal pathologies that accompany or cause voice disorders from the voice disorders per se (note that a vocal nodule or cancer is not a voice disorder but a cause of it)
- Distinguish between voice disorders associated with laryngeal pathologies (e.g., cancer, granuloma, endocrine disorders, hyperkeratosis, papilloma, leukoplakia, vocal nodules, polyps, contact ulcers) and functional disorders that are devoid of laryngeal pathologies (e.g., functional aphonia, functional dysphonia, puberphonia); note that many traditionally considered functional voice disorders are associated with laryngeal pathologies (e.g., vocal nodules, polyps, contact ulcers, thickening of the folds); base the distinction on positive evidence of laryngeal pathology and the results of careful procedures that rule it out
- Distinguish between the immediate cause of the voice disorder from its more remote cause; for example, the immediate cause of hoarseness (a voice disorder) may be physical—a vocal nodule; this hoarseness is not functional, whereas the cause of the nodule may be functional (vocal abuse)
- Distinguish between voice disorders with neurological involvement (e.g., those resulting from lesions of the vagus nerve, upper motor neuron lesions, cerebellar lesions, lesions of the basal ganglia, and such neurological diseases as amyotrophic lateral sclerosis and multiple sclerosis) and those without such involvement (e.g., functional aphonia or a voice disorder associated with vocal nodules); base the distinction on positive neurological findings and associated additional symptoms of dysarthrias

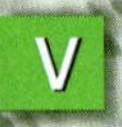

- Distinguish between voice disorders due to external trauma to the larynx and those with other causes; base the distinction on evidence of external trauma (e.g., accidents, assaults)
- Distinguish voice disorders due to hearing loss from those that are due to other causes; see Hearing Impairment for details
- Identify velopharyngeal incompetence by endoscopic and radiological findings

## Prognosis

- Prognosis is variable, depending on the voice disorder, associated medical condition, and client motivation; generally good unless the voice disorder is due to a neurodegenerative disease
- With treatment, prognosis is generally good for improvement in voice

## Recommendations

- Voice therapy for most clients
- No voice therapy for clients with inadequate velopharyngeal incompetence when there has not been necessary medical intervention
- When warranted, augmentative and alternative communication for clients with degenerative neuromuscular disorders
- Medical referral before initiating voice therapy
- See the following cited sources and the companion volume, *Hegde's PocketGuide to Treatment in Speech-Language Pathology* (3rd ed.), for details

Andrews, M. L. (2006). *Manual of voice treatment: Pediatrics through geriatrics* (2nd ed.). Clifton Park, NY: Thomson Delmar Learning.

Boone, D. R., McFarlane, S. C., & Von Berg, S. L. (2005). *The voice and voice therapy* (7th ed.). Boston, MA: Allyn and Bacon.

Case, J. L. (2002). *Clinical management of voice disorders* (4th ed.). Austin, TX: Pro-Ed.

Holland, R. W., & DeJarnette, G. (2002). *Voice and voice disorders*. In D. Battle (Ed.), *Communication disorders in multicultural populations* (3rd ed.), (pp. 299–333). Boston, MA: Butterworth-Heinemann.

Sataloff, R. T. (2005). *Clinical assessment of voice*. San Diego, CA: Plural Publishing.

Smith, E., Gray, S., Dive, H., Kirchner, L., & Heras, H. (1997). Frequency and effects of teachers' voice problems. *Journal of Voice, 11*(1), 81–87.

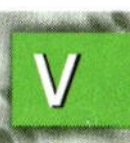

W

**Wernicke's Aphasia.** To assess this variety of fluent aphasia, see Aphasia and Aphasia: Specific Types.

**Wilson's Disease.** To assess motor speech disorders associated with this inherited, autosomal, progressive neurological disease with a gradual onset:

- Take note of late adolescent or early adult onset
- Review the medical records for evidence of copper deposits in the cornea of the eye, kidneys, liver, and basal ganglia
- Review the neurodiagnostic evidence of damage to the basal ganglia
- Observe such neurological symptoms as tremor in the outstretched arms, slow movement, and rigidity of muscles and drooling
- Assess Dysphagia
- Assess subcortical dementia in some cases
- Assess hypokinetic, spastic, and ataxic dysarthrias
- See Mixed Dysarthrias under Dysarthria: Specific Types and Dementia.

**Word Deafness.** Better known as Wernicke's aphasia; to assess this profound auditory comprehension deficit for spoken words, see Wernicke's aphasia under Aphasia: Specific Types.

**Word Fluency.** Assessment of fluency in rapidly producing words that start with a particular sound or words that belong to a certain category (e.g., animals or vegetables) is important in diagnosing Aphasia and Dementia; to assess:

- Ask the client to say as many words as rapidly as possible that begin with a particular sound (e.g., *Please say as fast as you can all the words that start with the s sound*); repeat the procedure with at least three letters or sounds
- Ask the client to name, as rapidly as possible, as many animals as he or she can
- Ask the client to name, as rapidly as possible, as many fruits as he or she can
- Ask the client to name, as rapidly as possible, as many furniture items as he or she can

**Word Fluency Measure.** A test of word fluency in which the client is asked to say as many words as possible that start with a given sound in one minute; the letters F, A, or S are specified in the test; proper names are not accepted; the total number of words produced in one minute is the score; norms are available for clients with aphasia and normal subjects.

Borkowski, J. G., Benton, A. L., & Spreen, O. (1967). Word fluency and brain damage. *Neuropsychologia, 5,* 135–140.

**Word-Retrieval Problems.** Assessment of difficulty in recalling specific words in conversation is important in diagnosing Aphasia, Dementia, and Traumatic Brain Injury; to assess:

- Engage the client in conversational speech
- Take note of the client's production of nonspecific words instead of specific words, circumlocution, silent pauses as the person searches for the missing word, repetitions and other kinds of dysfluencies, and neologistic speech (invention of words because the real words elude the client)
- See Aphasia for details

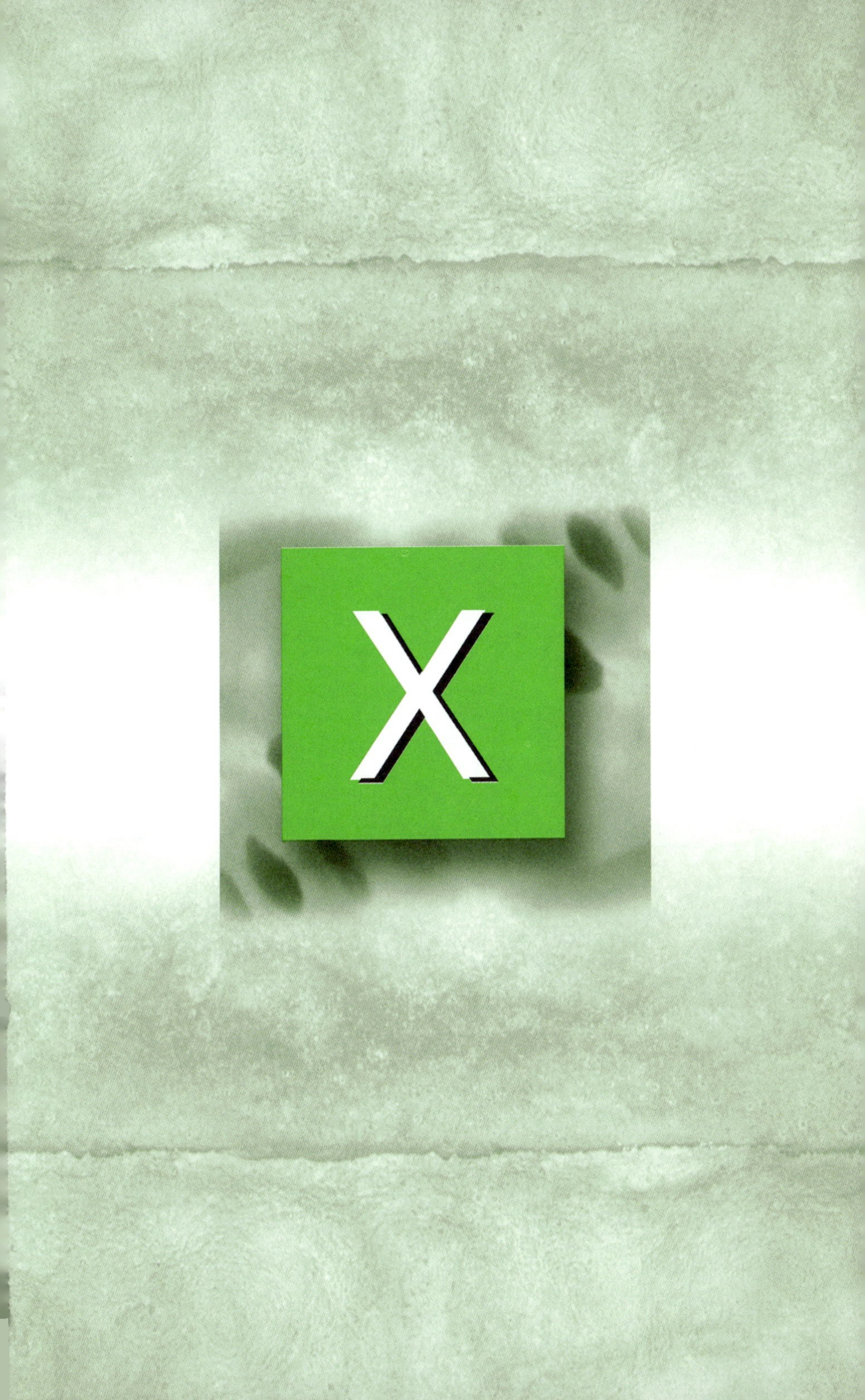
X

**XO Syndrome.** To assess this syndrome, also called the *Turner syndrome,* see Syndromes Associated With Communication Disorders.